The Wisdom of Menopause

Also by Dr Christiane Northrup

Women's Bodies, Women's Wisdom

Women's Bodies, Women's Wisdom is a groundbreaking and inspiring healthcare guide for women of all ages. Dr Christiane Northrup, a holistic physician trained in obstetrics and gynaecology, explains the workings of the female body and guides you through a comprehensive list of women's conditions and concerns. She powerfully demonstrates that when women listen to their body's own wisdom or change the basic conditions of their lives that lead to health problems, they heal faster, more completely and with far fewer medical interventions.

This important book offers important and relevant information on the entire range of women's health problems. This edition includes:

- A nutrition chapter emphasising individual dietary needs and body chemistry
- Information on improving fertility after the age of 35 – and how to cut the risk of a Caesarean section by 50 per cent
- A complete programme for menopause, including how to decide whether natural hormone replacement is right for you
- Holistic ways to prepare and heal faster if surgery is necessary
- Plus dozens of new natural treatments and a wealth of hard-to-find healthcare resources

Filled with helpful case histories, *Women's Bodies, Women's Wisdom* is contemporary medicine at its best, combining new technologies with natural remedies and the miraculous healing powers within the body itself.

The
Wisdom
of
Menopause

The Complete Guide to

Creating Physical and Emotional

Health and Healing

CHRISTIANE NORTHRUP, MD

PIATKUS

First published in USA by Bantam Books, 2001

Some of the material in this book was originally published in
Health Wisdom for Women, Phillips Publishing International

Copyright © 2001 by Christiane Northrup, MD

This edition first published in the UK in 2001 by
Piatkus Books Ltd
5 Windmill Street
London W1T 2JA
e-mail: info@piatkus.co.uk

Reprinted 2002 (three times), 2004

The moral right of the author has been asserted

A catalogue record for this book is available from the British Library

ISBN 0 7499 2222 2 hbk
ISBN 0 7499 2214 1 pbk

UK edition edited by Sara Miller
Illustrations by Judith E. Barrington, AMI, CMI

This book has been printed on paper manufactured with respect for the environment,
using wood from managed sustainable resources

Data manipulation by Phoenix Photosetting, Chatham, Kent
Printed and bound in Great Britain by CPI Bath

*This book is dedicated to the pioneering spirit
embodied in the women of the baby boom generation.*

Contents

List of Figures

Acknowledgements

Part of menopausal wisdom is knowing your limits and learning to accept help. I gratefully acknowledge the following individuals, whose help and support have made this book a reality.

My agent and friend, Ned Leavitt, who has shown me that solid contractual agreements are compatible with and essential to menopausal wisdom.

Irwyn Applebaum, president of Bantam Books, whose advice to write a good book set just the right tone of this whole process. Beth Rashbaum for her editing wisdom. Susan Warga, copy editor, for honing this material with her razor-sharp mind. My editor Toni Burbank, a literary legend whose roll-up-your-sleeves New England work ethic brought out the best in me. And Barb Burg of the Bantam publicity department for her continuing guidance and perspective.

Dr Karen Hayes, whose scientific background and can-do attitude in the initial months of this project provided me with the courage to begin and then continue this book in the first place.

Judy Barrington, my medical illustrator, for taking Mona Lisa's and my whimsically rough graphic ideas and perfecting them.

Marcella Sweet-Demetriou, my transcriptionist, who is also a creative designer whose style and artistry extend even to footnotes. My gratitude for your help is boundless.

The team at Phillips Publishing International, publishers of *Health Wisdom for Women*, my monthly newsletter. Special thanks to my editor Meg de Guzman, whose vision and skill are a major contribution to me and my newsletter subscribers.

Jack Wilson and Bill Heitz, who produced my television specials. Thank you for your vision, support, and delightful sense of fun.

Terah Kathryn Collins, whose feng shui skill and grace have helped me transform my home and office into environments that support me and my work on all levels.

Fern Tsao and her daughter Maureen, whose healing skills with acupuncture and Traditional Chinese Medicine keep my *chi* flowing freely.

Nancy Etnier, my Pilates teacher, for helping me stay strong, centred, and flexible. You've helped me prove to myself that age and physical decline don't have to be related.

To the warm and gracious staff of the Broad Arrow Tavern at the Harraseeket Inn for such consistent service and nourishing food during my many 'writing retreat' meals.

Dr Joel Hargrove, whose twenty-five years of research on the use of bioidentical hormones has provided hundreds of doctors with the right scientific information, and thousands of women with the right life-enhancing hormonal treatments.

Pamela Slye, who elevates domestic engineering to the level of a NASA scientist. Your help in my home continues to amaze and delight me.

Sharon Griffith, my highly skilled and practical bookkeeper, who also found Buddy, a very special cat, for me.

My family, especially my mother and brother John, who have known just how and when to support me the most during both the difficulties and celebrations of the past two years.

Charles Grover, whose good-hearted service, sense of humour, and willingness to help out with anything and at any time have set a new standard in my life.

Dr Mona Lisa Schulz, my research partner, colleague, and best friend. Your scholarship, friendship, and unfailing support and humour have transformed my life on every level. Thanks for having the strength to refuse to work on anything that isn't worthy of your attention and helping me do the same.

Diane Grover, my amazingly gifted administrative assistant and loyal friend, who has been there from the beginning. You have contributed to my well-being on all levels for over twenty years and I don't know what I'd do without you. I look forward to many more decades of co-creating together.

And finally, a thank-you to my daughters, Ann and Kate, for standing by me and providing me with living proof that the best way to access the wisdom of menopause while mothering you as teenagers is to learn how to care for myself and to stick with it.

The Journey Begins

*I*n the year or two before I actually started to skip periods, I began to experience an increasingly common feeling of irritability whenever my work was interrupted or I had to contend with a co-worker or employee who was not as committed to accomplishing the job as I was. Looking back, I recall that when I was in my thirties and my children were younger, their interruptions when I was in the middle of writing an article or talking on the phone were only mildly irritating to me. My love and concern for their welfare usually overrode any anger or frustration I might have felt.

But as I approached menopause, I found myself unable to tolerate distractions like my eighteen-year-old asking me, 'When is dinner?' when she could clearly see I was busy. Why, I wondered, was it always my responsibility to turn on the stove and begin to think about my family's food needs, even when I wasn't hungry and was deeply engrossed in a project? Why couldn't my husband get the dinner preparations started? Why did my family seem to be almost totally paralysed when it came to preparing a meal? Why did they all wait in the kitchen, as though unable to set the table or pour a glass of water, until I came into the room and my mere presence announced, 'Mum's here. Now we get to eat.'

The same thing occurred when it was time to get into the car and take off on holiday. Only when I myself made a definitive move towards the door did my family mobilise. It felt as though my presence caused them to lose their own personal initiative to take charge of a situation, be it dinner or a family trip. Still, during my childbearing years I accepted this, mostly good-naturedly, as part and parcel of my role as wife and mother. And in so doing, I unwittingly perpetuated it, partly because it felt so good to be indispensable.

During perimenopause, I lost patience with this behaviour on all levels, whether at home or at work. I could feel a fiery volcano within me, ready to burst, and a voice within me roaring, 'Enough! You're all able-bodied, capable individuals. Everyone here knows how to drive a car and boil water. Why is my energy still the organising principle around here?' My indignation grew as I mumbled to myself, 'If I were a man in the prime of life and at the pinnacle of his career, I wouldn't be interrupted like this. Everyone would be wondering how to help me, instead of the other way around!'

Little did I know that these little bursts of irritability over petty family dynamics were the first faint knocks on the door marked Menopausal Wisdom, signalling that I needed to renegotiate some of my habitual relationship patterns. Nor did I know that by the time I began to actually skip periods and experience hot flushes, my life as I had known it for the previous quarter of a century would be on the threshold of total transformation. As my cyclic nature rewired itself, I put all my significant relationships under a microscope, began to heal the unfinished business from my past, experienced the first pangs of the empty nest, and established an entirely new and exciting relationship with my creativity and vocation.

All of the changes I was about to undergo were spurred, supported, and encouraged by the complex and intricate brain and body changes that are an unheralded – but inevitable and often overwhelming – part of the menopausal transition. There is much, much more to this midlife transformation than 'raging hormones'. Research into the physiological changes taking place in the perimenopausal woman is revealing that, in addition to the hormonal shift that means an end to childbearing, our bodies – and, specifically, our nervous systems – are being, quite literally, rewired. It's as simple as this: our brains are changing. A woman's thoughts, her ability to focus, and the amount of fuel going to the intuitive centres in the temporal lobes of her brain all are plugged into, and affected by, the circuits being rewired. After working with thousands of women who have gone through this process, as well as experiencing it myself, I can say with great assurance that menopause is an exciting developmental stage – one that, when participated in consciously, holds enormous promise for transforming and healing our bodies, minds, and spirits at the deepest levels.

As a woman in midlife today, I am part of a growing population that is an unprecedented forty million strong. This group is no longer invisible and silent, but a force to be reckoned with: educated, vocal, sophisticated in our knowledge of medical science, and determined to take control of our own health. Think about it: forty million women, all undergoing the same sort of circuitry update at the same time. By virtue of our sheer numbers, as well as our social and economic influence, we are powerful – and potentially dangerous to any institution built upon the status quo. It's a safe bet the world is going to change, willingly or otherwise, right along with us. And it's likely to change for the better.

It's no accident that the current movement of psychospiritual healing is composed largely of women in their thirties, forties, and fifties. We are awakening en masse and beginning to deliver a much-needed message of health, hope, and healing to the world.

My personal experience tells me that the perimenopausal lifting of the hormonal veil – the monthly cycle of reproductive hormones that tends to keep us focused on the needs and feelings of others – can be both liberating and unsettling. The midlife rate of marital separation, divorce, and vocational change confirms this. I, for one, had always envisioned myself married to the same man for life, the two of us growing old together. This ideal had always been one of my most cherished dreams. At midlife I, like thousands of others, have had to give up my fantasies of how I thought my life would be. I had to face, head on, the old adage about how hard it is to lose what you never really had. It means giving up all your illusions, and it is very difficult. But for me the issue was larger than where, and with whom, I would grow old. It was a warning, coming from deep within my spirit, that said, 'Grow . . . or die.' Those were my choices. I chose to grow.

Midlife: Redefining Creativity and Home

For most women, identity and self-esteem are generated by our associations and relationships. This is true even for women who have high-powered jobs and for women who have chosen not to marry. Men, by contrast, usually get most of their identity and self-esteem from the outer world – the job, the income, the accomplishments, the accolades. For both genders, this pattern may change at midlife.

Women often begin to direct more of their energies towards the world outside of home and family, which may suddenly appear as a great, inviting, untapped resource for exploration, creative expression, and self-esteem. Meanwhile, men of the same age – who may be undergoing a sort of menopause of their own – are often feeling world-weary; they're ready to retire, curl up, and escape the battles of the workplace. They may feel their priorities shifting inwards, towards home, hearth, and family.

It's an ironic transposition: the man is beginning to look to relationships for his 'juice'; the woman is feeling biologically primed to explore the outer world. In married couples, this often produces profound role shifts. In the best of all worlds the man retires or cuts back on work, becoming the chief cook and bottle washer at home, and providing emotional and practical support for his wife's new interests. She, in turn, goes out into the world to start a business, get an education, or do whatever her heart dictates. If their relationship is adaptable and resilient, they adjust to their new roles. If not, he may become jealous of her success and independence, and put pressure on her to continue to care for him as she has always done. He may even get physically sick, often in the form of heart disease and/or clinically dangerous high blood pressure. It's important to note that this is not a wilful act; he's simply responding to the promptings of our lopsided culture.

A woman often finds herself in the difficult position, then, of having to choose between returning to the role of caretaker to nurture her husband at the expense of her own needs and pursuing her own creative passions. It's an old story, common to women in many cultures, not just our own. The woman in menopause, known mythologically as the 'crone', finds herself at a crossroads of life, torn between the old way she has always known and a new way she has just begun to dream of. A voice from the old way (in many cases it's her husband's voice) begs her to stay in place – 'Grow old with me, the best is yet to come.' But from the new path another voice beckons, imploring her to explore aspects of herself that have been dormant during her years of caring for, and focusing on, the needs of others. She's preparing to give birth to herself, and as many women already know, the birth process cannot be halted without consequences.

Caring for others and pursuing unexplored personal passions are not necessarily mutually exclusive choices, but our culture makes them seem so, always supporting the former at the expense of the latter. This is part of what makes the midlife transformation so much of a challenge – as I know only too well.

Why I'm Writing a Menopause Book Now

Though I have worked closely with menopausal women for over twenty years, I vowed that I wouldn't write a book on this subject until I entered the process myself. I knew that I would learn something through the direct experience of this transition that I couldn't possibly learn any other way. My personal approach to pregnancy and birth, for example, was completely transformed and deepened when I had my two daughters. The same has been true for the menopausal transition and its attendant challenges.

For some people, it's surprising to hear a doctor revealing anything of her personal life. But I've always been comfortable with the idea that what I have to offer as a woman, wife, and mother is every bit as valuable as what I have to offer as a trained medical professional – that they are equally valid as teaching tools, and that one can augment the other. In fact, I find the idea of dividing myself into a work persona and a home persona unimaginable. It's dishonest, and it creates a barrier to full communication on both fronts. This is why, throughout my professional career as a clinician, surgeon, and teacher of women's health issues, I've approached my patients and students from the fullness of who I am, in all my roles. And because this sharing has resulted in such an outpouring of warmth and acceptance from my patients and readers, I have once again found the courage to share some of my more recent experiences in this book.

Society in general, and the medical profession in particular, admonishes doctors to keep our personal stories to ourselves, especially when they involve difficult emotions like fear or anger – allegedly because to appear too human would undermine our authority. Yet I've found over the years that nothing illustrates a point quite as effectively or is as helpful to my patients as an honest personal story. Telling the truth of my own humanness and vulnerability is also helpful to me. This is, after all, one of the reasons why twelve-step programmes work so well to help people recover from the grip of addiction and denial. Honest stories help awaken the healer within us.

By sharing both the joy and the pain of my own transition, I hope that I can help to illustrate and also demystify the surges of creative energy that erupt in so many of us at midlife. I also bring many personal stories from my patients and my newsletter subscribers, whose experiences reveal how the emotional shifts that occur at menopause, which may at first feel uncomfortable or even frightening, ultimately help us do the work (and play) that await us on our journey.

The dilemma for me and women everywhere is that we often feel guilty about self-revelation, because by being true to ourselves and our own feelings, we feel that we are betraying others, especially family members. I assure you that I have shared the stories printed here with my family. For all other stories, I have sought the explicit permission of those concerned, except where so much detail has been changed that the subject cannot be identified.

Blazing a New Trail

Throughout most of human history, the vast majority of women died before menopause; for those who survived, menopause was experienced as a signpost of an imminent and inevitable physical decline. But today, with a woman's life expectancy averaging between seventy-eight and eighty-four years, it is reasonable to expect that she will not only live thirty to forty years beyond menopause, but be vibrant, sharp, and influential as well. The menopause you will experience is not your mother's (or grandmother's) menopause.

Women of our mothers' generation had an entirely different social and political environment in which to make their transition. Menopause (like menstruation, for that matter) was not discussed in public. Today this is no longer true. As we break this silence we are also breaking cultural barriers, so that we can enter this new life phase with eyes wide open – in the company of forty million kinswomen, all undergoing the same transformation at the same time. And, as you'll soon discover, the changes taking place in middle-aged women are going to act like the power plant on a high-speed train, whisking the evolution of our entire society along on fast forward, to places that have yet to be mapped. Whether you climb aboard this fast-moving train or step aside and let it pass will play a major role in how far you go and how you feel along the way.

Ultimately, I've found this journey bracing, exciting, and health-enhancing. And I'm certainly not alone. A 1998 Gallup survey, presented at the annual meeting of the North American Menopause Society, showed that more than half the American women between the ages of fifty and sixty-five felt happiest and most fulfilled at this stage of life. Compared to when they were in their twenties, thirties, and forties, they felt their lives had improved in many ways, including family life, interests, friendships, and their relationship with their spouse or partner. In other words, the conventional view of menopause as a scary transition heralding 'the beginning of the end' couldn't be further from the truth. So please join me – and the millions of others who have come before and will come after – as we transform and improve our lives, and ultimately our culture, through understanding, applying, and living the wisdom of menopause.

ONE

Menopause Puts Your Life Under a Microscope

*I*t is no secret that relationship crises are a common side effect of menopause. Usually this is attributed to the effects of the hormonal shifts occurring in a woman's body at this time of transition. What is rarely acknowledged or understood is that as these hormone-driven changes affect the brain, they give a woman a sharper eye for inequity and injustice, and a voice that insists on speaking up about them. In other words, they give her a kind of wisdom – and the courage to voice it. As the vision-obscuring veil created by the hormones of reproduction begins to lift, a woman's youthful fire and spirit are often rekindled, together with long-sublimated desires and creative drives. Midlife fuels those drives with a volcanic energy that demands an outlet.

If it does not find an outlet – if the woman remains silent for the sake of keeping the peace at home and/or work, or if she holds herself back from pursuing her creative urges – the result is equivalent to plugging the vent on a pressure cooker: something has to give. Very often what gives is the woman's health, and the result will be one or more of the 'big three' diseases of postmenopausal women: heart disease, depression, and breast cancer. On the other hand, for those of us who choose to honour the body's wisdom and to express what lies within us, it's a good idea to get ready for some boat rocking, which may put long-established relationships in upheaval. Marriage is not immune to this effect.

'Not Me, My Marriage Is Fine'

Every marriage, even a very good one, must undergo change in order to keep up with the hormone-driven rewiring of a woman's brain during the years leading up to and including menopause. Not all marriages are able to survive these changes. Mine wasn't, and nobody was more surprised about that than I. If this makes you want to hide your head in the sand, believe me, I do understand. But for the sake of being true to yourself and protecting your emotional and physical health in the second half of your life – probably a full forty years or more – then I submit to you that forging ahead and taking a good hard look at all aspects of your relationship (including some previously untouchable corners of your marriage) may be the only choice that will work in your best interest in the long run, physically, emotionally, and spiritually.

From the standpoint of physical health, for example, there is plenty of evidence to suggest that the increase in life-threatening illnesses after midlife, which cannot be accounted for by ageing alone, is partly rooted in the stresses and unresolved relationship problems that simmered beneath the surface during the childbearing years of a woman's life, then bubbled up and boiled over at perimenopause, only to be damped down in the name of maintaining the status quo. The health of your significant other is also at stake. Remaining in a relationship that was tailor-made for a couple of twenty-somethings without making the necessary adjustments for who you both have become at midlife can be just as big a health risk for him as it is for you.

This is not to say that your only options are divorce or heart attack. Rather, in order to bring your relationship into alignment with your rewired brain, you and your significant other must be willing to take the time, and spend the energy, to resolve old issues and set new ground rules for the years that lie ahead. If you can do this, then your relationship will help you to thrive in the second half of your life. If one or both of you cannot or will not, then both health and happiness may be at risk if you stay together.

Preparing for Transformation

At midlife, more psychic energy becomes available to us than at any time since adolescence. If we strive to work in active partnership with that organic energy, trusting it to help us uncover the unconscious and self-destructive beliefs about ourselves that have held us back from what we could become, then we will find that we have access to everything we need to reinvent ourselves as healthier, more resilient women, ready to move joyfully into the second half of our lives.

This process of transformation can only succeed, however, if we become proactive in two ways. First, we must be willing to take full responsibility for our share of the problems in our lives. It takes great courage to admit our own contributions to the things that have gone wrong for us and to stop seeing ourselves simply as victims of someone or something outside of ourselves. After all, the person in the victim role tends to get all the sympathy and to assume the high road morally, which is appealing; none of us wants to feel like the bad guy. But even though taking the victim role may seem a good choice in the short run, this stance is ultimately devoid of any power to help us change, heal, grow, and move on.

The second requirement for transformation is more difficult by far. We must be willing to feel the pain of loss and grieve for those parts of our lives that we are leaving behind. And that includes our fantasies of how our lives could have been different *if only.* Facing up to such loss is rarely easy, and that is why so many of us resist change in general and at midlife in particular. A part of us rationalises, 'Why rock the boat? I'm halfway through my life. Wouldn't it just be easier to accept what I have rather than risk the unknown?'

The end of any significant relationship, or any major phase of our lives, even one that has made us unhappy or held us back from our full growth and fulfilment, feels like a death – pure and simple. To move past it, we have to feel the sadness of that loss and grieve fully for what might have been and now will never be.

And then we must pick ourselves up and move towards the unknown. All our deepest fears are likely to surface as we find ourselves facing the uncertainty of the future. During my own perimenopausal life changes, I would learn this in spades – much to my surprise.

By the time I was approaching menopause, I had worked with scores of women who had gone through midlife 'cleansings'; I had guided and counselled them as their children left home, their parents got sick, their marriages ended, their husbands fell ill or died, they themselves became ill, their jobs ended – in short, as they went through all the storms and crises of midlife. But I never thought I would face a crisis in *my* marriage. I had always felt somewhat smug, secure in my belief that I was married to the man of my dreams, the one with whom I would stay 'till death do us part'.

Delirious Happiness and Shaking Knees

I will always remember the happiness of meeting and marrying my husband, a decision we made merely three months after we met. He was my surgical intern when I was a medical student. He looked like a Greek god, and I was deeply flattered by his attention, especially since I wasn't at all sure I had what it took to attract such a handsome man with such a country club background. Something deep within me was moved by him beyond all reason, beyond anything I'd ever felt before with any other boyfriend. For the first five years of our marriage my knees shook whenever I saw him. There wasn't a force on this planet that could have talked me out of marrying him. I remember wanting to shout my love from the tops of tall buildings – an exuberance of feeling that was very uncharacteristic of me.

He, however, was considerably less eager to display his feelings. I couldn't help but notice during the years we were both immersed in our surgical training that my husband seemed uncomfortable relating to me when we were at work, and often appeared cold and distant when I'd try to show affection in that setting. This puzzled and hurt me, since I was always proud to introduce him to my patients when we happened to see each other outside of the operating room. But I told myself that this was because of the way he had been brought up, and that with enough love and attention from me, he would become more responsive, more emotionally available.

The Childbearing Years: Balancing Personal and Professional Lives

My husband's life didn't change much when we had our two daughters. Mine, however, became a struggle – one that millions of women will recognise from their own experience – as I tried to find satisfying and effective ways to mother my children, remain the doctor I wanted to be, and at the same time be a good wife to my husband. Nonetheless, these were happy years, for both of us adored our daughters from the beginning and enjoyed the many activities we shared with them – the weekend walks, the family vacations, the simple daily contact with two beautiful, developing young beings.

I did sometimes resent the disparity between what I contributed to the upkeep of our family life and what my husband did. Once, when the children were still young, I asked him if he'd consider working fewer hours so that I wouldn't have to give up delivering babies, an aspect of my practice that I dearly loved. He replied, 'You've never seen a part-time orthopaedic surgeon, have you?' I admitted that I hadn't, but suggested that this didn't mean it couldn't happen with a little imagination on his part. It was not to be, however. It was I who, like so many other women, became the master shape-shifter, adjusting my own needs to those of everyone else in the family.

In the early years of our family life, I was also becoming increasingly aware that the inequities that bothered me in my marriage were a reflection of inequities that existed in the culture around us. I saw many people like my husband and me – people who had started their marriages on equal grounds financially and educationally, even people who, like us, did the same work – and always, once the children arrived, it was the wife who made the sacrifices in leisure time, professional accomplishment, and personal fulfilment.

Change Yourself, Change the World

During those often exhausting years, I began to put into action some of the ideas I'd been developing about women's health – while always being careful not to say much about those ideas at home, where I knew they would not be welcomed by my husband. Inspired by my own experiences as well as those of my patients, and buoyed by the conviction that my ideas could make a difference in people's lives, in 1985 I joined three other women in the venture of establishing a health care centre we called Women to Women. The idea of a health centre run by women for women was virtually unheard of at that time. Our central mission was to help women appreciate the unity of mind, body, and spirit, to enable them to see the connection between their emotional health and their physical well-being. I wanted to empower women, to give them a safe place in which to tell their personal stories so that they could discover new, more health-enhancing ways of living their lives.

I knew that sometimes this would involve challenging the status quo, because the inequities of the culture take a terrible toll on women's bodies as well as their spirits. But as I practised this new, holistic form of medicine, which was quite revolutionary for its day, I realised that the fact that I had a normal, happy family life, as well as a husband with conventional medical ideas who practised in the same community, provided a kind of cover for me. It made me appear 'safe' at a time when my ideas were considered unproven at best, dangerous at worst.

My three partners in Women to Women and I bought an old Victorian house that we could convert into a centre for our new practice. We all agreed that we wanted to keep our husbands out of our new venture, lest their participation undermine our enthusiastic but still tender confidence in ourselves as businesswomen.

Of course, in my case, at least, that didn't necessarily mean that I didn't want my husband's support. I clearly remember a day at the beginning of the building and site renovation. Two bulldozers sat on the lawn, workers were everywhere, and the existing building had been torn apart. At that moment the whole project suddenly became real for me, and I realised that my colleagues and I were now responsible for paying for all of this. This was an overwhelming thought. When I came home that evening, I uncharacteristically reached out to my husband for help in calming my fears. 'I'm scared,' I told him. 'I'm not sure I can do this.' He replied, 'I hate it when you're disempowered like this.' I quickly realised that I'd been foolish to expect anything from him.

His response to my uncharacteristic and risky moment of emotional vulnerability simply reinforced the coping style I'd developed in childhood, a stoicism that was a necessity in a household where emotional neediness was frowned upon and we were told to 'keep a stiff upper lip'. Another favourite saying in my family was 'Don't ask for a lighter pack, ask for a stronger back.' So, as usual, I pulled myself up by my own bootstraps, dug into my inner resources, and pretended that I wasn't afraid.

As it turned out, Women to Women became a great success. Our work struck a resonant chord with our patients, and the centre grew steadily by word of mouth. As excited as I was about what I was doing, I could never interest my husband in any of the ideas about alternative medicine that were at the core of my new clinical practice. We did, however, have enough other areas of mutual interest that I didn't think his attitude towards my work mattered. In fact, I was rather proud of myself for being able to sustain a loving relationship with a card-carrying member of the American Medical Association.

Marrying My Mother

Looking back, I see that in marrying my husband I had made a secret and mostly unconscious vow that I would do whatever it took to make this marriage work and be the woman I thought he wanted – as long as I could also pursue the work that I loved. Unbeknown to me, I was re-creating with my husband many aspects of the unfinished business I had carried over from my relationship with my mother, a fact that would only begin to dawn on me some twenty-two years later, as I entered perimenopause.

Until then, in my marriage I would continue to play the role of the eager-to-please child I had once been, while my husband would fill the role of my remote, emotionally unavailable mother. As the quiet, sensitive child in a family of outgoing, athletic siblings who loved to spend every moment of life charging full speed ahead up mountains and down ski slopes, I had always been the type who tended to disappear, going off by myself into a quiet room where I could listen to music, read fairy tales, sit dreamily by a fire, or gaze out onto the ocean. Much more tuned in to the other members of our large, bustling family, my mother always seemed too busy to notice me. And although my father supported my studious side, he, like most men of his era, left the hands-on parenting to my mother.

Longing for my mother's approval, I tried to win her love by being good. So I worked and studied hard, never got into trouble, and made myself into my mother's little helper, cooking, cleaning, creating centrepieces for holiday dinners – whatever I could think of that would prove my worth. Intuiting that my mother was in some pain – though it would be many years before I understood the nature of that pain – I tried to be a comfort as well as a help to her, just as I would later try in my marriage to heal my husband's childhood wounds, to give him enough love to make it possible to overcome his early fears and hurts.

Meanwhile, I looked to my teachers for the applause I couldn't get at home. My search for acknowledgement made me a classic over-achiever at school, a pattern that would continue all the way through medical school and into my marriage.

Eventually, just as I had turned to my schoolteachers for the support and approval I didn't get at home, I would one day turn to people other than my husband to meet my emotional needs. But until I began the process of self-knowledge that culminated in the dismantling of my marriage, I simply accepted the fact that, like my mother, my husband could not really see or appreciate me for who I was. In fact, I never expected him to. I was operating under the assumption that I was fundamentally unworthy of being cherished by such a special person.

Had I felt more worthy of love, I never would have chosen someone like my husband. Several of the boyfriends I was involved with before I met him did admire and value me. But when your working belief about yourself is that you have to earn love – earn it both by overachieving in your own life and by rescuing someone from the pain of their own – then you will attract a person who reflects those beliefs back to you. Inevitably the young men who were supportive of me were not the ones I wanted. I wanted precisely the kind of emotional unavailability that felt most like home to me – and I got it.

In this way my husband was a true soul mate, and I cannot blame him for what happened between us. It was only when I was able to change my soul – to change from the inside out, in the most fundamental of ways – that we ceased to be life partners.

My mother and I, on the other hand, have worked through most of our old conflicts and are now closer than ever before.

Why Marriages Must Change at Midlife

When we look at the typical dynamics of intimate family relationships in this culture, it's reasonably safe to say that the vast majority of the nurturing, supportive, subordinate roles fall to the women, as does most of the self-sacrifice. Yes, it has become somewhat more common for women to achieve high-ranking positions in corporate, political, and scientific arenas. But whenever career concessions must be made for the sake of the family, it's still likely to be the woman who steps down or cuts back.

It's true that a woman's biology tends to encourage her involvement with her family at the expense of other interests during the childbearing phase of her life. But it's also true that the culture's atmosphere of gender inequity exploits this tendency to an extreme. This can lead to an incredible surge of pent-up resentment when the hormonal veil lifts and a woman suddenly sees with clarity what has happened in her life.

The emotional changes that come about in the years leading up to and during menopause can feel earthshaking and even terrifying, particularly for those of us who are accustomed to thinking we're in control. It's one thing to resist change from some external force. It's quite another when the change is coming from within, and everything you cling to that's comfortable in its familiarity, including your very identity, is metamorphosing from the inside out. There are only two ways to avoid this abrupt, jolting level of change: defy social and cultural dictates throughout your childbearing years, so that by the time you approach menopause you will already have put into effect many of the changes that cry out to be made at midlife, *or* defy your body's wisdom at perimenopause and ignore its call for truth and creative expression. The latter course can have disastrous consequences for your own health as well as the health of your significant other, not to mention your relationship, which would then be based on something other than mutual respect and love.

How Your Brain Is Hardwired
for Relationships

Nothing in our lives can affect us more profoundly, both physically and emotionally, than our relationships with others. The neural pathways that enable us – that actually compel us – to relate to other human beings are laid down in our brains in early childhood. The experiences we have at this critical stage will influence the circuitry that develops and stays with us for life. If, for example, our needs as infants are met by a loving caretaker who responds to our cries by feeding or changing or stroking or rocking us when we are hungry or cold or wet or scared, then we will feel good about ourselves, and trusting of the outside world. Our needs have been validated, our emotional cravings met, with our relationship with another human being serving as confirmation of our worthiness. And certainly the biochemistry of motherhood supports this outcome. The hormones associated with birth and nursing in a happy, healthy, well-supported mother predispose her to fall in love with her baby and to fill the child with a sense of being loved and accepted unconditionally.

Sometimes, however, our parents did not themselves experience this kind of unconditional love and may therefore be unable to give it to us. Then our cries may go unheeded or, worse, meet with active disapproval or resentment, and we will feel that the universe is not a safe place. Our relationships with others will seem undependable, even threatening.

The feelings we develop about ourselves and others as children become etched into the circuitry of our brains, where they will continue to affect our relationship choices and responses throughout life. They are part of our basic emotional portfolio, easily accessible and freely expressible, sometimes excessively so. On the other hand, those feelings that were not reinforced by early experience tend to wither away, to become unavailable to us without the expenditure of a great deal of effort – or the help of a psychotherapist.

Your ability to live successfully, however you might define success, depends to a great degree on how you relate to other people. If that part of your life is unsatisfactory, the only way you can revise the old relational circuits that determine your current relationships is to expose them, to learn how your brain was wired in your youth. Once you have a better understanding of the environment in which you were born and brought up, it becomes possible – though never easy – to change some of the choices you usually make automatically, as a consequence of that old wiring.

But change can occur only when you understand what it is you need to change. You must ask yourself why you feel the emotions you feel, choose the mates you choose and act the way you act. The answer is in those early life experiences that served as the architects of your neural circuits and live on today in your very cells.

During and after adolescence we almost invariably find ourselves attracted to mates who enable us to revisit and perhaps heal the unfinished emotional business of childhood. In our culture, romantic love is where we express our deepest longings. Thus each romantic relationship we enter into can serve as a microscope into our emotional circuitry. More than any other aspect of our lives, our intimate relationships bring to light the old wounds still begging for closure.

In retrospect, I can see that this was true of my feelings towards the man who became my husband. I was acting out with him a family drama that was still ongoing for me. And although I can't speak on his behalf, in all likelihood I served a similar purpose for him. It took the hormonal and developmental changes of the climacteric to help me see that the role I played in my marriage was based on old beliefs about myself and my worth, beliefs that no longer served me well and were no longer valid.

Menopause to the Rescue

It may not feel like a rescue at the time, but the clarity of vision and increasing intolerance for injustice and inequity that accompany the perimenopausal changes are a gift. Our hormones are giving us an opportunity to see, once and for all, what we need to change in order to live honestly, fully, and healthfully in the second half of our lives. This is the time when many women stop doing what I call 'stuffing' – stifling their own needs in order to tend to everybody else's. Our culture expects women to put others first, and during the childbearing years most of us do, no matter the cost to ourselves. But at midlife we get the chance to make changes, to create lives that fit who *we* are – or, more accurately, who we have become.

If, however, a woman cannot face the changes she needs to make in her life, her body may find a way to point them out to her, lit up in neon and impossible to ignore. It is at this stage that many women reach a crisis in the form of some kind of physical problem, a life-altering or even sometimes life-threatening illness.

One very common physical problem in the years leading up to menopause, for example, is fibroid tumours in the uterus. Forty per cent of all perimenopausal women in our culture are diagnosed with one or more fibroid tumours, and many of them will undergo midlife hysterectomies to deal with the problem. In conventional medicine, we doctors are content to explain that the reason fibroids occur so frequently in women in their forties is because of changing hormone levels, with too much oestrogen being produced compared to progesterone.

Though this is true as far as it goes, it is not the whole truth. I know this both personally and professionally, through the experience I had with a fibroid tumour that was first diagnosed when I was forty-one. Bodily symptoms are not just physical in nature; often they contain a message for us about our lives – if only we can learn to decipher it. Sometimes, as happened with me, the message becomes clear only in stages, with its full meaning available only in retrospect. But what I learned first hand over the course of the eight years during which I was processing the experience of my fibroid is that we attract precisely the illness or problem that best facilitates our access to our inner wisdom – a phenomenon that is both awe-inspiring and sometimes terrifying. Though this is true throughout our lives, it hits us harder and more directly during perimenopause and menopause, as though nature is trying to awaken us one last time before we leave our reproductive years, the era when our inner wisdom, mediated in part by our hormones, is loudest and most intense.

I had a fibroid as my wake-up call. Another woman might have had a flare-up of migraine headaches, or PMS, or breast symptoms, or any of the several other conditions so common at perimenopause. Your body's message to you will be in the language that best breaks through your particular barriers and speaks most specifically to the issues you need to change in your life. The wisdom of this system is very precise.

My Personal Fibroid Story: The Final Chapter

My fibroid was initially diagnosed in 1991, several years before my first book, Women's Bodies, Women's Wisdom, was published. By then I had been working on the book for over three long years, and for a while it felt literally like a stuck creation. In my darkest moments I sometimes doubted that the book would ever be published. I assumed at the time that my fibroid was related to my frustration at how long it was taking me to finish the book and get it out into the world. Fibroids can often represent blocked creativity, or creativity that hasn't been birthed yet, usually because it is being funnelled into dead-end relationships, jobs, or projects. (Blocked creative energy can also express itself in other locations, such as the ovaries, Fallopian tubes, lower intestines, lower back, bladder, and hips, as well as the uterus – all of which are part of the second female energy centre, or what Eastern medical practitioners call the second-chakra area.)

When Women's Bodies, Women's Wisdom was finally published, it was well received, much to my surprise. I had secretly feared that I'd be vilified by my beloved profession for writing the truth as I saw it about the profound connection between women's lives and their health. Though the book wasn't exactly embraced with open arms by my fellow obstetricians and gynaecologists, it wasn't rejected, either. And the women for whom I had written it received it with great enthusiasm.

I was happy and relieved about the response I got, and my fibroid remained quiescent. It didn't go away, but it didn't get much larger, either. It remained as a kind of semidormant whisper from my inner wisdom. I knew the fact that it was there was not a fluke. It meant something. So I vowed to remain open to its message.

Over the next few years I continued to heed my inner voice – as far as I was able to understand it. I tried to change relationships that weren't working for me, I found new ones that were more reciprocal, more of a partnership, and I tried to follow my creative instincts wherever they led me. Thus, after more than a decade of what had been deeply fulfilling work with my colleagues at Women to Women, I found that my heart was increasingly drawn to writing and teaching. Because I was eager for my message to reach a larger audience than ever before, I began to reduce my involvement in the clinic.

I gave up my surgical practice and gradually, ever so gradually, cut back on direct patient care, too. Though I was very excited by the new direction my life was taking, I felt conflict about losing this close connection with my patients. I loved having a regular practice in which I saw the same women year after year, helping them in times of illness, celebrating with them as they learned the skills of creating health. But the pile of charts requiring my attention at the end of each day was increasingly giving me a knot in my stomach.

Meanwhile, *Health Wisdom for Women,* the monthly newsletter that I had started in 1994, was doing well, and I was spending a great deal of time researching and writing it each month. I also began travelling around the country teaching and lecturing. All during this time of change I was trying to understand what my fibroid was trying to teach me – especially when, after having been stable for almost four years, it began to grow larger, until finally it was the size of a football. Although I didn't feel that my life was acutely out of balance in any way, I was aware that the various changes I was making were accompanied by a lot of guilt, and that guilt about doing something we love is always a clue that points to blocked energy. But since I was feeling so fulfilled in my work life, I did not understand what the blockage could be.

On Thanksgiving Day 1996, while trying to find something to wear for dinner that would conceal the now visible swelling in my belly, I finally realised that I was tired of trying to dress around my fibroid, tired of the discomfort it caused me whenever I lay down on my abdomen. I decided that it was time to give up my attempts to shrink it through visualisation, homeopathy, diet, and acupuncture. I was ready to ask for help and have my fibroid surgically removed.

After agreeing a date for the surgery, I started to take a GnRH agonist, a medication that decreases oestrogen levels and therefore shrinks fibroids. This creates an artificial menopause, with many of

the same side effects experienced by women in real menopause, such
as memory change, hot flushes, and bone loss. Nonetheless, I decided
that the benefits I would get from shrinking the tumour – the smaller
the tumour, the smaller the incision, and the lower the risk of excessive blood loss – were worth the inconvenience, especially since I was
only going to be taking the drug for two months.

Little did I know that the benefits would extend far beyond the
shrinking of the tumour. Looking back on this period now, I see that
the two months of artificial menopause brought on by the drug jump-
started the changes in my brain – and my life – that set the stage for a
complete cleansing and reorganisation of some of my closest
relationships, including, ultimately, my marriage.

Fired Up and Having My Say

One evening, a couple of weeks after I started taking the GnRH agonist, all of the family, including our household manager and former
nanny, whom I shall refer to as Lida, was gathered before the television set watching an episode of *ER*. At the end, one of the nurses was
telling a visitor that he should come in and talk to his friend, a man
who had been so badly burned that he was near death. Observing that
the nurse was not telling the visitor the truth about how serious his
friend's condition was, Lida said to me, 'Do they teach you to be like
that in your medical training?' 'Be like what?' I asked her. 'Do they
teach you to withhold the whole truth when the situation is very
dire?' she clarified. After thinking about her question for a minute, I
replied that there was indeed an unspoken belief among our teachers
in medical school that patients (and their family and friends) were not
really able to handle the truth, and that this belief resulted in many
things being left unsaid – a fact that was beautifully illustrated in what
we had seen on television.

My husband stood just then, drawing himself up to his full, quite
impressive height, and proclaimed, 'Of course they don't teach you
that. I don't know what you're talking about!' Something within me
snapped. After years and years of down-regulating my personal truth
to make myself acceptable to my husband and to every authority
figure like him in medical school, I simply couldn't keep still another
moment. I told him that I felt that I – and everybody else – had been
socialised in a thousand non-verbal ways to talk with my patients in a
certain way, and that this way left out a lot of the truth of their
experience and mine. Of course there was no Don't Talk to Patients

101 course, I said, but I'd learned by example that a hand on the door-knob, the sight of a doctor racing from bed to bed on rounds, conveyed a world of information to patients about what they could and couldn't expect in the way of communication and contact with their physician.

As the conversation heated up, my husband and I retired to the bedroom to spare the others our anger. And for the next forty minutes I felt myself grow taller and taller with my own truth. I told my husband what I believed – about medical practice, about our relationship, about the inequity in the way we'd been living all these years – and I offered no excuses for what I said, nor any attempt to make it easier to hear. This was one of those amazing volcanic eruptions that occur from time to time when the lid finally blows on the container overstuffed with things we know but can't talk about because we are female and have to survive by making authorities like us. Everything we've tried to ignore and struggled to keep beneath the surface bursts forth in all its unedited glory. At the end, my husband did not look as tall as he had at the beginning, and he was speaking softly and apologising to me. That was the turning point in our marriage. There was no going back.

What had happened in that moment when I suddenly opted to speak out instead of remaining silent was a direct result of my artificial menopause. Usually menopause comes on gradually, of course. But when it happens more or less instantly because of medication, as it did for me, or because of surgery or radiation, as it does for other women, the sudden hormonal changes can result in insights about our lives that are as dramatic and unexpected as the hot flushes that often plague us at this time. Though my own premature menopause was not permanent and the hot flushes ended as soon as I stopped taking the medication that caused them, the inner change brought about by that brief menopausal interlude *was* permanent. It brought to the surface all the hidden conflicts in myself and my marriage.

Feeling the Joy of Co-creative Partnership

Although until that time I had been in a marriage that had silenced my voice at home, it had not stopped me from becoming increasingly vocal in my work, and I was now being heard by people far beyond my immediate circle. My career star was definitely on the rise. I had co-founded a very well-known women's centre, become president of the American Holistic Medical Association, and written a book that had brought me enormous validation for my work and my ideas. My faith in my own work was growing all the time.

I was also proud of the fact that I was contributing more and more to the family finances, and as usual had looked to my husband for approval – but that was not to be.

As happens for so many women at midlife, around this time I found a new model for partnership. I first met Dr Mona Lisa Schulz when I was finishing writing *Women's Bodies, Women's Wisdom*. With both an MD (doctor of medicine) and PhD (a doctorate) in neuroscience, Mona Lisa eventually became my research partner as well as one of my closest friends. She appraised my work from the viewpoint of pure science and found scientific validation for it. Up until then, my training had led me to believe that hands-on clinicians weren't really scientists. Scientists were people who didn't dirty their hands with the messy details of patients' actual lives, preferring instead to gather data under perfectly controlled conditions. The kind of medicine I was practising was anything but controlled, given that I was helping women choose individual solutions to their health care problems based on a partnership between doctor and patient, and between the patient and her own inner wisdom. This, surely, was not science.

But Mona Lisa helped me see myself and my contribution more clearly. Until I met her, I had found precious few local doctors who took the same approach to medicine that I did, and fewer still who were willing to talk about it publicly. That was a time when it still wasn't safe to call yourself 'holistic', so there weren't too many other volunteers for possible professional martyrdom. But Mona Lisa was one of them. She shared my vision as well as my willingness to take risks, to speak out.

Mona Lisa's approach to science isn't limited to the conventionally acceptable. In addition to being a neuroscientist, she is a practising medical intuitive. She is able to ascertain the emotional and mental patterns associated with a person's illness, knowing only their name and age, and without ever having seen them. Her scientific validation of intuition – defined as the capacity to know something directly without sufficient objective data – contributed to my growing faith in my own inner guidance. I could share with her my lifelong interest in mysticism, astrology, and angels. She also taught me how to use tarot cards as a tool to focus my intuition. I, in turn, provided her with a role model of a physician who had successfully combined right-brain intuitive wisdom with left-brain diagnostic and surgical skills.

Our work together became an exquisite working model for a partnership between two people who are both peers and friends. Besides ideas and values, we shared many of the same attitudes towards life. We had the same sense of humour, loved going to films together, enjoyed putting on parties for my daughters, giggled while we helped each other choose 'speaking costumes' for the public appearances both of us were making ever more frequently in those days. This experience of working with someone who was fun, happy, fulfilled, and ambitious set a whole new standard for the kind of person I wanted to spend time with.

More Validation:
My Message Goes out on Television

Early in 1997 I began working on my first two public television specials. Soon after GnRH had jump-started my brain, I met Jack Wilson and Bill Heitz, two producers from Chicago whose wives had suggested they track me down and put my work on television. Co-creating what eventually turned out to be four successful television specials with Jack and Bill also boosted my self-confidence. Now I had the experience of being truly seen and highly valued not only by a rigorous scientist, but by two people who had believed in me even when I was a complete novice as a television personality.

This was an enormously exciting time for me. However, by this time I was out of the office more often than I was in it. My dream of teaching and writing, of bringing my message to an ever wider audience, had become a full-time reality – and even more. Reluctantly I cut the cord with Women to Women completely, selling my share of both the business and the building to my partners. The work I was doing no longer fitted the model that we had started together. I knew it was time to go out on my own.

The Forces That Change the Goose
Also Change the Gander

As I was making and experiencing all these changes in my life, my husband was going through changes of his own. His midlife re-evaluation started with questioning his career goals. The era of managed care was forcing him to change the way he practised, and he found himself increasingly unhappy in his work. He was also becoming very anxious about money, a fear that my own success seemed only to intensify, rather than to soothe. I couldn't understand why he worried so much about our finances. After all, I thought, I was making good money, and we were in this together.

One reason for his anxiety was that he was thinking about retiring when our younger daughter left school – which was just two short years away. In contrast, I felt as though I was just hitting my stride, and I had no intention of retiring, then or ever. During the retirement planning sessions my husband scheduled with our accountant, I felt as though we were in two different worlds. There didn't appear to be any computer programs designed to take into account two sets of goals as different as the ones my husband and I described in these meetings.

Like many other men at midlife, my husband seemed to deal with his anxiety about change by trying to exert more and more control over our financial resources – resources that were increasingly from my earnings. Or perhaps he had always exerted that kind of control and I was just now waking up to it. For, like many women, I had always been convinced that my husband was better at money management than I was, so I had turned it over to him. He did all the planning and paid all the bills, spending hours at his computer each week doing so. As he went through his midlife crisis, this task seemed to fill him with ever more dread and worry every time he did it, with the result that he tried to micromanage my own expenditures. A part of me was convinced that we were indeed overspending, and I was always on the verge of succumbing to the same fears that plagued him.

But no matter how hard I tried, I could never live within the budget he considered appropriate to our circumstances. I found myself hiding purchases from him, in case he blew up at me. Of course, the conflict between the ideals I had been promoting all these years to my patients and the reality I was living was not lost on me. But my fear of my husband's anger was very real. I let myself be controlled by it, and silenced by it, for years. Even then I was still in some ways the person who wanted more than anything to please, to appease.

Real Menopause Hits

Two weeks after leaving the centre I had co-founded nearly fifteen years before, my 'official' hot flushes began. They were much less intense than the drug-induced hot flushes I had experienced earlier – flushes so extreme that I routinely removed my winter coat and stripped down to a T-shirt in the middle of winter. Nonetheless, they were eloquent enough to make me realise that I was finally entering menopause for real.

It was 18 December 1998 – the end of a year and, as it turned out, the end of an era. The separation I had just negotiated from Women to Women was only a warm-up for what was about to happen on the home front – though on the surface things looked fine, even festive. The day my hot flushes started was also the day I, my husband, and our daughters embarked on a long-awaited family ski trip to Austria, where we would spend Christmas with my mother and my siblings. This was something I had dreamed for years about doing.

The trip was wonderful in many ways, and I was very happy to be with my extended family in such a magical place, but I felt the strain in my marriage as never before. When I looked around at other couples around us, men and women who were clearly engaged with and enjoying each other, I felt very alone. I found that I was avoiding my husband on that trip, skiing mostly with my daughters, my sister, and my mother. I simply didn't want to use my energy to try to soothe my husband and keep him comfortable, as I had always done before. The coming of my hot flushes had signalled another stage in my own midlife re-evaluation – a commitment to setting healthier boundaries, to taking better care of myself, to speaking the truth.

In case I had any doubts, my body reinforced my decision to honour my own needs. I broke out in adult acne, a sign that something had 'got under my skin' and was now about to erupt. When I turned to the Motherpeace tarot cards I had used at many other moments of uncertainty in my life, I kept drawing the Shaman of Swords card, whose message is about saying what you know to be true. The universe was speaking to me in many guises. I was now ready to hear.

My Marriage Goes Bankrupt

Soon after the New Year, at the beginning of 1999, a series of over-draft notices that arrived from our bank seemed to me to symbolise the degree to which my husband and I had failed to create a viable partnership. Our household account had insufficient funds. So did our marriage. When I suggested that I needed my own space for a while and wanted us to consider separate bedrooms during this period, my husband left in a fit of rage. He did not return.

Almost overnight I was handed the opportunity – and the responsibility – to assume complete financial dominion over both my business and my household.

Up until the moment my husband left, it had never occurred to me in all my years of marriage that I would ever end up divorced. My fantasy was always that my husband would change or that I would change or that something would change so that the two of us could become the team I thought we were capable of being. For years psychics and astrologers had been telling me we were meant to be together. This couldn't be happening.

And yet despite what seemed to be in the stars, and despite our three years of couples therapy, I had reached the end of the road. I could no longer allow myself to be in what I perceived was an unbalanced relationship. I needed to come into my own. I was no longer willing to be controlled by another person, emotionally, financially, or physically. I had come too far.

Finally I was ready to do the last part of the self-healing that I'd spent half a century preparing for. Menopause had spurred me to make the ideals I'd been promoting in my work a reality. I knew I now had two choices: to mute my voice so that I could stay in my marriage, or to find the courage I needed to take steps towards getting a divorce. But what a hard choice it was.

Perhaps one reason it was so hard was that the 1950s was the period in which my brain had been wired for relationships. If my marriage had broken up in that era, it would have been widely agreed that I had wrecked our relationship with my ambition. Why couldn't I have just put my husband's needs before my own? Why did I insist on being fully supported and fully met in my marriage relationship? Why did I insist on pushing my husband past where he felt comfortable going? I did it because I had no other choice. Something within me, some voice from my very soul, was urging me on, and I had to trust it.

Nonetheless, I was frightened of what it would be like to live without my longtime mate. And then one day I remembered something one of my daughters had said to me several months before: that things were so unpleasant in our house, she doubted she would come home for holidays once she had left for college. That gave me courage to move forwards.

Healing Through Pain

Even though I could see, in retrospect, that I had started the process of letting go of my marriage several years before, I was still not prepared for the deep sense of loss I felt when it ended. Initially I felt as though one of my limbs were missing. For weeks I awoke before dawn, feeling an acute ache in my throat and in my heart as soon as the realisation hit me, once again, that my husband was not next to me in bed.

Once out of the house, I found I could sometimes get along OK for days at a time. Then I'd go somewhere and have to fill out one of those forms that are ubiquitous in our lives, and I'd think about how the day was going to come when I would have to tick the box that said 'divorced'. I dreaded that day.

I remembered how hard it was for my mother after her marriage ended. But hers was a happy marriage, cut short when my father died suddenly on the tennis court at the age of sixty-eight. That had been a terrible blow for her. Still, in the early months of my separation, I remember thinking that my own pain was in some ways even worse, because it made me question the most central fact of my life for the past twenty-four years. Even though I knew that 50 per cent of all marriages ended in divorce, I felt like an incredible failure. I was becoming the kind of woman I'd always heard no one wants to invite anywhere in case she might steal another woman's husband: a woman alone at midlife, unclaimed, unwanted, and dangerous to the status quo.

Loss is a recurrent theme at midlife. Even women who don't go through divorce at this time often face other losses – the death of parents or spouse, estrangement from a child, being let go from a job, changes in physical appearance, or the realisation that the reproductive years are over. For a woman who has never borne a child and had always hoped that that was in her future, the end of her fertility can be a terrible loss. But no matter what the circumstances, nearly every woman has to give up *some* dream about what she thought her life would be like.

And when that realisation hits, it is very painful. Gradually I allowed myself to feel all my grief and pain, secure in the knowledge that it would not destroy me. I knew that only then could I move forwards with my life.

Healing Through Anger

I would be lying to you, and perpetuating a grave disservice to midlife women, if I allowed you to believe that my feelings at this time were solely about grief and loss. There was also another feeling brimming up from my depths, and this emotion saved me from the paralysis that I might otherwise have felt.

It was the emotion of anger that gave me the energy to proceed with the onerous task of dismantling twenty-four years of married life – and building another kind of life. I used the volcanic energy of my anger to guide me towards identifying my needs and then getting them met. Having experienced my husband's departure as an abandonment of me and our daughters, I was determined to do whatever I had to in order to make our lives whole again.

At first I wasn't sure I could do it. My anger was tempered by a liberal dose of fear. But every time I teetered on the brink of despair or terror, some piece of evidence would arrive in the post that compelled me to see the truth: overdraft notices from the bank, credit card bills, and solicitors' letters were appearing with great regularity. Like it or not, I was on my own, financially and in every other way. I was going to have to give up my sentimental fantasies that our marriage could still be saved. My focus would have to be on ensuring my own and my daughters' well-being.

I also had another source of energy during this hard time. My brother had gone through a divorce himself some years before. He seemed to know instinctively when to ring me and what to say to give me encouragement. His clear-sightedness proved to be invaluable to me.

Healing Through Acceptance

I began a daily prayer practice to give me the courage to continue the process of letting go of my marriage and my identity as a married woman. This involved taking a walk every morning and stopping halfway through to look out over the harbour. There I would think about all that I had to be grateful for in my life – which was a lot.

Then I would say a prayer of thanks out loud, sending the words down the river to its source. Each day as I stood there I watched the ice on the river receding, the tides changing. Spring would come soon, I knew, and with it the healing energy of rebirth and renewal. I was grateful for winter and the time it gave me to grieve, grateful for having spring to look forward to.

On the weekend just before our twenty-fourth wedding anniversary, about three months after our separation, I felt especially bereft, my feelings of loss temporarily obliterating all my intellectual and emotional reasons for proceeding with divorce. A friend of mine had telephoned that morning and told me how sad she felt about our split, since she could feel that there was still so much love between my husband and me. She told me she would spend part of the weekend burning prayer sticks for us in the ashram where she worships.

On Monday, the day of our anniversary, I felt filled with longing. I spent the whole day wanting to ring my husband. Then, as I was sitting down to dinner with the girls, the doorbell rang. It was the florist, delivering a dozen white roses accompanied by a card that read, 'Thanks for almost twenty-four years together. And our two daughters.' I wept and said to the girls, 'Never doubt that your father and I have always loved each other.'

Armadillo Medicine: The Power of Vulnerability

During the weeks just after my separation, a newspaper reporter interviewed me for a story she was doing about my work. 'I have only one more question,' she said at the end. 'Has Chris Northrup ever really suffered?'

I was shocked. At that very moment I was feeling the loss of the most significant relationship of my life, and feeling it in every cell of my body. How could she assume my life was easy? But I said nothing. It was too soon to discuss my situation publicly. The wounds were too new, too raw.

Earlier that same month Mona Lisa had said to me, 'You're not vulnerable enough, so no one feels drawn to take care of you. I, on the other hand, have had so many health problems that everyone feels drawn to take care of me. I attract "mothers" wherever I go.'

This made me furious. It hadn't felt safe to allow myself to be

vulnerable with my husband, or before that with my mother. Somewhere along the line I had lost the ability. Besides, it hadn't been an
ability I admired. I'd watched far too many women milk the victim
role, playing on the sympathy of others to get their needs met. I had
never wanted to be such a woman. But I knew that our culture identified so deeply with victims that it doubted the humanity of those who
didn't assume that role. That was really what the newspaper reporter
had been saying to me with her question.

For two nights in a row after my conversation with Mona Lisa I
sought guidance in a set of animal 'medicine cards' that worked something like a tarot pack. Each time I drew I picked the card known as
Armadillo (in the reversed position), whose message is this:

> You may think the only way to win in your present situation is
> to hide or to pretend that you are armour-coated and invincible,
> but this is not the way to grow. It is better to open up and find
> the value and strength of your vulnerability. You will experience
> something wonderful if you do. Vulnerability is the key to en-
> joying the gifts of physical life. In allowing yourself to feel, a
> myriad of expressions are made available. For instance, a true
> compliment is an admiration flow of energy. If you are afraid of
> being hurt and are hiding from anything, you will never feel the
> joy of admiration from others.[1]

This message was right on target for me. And once again I was
reminded of how well I had learned from my stoic mother to hide my
vulnerability. It was now time to change this pattern, as part of letting
go of my past.

At midlife, some women seek new satisfactions in the world
beyond that of home and family life. They may need to don some
armour. But other women need to let the armour down a bit. That
was the case for me. And it's also true for many men, who traditional-
ly spend the years leading up to midlife focused on achieving success
in the workplace. The point is that at midlife, more than at any other
time, the aspects of your personality that kept you alive and functional for the first half of your life may actually put you at risk in the
second half. All of us must find the courage to make the changes that
will enable us to live our lives in an empowered fashion.

Celebrating the Past While Creating a New Future

Our household became much more relaxed once my husband left. The tension was gone. I adopted a couple of kittens from our local animal shelter and found that they brought me and my daughters a great deal of comfort and enjoyment. We had never had pets before, because a dog had always seemed like too much trouble, and my husband was allergic to cats.

Surprisingly, I also found that I was sleeping better than I had in years, waking up easily every morning without the alarm clock. This had never happened before. Looking back now, I can finally appreciate how much energy I had been using in the effort to keep my marriage going.

As the weeks went by, I began the slow process of feeling what it was like to have myself to myself. And on some very deep level I began to feel, ever so gradually, that I was recharging my inner batteries from a source deep within me. As with all grieving and letting go, there were ups and downs to this process. One week, for example, I found myself crying while watching the Thursday night TV shows I used to watch with my husband and daughters as a weekly ritual. But then one week later I was able to spend the evening alone, away from the TV, revelling in the beautiful light on the river outside my home. I was alone, but I was not lonely. I knew I was going to make it. I was happy.

The kind of marriage I had worked well for me for many years, and I am very grateful for having been able to experience all the joys and pleasures of family life with my husband and our two children. Those joys were very real, as I was reminded the day my husband came to claim his share of the paintings that were hanging on our walls. After he removed them, I was left with that awful feeling of loss that newly bare walls give you at such times. To get me past this latest milestone in grief, two friends and I spent an afternoon creating an entire wall of family photos in the dining room – providing concrete and comforting evidence of the good times in my past. A year later I replaced the photos of my husband with those of my daughters and me. I have learned that letting go is a process, not an event.

I have also learned that part of the process is acknowledging the past value of the relationship you are leaving behind, and doing this not just silently, to yourself, but, when appropriate, to the person who was part of that relationship.

I did this myself five months after our separation, when my husband and I were nearing a settlement. As we were leaving one of our mediation sessions, I asked him to meet with me privately, and then I poured out everything that was in my heart. I apologised for trying to change him. I said how glad I was that neither of us had used an affair to get out of the marriage. I thanked him for the safe haven of the family we had created together, and for the wonderful children who would not have existed without our love for each other. I told him I was grateful for the support and structure he provided for me when I was out blazing new trails in women's health. I also told him that I loved him.

My feelings were so poignant during that outpouring of gratitude that I could easily see why estranged couples might want to keep their anger and resentment alive. That way they wouldn't have to feel all the pain of what they are losing. But I could also see how damaging this could be to their children, themselves, and everyone else involved, and I was glad I had found the courage to express what was in my heart.

I let go of so much that year, including my feelings of failure. Margaret Mead, the renowned anthropologist, once pointed out that in the past, most marriages continued until 'till death do us part' because after twenty-five years of marriage, one or both members of the couple had died! In other words, at the same age that most of us are going through the changes of menopause, our ancestors were falling ill and dying – or were already dead. 'Till death do us part' was much easier to accomplish when lives were shorter. Mead's observation helped me feel less of a failure for being unable to preserve my marriage.

My health remained good throughout the difficult and painful year of my divorce. I allowed my tears to flow freely, my anger to erupt and dissipate. I also called on spiritual guidance unceasingly, and this, together with my new emotional openness, helped me negotiate a period characterised by significant hormonal change with minimal symptoms. I also used a variety of natural approaches to hormonal balance, as I will discuss in chapter 6.

Now it is time for me, as for so many other women of the baby boom generation, to be pioneers in re-creating the second half of our lives on our own terms. As we do so, we must keep in mind that physical and emotional health is our natural state, even during this time of transition. And although the life ahead of us is uncharted territory, fraught with all the uncertainty that accompanies change, it is no less precious and need be no less joyous than the life that is receding quickly into the pages of our personal history.

Have no regrets, whatever you decide. Take advantage of the clarity of vision that is the gift of menopause, and use that gift to let the second half of your life be truly your own.

TWO

The Brain Catches Fire at Menopause

A woman recently told me that when her mother was approaching the age of menopause, her father sat the whole family down and said, 'Your mother may be going through some changes now, and I want you to be prepared. Your uncle Ralph told me that when your aunt Carol went through the change, she threw a leg of lamb right out of the window!' Although this story fits beautifully into the stereotype of the 'crazy' menopausal woman, it should not be overlooked that throwing the leg of lamb out of the window may have been Aunt Carol's outward expression of the process going on within her soul: the reclaiming of self. Perhaps it was her way of saying how tired she was of waiting on her family, of signalling to them that she was past the cook/chauffeur/dishwasher stage of life. For many women, if not most, part of this reclamation process includes getting in touch with anger and, perhaps, blowing up at loved ones for the first time. The events that evoke anger are never new. What is new, however, is our willingness and energy to let that anger be acknowledged and expressed, both to ourselves and to others. This can be the first step towards much-needed change in our lives . . . change that is often long overdue.

Our Cultural Inheritance

Regardless of where you currently stand in your menstrual or perimenopausal transition, chances are you've inherited a few beliefs about your cycle that boil down to a variation of the following: 'The issues that arise premenstrually have nothing to do with my actual life. They are strictly hormonal. My hormones exist in a universe that is completely separate from the rest of my life.' I found a superb example of this culturally sanctioned unconsciousness about premenstrual syndrome (PMS) in a popular women's magazine:

> I love PMS! It gives me so much perspective! It makes me cry in the supermarket aisle because they're out of Calamata olives – a deliberate plot . . . to sabotage the new recipe I'm dying to try on my one day off! It makes me pick fights with my husband over incredibly important stuff – like the fact that he's forgotten to put out my morning coffee cup alongside his, which is incredibly symbolic of something deeper, don't you think? . . . And then, POOF! My period arrives and I wake up to a world that looks rosy. Gone is the pressure to get a divorce, send my kids to reform school, and move to another country. In fact, compared to how I felt the previous week, I feel pretty good indeed.[1]

The writer goes on to explain that her PMS has only intensified as she has got older and that her gynaecologist has suggested that she go back on the pill, or try Prozac before her period. In other words, she needs to get 'fixed'. But she's ignoring potentially important messages from her body. PMS and the escalation of symptoms that are so common during perimenopause are really our inner guidance system trying to get us to pay attention to the adjustments we need to make in our lives, adjustments that become particularly urgent during perimenopause.

If we don't pay attention to the issues that come up for us every month during the years when our periods are regular, our symptoms will escalate as we get older. Every premenstrual issue that this writer blames on PMS is potentially related to a larger and deeper need that is not being met. The issues she raises may appear superficial or even silly at first glance. But if she were to be completely honest with herself, she would realise that the lack of olives at the supermarket and the fact that her husband doesn't put out her coffee cup in the morning may be doorways to deeper needs that she has been ignoring: the need for more time off, a longing for the sensual satisfaction of cooking, a longing to be cherished daily by her husband. When these needs aren't acknowledged, the body ends up screaming louder and louder to get our attention.

By reducing her body's signals to physical symptoms, the writer has bought into the dualistic belief system that pervades Western medicine. Her attitude – one that is all too common – is that troublesome hormones are a woman's cross to bear, but with a variety of remedies and a sense of humour, they can be kept to a low roar, so they're at least tolerable. Instead of seeing an opportunity for insight here, she has diminished and dismissed her inner guidance.

Our Brains Catch Fire at Menopause

Our brains actually begin to change at perimenopause. Like the rising heat in our bodies, our brains also become fired up! Sparked by the hormonal changes that are typical during the menopausal transition, a switch goes on that signals changes in our temporal lobes, the brain region associated with enhanced intuition. How this ultimately affects us depends to a large degree on how willing we are to make the changes in our lives that our hormones are urging us to make over the ten years or so of perimenopause.

There is ample scientific evidence of the brain changes that begin to take place at perimenopause. Differences in relative levels of oestrogen and progesterone affect the temporal lobe and limbic areas of our brains, and we may find ourselves becoming irritable, anxious, and emotionally volatile. Though our culture leads us to believe that our mood swings are simply the result of raging hormones and do not have anything to do with our lives, there is solid evidence that repeated episodes of stress (due to relationship, children, and job situations you feel angry about or powerless over, for example) are actually behind many of the hormonal changes in the brain and body. This means that if your life situation – whether at work or with children, your husband, your parents, or whatever – doesn't change, then unresolved emotional stress can exacerbate a perimenopausal hormone imbalance. In a normal premenopausal hormonal state it's much easier to overlook those aspects of your life that don't really work, just as you can overlook them more easily in the first half of your menstrual cycle – the time when you're more apt to feel upbeat and happy and able to sweep difficult material under the carpet. But that doesn't mean the problems aren't there.

Learning to Recognise and Heed Our Wake-up Calls

Whether you are in early perimenopause at thirty-five or standing at the threshold of menopause, your body's inner wisdom will attempt to catch your attention through four kinds of escalating physical and emotional wake-up calls.

Our First Wake-up Call: PMS

What happens if, during our childbearing years, we ignore our cyclic nature, disconnect from the body's wisdom, and attempt to function as though we were linear beings, with the same drives, the same focus, and the same aptitudes day after day? Very often PMS happens. With its physical and emotional discomfort, PMS is one way a woman's body elbows her every month to remind her of the growing backlog of unresolved issues accumulating within her. Everything from unbalanced

FIGURE 1: THE FIRST TWO WAKE-UP CALLS: PMS AND SAD

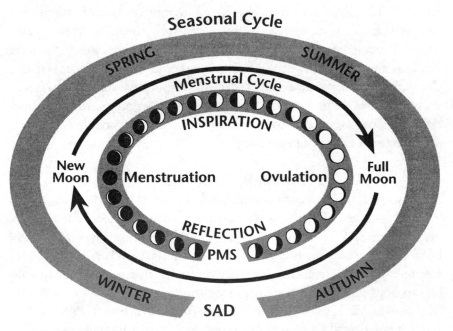

PMS is to the monthly cycle as SAD is to the annual cycle.
Both conditions respond to the same treatment while asking us to
deepen our connection to our cyclic wisdom.
© 2001 by Northrup and Schulz

nutrition to unresolved relationships can disrupt the normal hormonal milieu, wreaking physical and emotional havoc during the childbearing years. Ignoring these early, relatively gentle nudges month after month sets her up for sharper and more urgent messages. Inconvenient as they are, these pains are our allies, begging us to look up and see what's not working in our lives. Often we don't, however. Most of us are too busy, and the discomfort isn't that bad, after all. It's easier to just ignore it. But the body is insistent!

A Poignant Wake-up Call: Postpartum Depression

It is well documented that women who have significant PMS are also more apt to suffer from postpartum depression in the first days or weeks after giving birth. Or sometimes those who suffer from postpartum depression will go on to develop PMS when their menstrual cycles resume. Because new mothers often feel far too vulnerable to complain, postpartum depression is underdiagnosed and undertreated in our culture, even though between 10 and 15 per cent of all women experience some form of mood disorder following childbirth, ranging from major depression to anxiety disorders such as panic attacks. As with all illness, there are genetic, environmental, and nutritional factors that are associated with postpartum depression. But it is also true that postpartum depression is often a sign from a mother's inner wisdom that she isn't getting the support and help she needs at this time, and that certain areas of her life, especially her relationships with one or both parents or with her partner, require some attention. If these issues aren't resolved, they are very likely to resurface during the hormonal shifts of perimenopause.

An Annual Wake-up Call: SAD

If the monthly messages go unheeded, a woman's body may send a louder wake-up call on a yearly basis, in the form of seasonal affective disorder, or SAD. It begins with an intensification of the symptoms of PMS during the autumn and winter of the year, when the days are shortest and darkness dominates. Eventually it can evolve into full-blown depression and despair during the time of year when daylight is abbreviated. It is well known that providing two hours of full-spectrum artificial light in the evening, to trick the body into thinking the days are longer, can reverse the weight gain, depression, carbohydrate craving, social withdrawal, fatigue, and irritability of SAD.

But studies have shown that without continued use of the artificial lights, the symptoms return the following autumn . . . unless the wake-up call is heeded. The link between PMS and SAD is a profound example of how women's wisdom is simultaneously encoded into both our monthly cycles and the annual cycle of the seasons.

Perimenopause: The Mother of All Wake-up Calls

For many women perimenopause can be, as one of my patients described it, 'PMS times ten' – and this is particularly the case for those who, for one reason or another, hit the snooze button instead of heeding their monthly and seasonal wake-up calls. This is not to discount the direct physical effects of changing hormone levels. However, it is a safe bet that any uncomfortable symptoms that reveal themselves during times of hormonal shift will be magnified and prolonged if a woman is carrying a heavy load of emotional baggage. These symptoms are the body's wisdom, pleading yet again that unresolved life issues be attended to. Throughout a woman's childbearing years, a kind of 'debt account' is established where existing and future issues accumulate, compounding interest with each passing month that the debt goes unpaid.

Thus the average woman, blessed with approximately 480 menstrual periods and 40 seasonal cycles to bring her to the threshold of her menopause, gets about 500 progress reports. How is her physical health and nutrition? How are her emotions? What's happening in her relationships and her career? There have been approximately 500 opportunities to resolve those issues . . . or sweep them under the carpet. At perimenopause the process escalates. The earnest, straightforward inner self, which has tried for years to get our attention, makes one final hormonally mediated attempt to get us to deal with our accumulated needs, wants, and desires. This is likely to turn into a period of great emotional turmoil, as each woman struggles to make a new life, one that can accommodate her emerging self. Externally and internally, this period is a mirror image of adolescence, a time when our bodies and brains were also going through major hormonal shifts that gave us the energy to attempt to individuate from our families and become the person we were meant to be. At menopause we pick up where we left off in adolescence. It is now time to finish the job.

It should be no surprise, then, that research has documented that those women who experience uncomfortable – even severe –

symptoms of PMS are often the same women who have a tumultuous perimenopause, with physical and emotional symptoms that become increasingly impossible to ignore.[2]

As a woman makes the transition to the second half of her life, she finds herself in a struggle not only with her own aversion to conflict and confrontation, but also with the culture's view of how women 'should' be. The body's inner wisdom gets its last, best chance of breaking through culturally erected barriers, while shining a light on aspects of a woman's life that need work. To resolve the situation, then, it is up to the individual woman to meet her body's wisdom halfway.

Is It Me or Is It My Hormones? Debunking the Myth of Raging Hormones

The fluctuating hormone levels that most women experience during perimenopause and during menopause do not, in and of themselves, cause the distressing emotional and psychological symptoms (such as anger and depression) that so many women suffer with PMS and at midlife. But if there is an underlying susceptibility to distress in the first place, there is no doubt that hormonal swings will help bring that distress to the surface.

Though hormone levels and mood do tend to fluctuate widely during our reproductive years, and even more widely still during our perimenopausal years, research has failed to show any appreciable differences between the hormone levels of those women who suffer from PMS-like symptoms and those who don't. What has been well documented, however, is that the *brains* of women who suffer the most from PMS-like symptoms are more susceptible to the effects of fluctuating hormone levels.[3] In other words, it is not the hormone levels per se that are the problem. Rather, it is the particular combination of a woman's hormone levels and her pre-existing brain chemistry along with her life situation, that results in her symptoms. It is estimated that 27 per cent of all women who experience agitation and depression during their periods, and 36 per cent of all women who become depressed premenstrually, will be very sensitive to the hormonal changes that occur at menopause.[4]

Though we tend to blame perimenopausal symptoms on hormonal shifts in the body, their origins are far more complex. Several women in my practice, for example, have experienced symptoms such as hot flushes and mood swings in their later forties – despite having been on full hormone replacement for over twenty years as a result of having undergone hysterectomies and removal of their ovaries while still in their twenties. Clearly, changes in reproductive hormones alone do not account for these symptoms. They are signals from our mind and body that we have reached a new developmental stage – an opportunity for healing and growth.

ANATOMY OF MENOPAUSAL WISDOM **Menopause combines the wisdom of the prior stages and brings it to a new level.**	
Body Process	**Encoded Wisdom**
MENSTRUAL CYCLE	Cyclic intuitive wisdom and emotional recycling and processing
PREGNANCY/FERTILITY	Capacity to conceive an idea or a life with another, hold it, nurture it, and allow it to be born
MENOPAUSE	Passage into the wisdom years Capacity to be open to constant intuitive knowing Reseeding the community

Moving Inwards

Until midlife, it is characteristic for a woman's energies to be focused on caring for others. She is encouraged to do so, in part, by the hormones that drive her menstrual cycles – the hormones that foster her instincts for nurturing, her devotion to cohesion, and harmony within her world. But for two or three days each month, just before or during our periods, there is a hormonal interlude when the veil between our conscious and unconscious selves is thinner and the voice of our souls beckons to us, subtly reminding us of our own passions, our own needs, which cannot and should not always be subsumed to the needs of those we love.

This fluctuation between inner and outer worlds and the way it is influenced by our hormones was revealed in a fascinating study done in the 1930s by a psychoanalyst and a physician. Dr Therese Benedek studied the psychotherapy records of patients, while Dr Boris Ruben-stein studied the ovarian hormonal cycles of the same women. By looking only at a woman's emotional state, Dr Benedek was able to identify where she was in her menstrual cycle with incredible accuracy. The two doctors found that just before ovulation, when oestrogen levels were at their highest, women's emotions and behaviour were directed towards the outer world. At ovulation, women were more relaxed and content and quite receptive to being cared for and loved by others. During the postovulatory and premenstrual phase, when progesterone is at its highest (and PMS symptoms are also at their peak), women were more likely to be focused on themselves and more involved in inward-directed activity.[5]

I like to think of the first half of our cycles as the time when we are both biologically and psychologically preparing to give birth to some-one or something outside of ourselves. In the second half of our cycles, we prepare to give birth to nothing less than ourselves. It is at this time that the more intuitive parts of our brain become activated, giving us feedback and guidance about the state of our inner lives. One of my newsletter subscribers, Lucinda, describes the process eloquently.

LUCINDA: HEALING PMS

PMS has been an issue for me that has severely limited my life, distorted my children's experience of their mother, and made my husband's life with me very scary. He insisted for years that an alien must take over my body when my hormones fluctuated in prepara-tion for my menstrual cycle! Migraines were part of this pattern, too. I insisted that it was the 'true ugly me' that surfaced at a weakened time! One minute I would be rational and peacefully attending to my life tasks, the next I would be argumentative until war broke out!

Then I would cry and feel like the worst person on the planet. This didn't happen every month, but when it did it was on schedule, around the seventeenth day of my cycle. The consequence of this pattern was that I feared I was crazy, and I could not count on myself for normal planning of life events, making me an unreliable family member. While I longed for intimacy, I was too scary a person to approach. I was caught in the busy schedule of a working wife and mother and couldn't figure out this problem in my life. I limped along, trying to appear normal to the outside world but becoming more and more exhausted.

As the years passed I was introduced to new theories about the mind–body connection and information about the benefits of physically releasing emotional distress, past as well as present, through crying, yawning, sweating, shaking, and so on. These things remained a concept for a long time. I knew the information in my head, but I had not assimilated it into my being for use. I was still fighting the monthly disability of PMS and internally asking why – why did I, who was creative, intelligent, and loving, have this condition that was ruining my life?

Insight came one day as I was getting a migraine and knew what would follow. I consciously asked myself what would happen if, instead of fighting the feeling and judging myself as a defective person, I instead allowed myself to feel fully what was happening in my body. I surrendered my control and focused on just being present with my body for the first time ever.

I felt vulnerable. The shift in my hormones left me feeling vulnerable. That was not a state of being I could tolerate. I was a warrior, not a maiden. I cried, acknowledging my defencelessness. I experienced my feminine side for the first time. In fear, I had raged against it in the past. No wonder I felt like a victim. I was battering my own feminine side – my internal goddess.

I stayed with the feeling. I didn't die. I needed her softness and wisdom. The migraine faded. I eased up on my self-judgement and embraced that part of myself long hidden – even from my own view.

The physical symptoms that had accompanied my PMS lessened. I use the increased energy to do some other things for myself. I have a holistic nutritionist and am improving my diet slowly. I use a good massage therapist. I continue to discharge my past and present feelings. I have fun at whatever I am doing because I see it as important, as my own creative expression. I talk before crisis occurs.

I have continued to be challenged by my body's response to my poor choices. I am grateful for its ability to do so, and now when I wonder, it is more a question of what than of why. What am I doing that denies my feminine inner wisdom and goes against my true spiritual identity?

As I sit present with that question, the answer bubbles up from within. We do come with an instruction kit, if we will just quiet ourselves to receive the information and learn some new skills.

Moving from an Alternating to a
Direct Current of Wisdom

At midlife, the hormonal milieu that was present for only a few days each month during most of your reproductive years, the milieu that was designed to spur you on to re-examine your life just a little at a time, now gets stuck in the on position for weeks or months at a time. We go from an alternating current of inner wisdom to a direct current that remains on all the time after menopause is complete. During peri-menopause, our brains make the change from one way of being to the other.

Biologically, at this stage of life you are programmed to withdraw from the outside world for a period of time and revisit your past. You need to be free of the distractions that come when you are focusing your mothering efforts solely on others. Perimenopause is a time when you are meant to mother yourself.

It may be no accident that the word *menopause* invites the association 'pause from men'. In truth, you are being urged, biologically, to pause from everyone – from mankind in general – in order to do important work on yourself. Perhaps as a result of this, one of the most common threads running through women's descriptions of how they feel during the menopausal transition is the longing for time alone, for a refuge that provides peace, quiet, and freedom from distractions and demands.

It's a wistful dream, seemingly out of reach in this busy age of multidirectional tugs-of-war. But those who have the yearning often believe nonetheless that their uncomfortable menopausal symptoms would simply dissolve if only they had the luxury of shutting out the world so they could tune in to the growth process occurring within themselves. This wistful dream is real. It comes from your soul. I've come to realise that you can trust it and believe in it – and that you must do its bidding.

Even if this dream seems out of reach, the simple truth is that every woman *can* find refuge within her existing environment. Even if you can't charter a plane to a deserted island, odds are that if you acknow-ledge and validate your need for solitude, then you can clear some time and find a private corner to which to retreat daily. You can insulate yourself from noise, telephones, and interaction with others. I encourage every woman to find a way to do this on whatever level is possible. When we commit to taking this first step, we have the chance to develop a newfound sense of ourselves and our life's

FIGURE 2: CURRENTS OF WISDOM

FSH and LH stimulate ovulation and are released cyclically each month up until the years before menopause. They then undergo a change during which ovulation gradually ceases and FSH and LH levels gradually increase. I believe that these high levels have to do with moving from 'AC current' to 'DC current'. The intuitive wisdom that was once available most clearly during only certain parts of the menstrual cycle is now potentially available all the time.

purpose, which gives us an exhilarating sense of what is possible for us during the second half of our lives.

The Multiple Roles of Your 'Reproductive' Hormones

It has long been known that our female hormones are not involved solely with reproduction. They are connected with our moods and with the way our brains work. Boys and girls have the same rate of depression up until puberty. After that, when ovarian hormones surge and cycling begins, depression increases in females, with the highest incidence reached between the ages of twenty-two and forty-five. The lifetime incidence of depression in males is only one in ten, while in females it is one in four. After menopause, the rates of depression in men and women reach gender parity once again. Cross-cultural studies have shown that women have a higher lifetime incidence of depression in other cultures as well.

I believe that this gender-wide susceptibility to depression is in part related to the subservient roles that most women in most cultures have been forced to play for millennia. That said, it is also true that the menstrual cycle, pregnancy, the postpartum period, and the perimenopausal period are all associated with depression in many women. And those who are susceptible to PMS are also the most susceptible to postpartum depression and perimenopausal mood problems. Part of the reason for this has to do with the complex interaction between the hypothalamus, the pituitary gland, the ovaries, and the multiple hormones that are produced in and interact within these key areas. These key hormones are:

- *GnRH* (gonadotropin-releasing hormone), which is produced in the hypothalamus

- *FSH* (follicle-stimulating hormone) and *LH* (luteinizing hormone), which are produced in the pituitary and stimulate, in turn, the rise of oestrogen and progesterone during the monthly menstrual cycle

- *Oestrogen,* produced in the ovaries, body fat, and other areas

- *Progesterone,* produced primarily in the ovaries – which, together with oestrogen, prepares the lining of the uterus for implantation and growth of an embryo.

The hypothalamus regulates the production of all of these hormones and is in turn regulated by them – and by many others. It has receptors on it not only for progesterone, oestrogen, and androgens (eg DHEA, testosterone), but also for noradrenaline, dopamine, and serotonin, neurotransmitters that regulate mood and that are affected in turn by our thoughts, beliefs, diet, and environment.

If oestrogen, progesterone, and androgen had no other role in the body besides driving reproduction, your levels of these hormones would drop to zero after menopause. But they don't. Similarly, if GnRH, FSH, and LH suddenly were without purpose after menopause, one might expect that there would cease to be any of these hormones circulating in your system after that time. In fact, quite the contrary is true.

During perimenopause, GnRH levels begin to rise in the brain, causing FSH and LH to surge to their highest levels ever. A popular explanation is that this is the body's attempt to 'kick-start' the ovaries into resuming their original function, which might make sense if it weren't for one eloquent fact: those elevated FSH and LH levels *stay* elevated, permanently, well after it is physiologically obvious that the ovaries (which have, essentially, run out of eggs) have no intention of jumping back onto the reproductive bandwagon. It would seem that your body, in its wisdom, has ulterior motives for continuing to produce the so-called reproductive hormones, and reproduction no longer is the point. In fact, evidence is mounting that at least one of the roles for this off-the-charts production of FSH and LH, and of the GnRH that precipitates this rise, is to drive the changes taking place in the midlife woman's brain.

For biological reasons, females of the human species are often easier to control – intellectually, psychologically, and socially – during their childbearing years than they are before puberty (from birth to the age of eleven) or after menopause. When we are creating a home and building a family, our primary concern is to maintain balance and peace. We seem to know instinctively that when we're bringing up a family, it's better for all if we compromise and maintain whatever support we have, even if it's less than ideal, rather than risk going it alone. Though this may mean we lose sight of our individual goals, our ability to 'go with the programme' is in fact protective. A recent

FIGURE 3: THE HYPOTHALAMUS-PITUITARY-OVARY CONNECTION

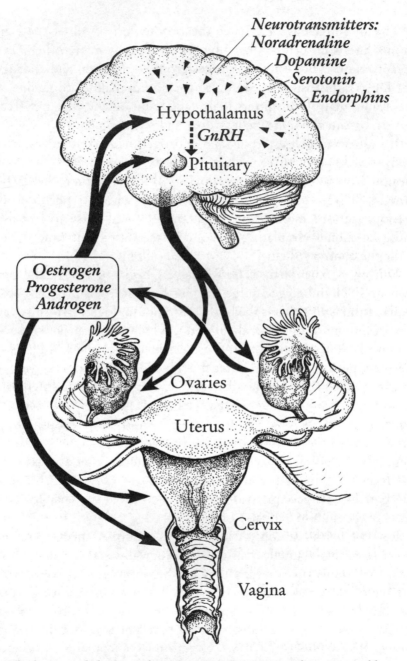

Neurotransmitters:
Noradrenaline
Dopamine
Serotonin
Endorphins

Hypothalamus
GnRH
Pituitary

Oestrogen
Progesterone
Androgen

Ovaries

Uterus

Cervix

Vagina

The brain and the reproductive organs are intimately connected by a complex series of feedback loops.
© 2001 by Northrup and Schulz

medical study done in Sweden, for example, demonstrated that single mothers had an almost 70 per cent higher risk of premature death than did mothers with partners. And, surprisingly, this increase in the rate of premature death was the same regardless of socioeconomic or health factors. In other words, even single mothers with adequate economic resources who were physically and psychologically healthy were at greater risk.[6]

This process of sublimating our truest selves begins early, in adolescence. The 'activist' mind-set of the prepubescent girl, her childlike forthrightness and honesty, and her tendency to jump in when there is conflict all become hormonally sublimated. Though an adolescent girl may be concerned with social injustice, she is likely to be even more preoccupied with her body image and attractiveness to potential mates. To put it another way, while a woman is being biologically primed for childbearing, child rearing, and nurturing of others – all vital and species-enhancing roles – the conflicts in the world at large become somewhat blurred to her. Her concern with personal injustices and childhood traumas may also fade or be suppressed. She is likely to give minor offences no more than cursory attention, for to lick her own wounds, analyse old hurts, or confront long-standing abuses would demand precious energy. She needs to fulfil her primary role, which, biologically speaking, is to reproduce and nurture.

She is rewarded handsomely for complying with this biological agenda. Reproductive hormones are directly responsible for stimulating opioid centres in the brain. These areas actually produce narcotic-like chemicals that swirl into the bloodstream and provide a feel-good sensation, a natural high. Oestrogen, for example, is richly provided during the high-fertility phase of the menstrual cycle, when a woman is most 'electric' to men and most receptive to their advances. Hormones such as prolactin also flood the system while she is in mothering mode, breast-feeding her baby or nurturing her loved ones. Those strong feelings of attraction, that deep sense of satisfaction, that mantle of loving warmth and purpose that a woman feels when nurturing – all are due in part to natural, narcotic-like chemicals produced by the brain in response to reproductive hormones. Since it feels wonderful, she is encouraged to continue. This is one of the reasons why women are extraordinary caretakers.

Women who are lesbians and/or who choose not to marry or bear children are not exempted from this built-in incentive system, because it is stamped into their circuits within the first few days of life as a

FIGURE 4: REWARD ACROSS THE LIFE CYCLE

Premenopausal Years

Goals and Behaviour driven by Society's demands

Goals and Behaviour driven by Soul's demands

Menopause Years

© 2001 by Northrup and Schulz

female embryo. Whether the nurturing behaviour is related to pregnancy and child rearing or to other forms of caregiving, the biological feedback is unavoidable, powerful, and very, very positive.

How Menopausal Hormonal Changes Facilitate Your Brain Rewiring

As a woman enters menopause, she steps out of the primarily childbearing, caretaking role that was hormonally scripted for her. This is not to say that the postmenopausal woman is no longer an effective nurturer. Rather, she becomes freer to choose where she will direct her creative energies, freer to 'colour outside the lines'. Many of the issues that had become blurred to her when the hormones of puberty kicked in may suddenly resurface with vivid clarity as those hormones recede. This is why so many midlife women recall, and decide to confront, past abuses. The concern with social injustices, the political interests, and the personal passions that were sublimated in the childbearing years now surface in sharp focus, ready to be examined and acted upon. Some women funnel this heightened energy into new businesses and new careers. Some discover and cultivate artistic talents they never knew they had. Some women note a surge in their sexual desire, to heights never before experienced in their lives. Some report changes in sexual preference.

Embracing the Message Behind Our Menopausal Anger

The GnRH pulses associated with menopause prime the brain for new perceptions – and, subsequently, for new behaviour. It is very common for women to become more irritable, even downright angry, about things that were more easily overlooked before. Long before we begin to feel hot flushes from changing hormonal levels, our brains undergo changes in the hypothalamus, the place where GnRH is produced. This same brain region is key for experiencing, and ultimately expressing, emotions such as anger.[7] It is well known that hormones modulate both aggression and anger. Our midlife bodies and brains fully support our ability to experience and express anger with a clarity not possible prior to midlife.

GnRH is just one of several hormones that support the changes occurring in the brain. Oestrogen and progesterone molecules bind themselves to areas such as the amygdala and hippocampus, which are important for memory, hunger, sexual desire, and anger. Changing levels of these and other hormones may well help to bring up old memories, accompanied by strong emotions, especially anger. This is not to say that anger is caused by hormonal change. Rather, it means that the hormonal changes simply facilitate remembering and clearing up unfinished business.

Many women are disturbed or frightened when they feel this anger arising. Maybe you don't feel angry. Maybe you're 'just' irritable, grouchy, aggravated, envious, overwhelmed, or depressed, or you 'just' have high cholesterol or high blood pressure. Believe me, all these emotions and physical conditions are associated with the same thing: anger. Anger in women has a bad press in general unless that anger arises in the service of others. This probably accounts for the fact that although anger has been studied exhaustively in men, the gender in which it is acceptable, the only kind of female anger that has received a great deal of study is maternal anger, the function of which is to protect a child who is threatened. It is also culturally acceptable for women to express their personal anger by fighting for social justice, which too often becomes a platform for releasing personal anger. Though we're socialised to believe that our anger arises from observing the injustice done to others, the political is always personal: our anger is ultimately about ourselves, and its energy is always urging us towards self-actualisation.

That doesn't mean we should abandon social protest, reform, and a quest for justice. It simply means that we must bear in mind our personal motivation for participating in these arenas, not allowing them to distract us from self-transformation and self-healing – processes that always render us even more effective as agents for social change.

We need to claim our anger. Especially during midlife, it can play an important role in improving the quality of our lives and our health. It is a powerful signal from our inner wisdom – one we should learn to listen to and act on. It often arises from:

- Being unable to count on promises or commitments made to us

- Losing power, status, or respect

- Being insulted, undermined, or diminished

- Being threatened with physical or emotional pain

- Having an important or pleasurable event postponed or cancelled to suit someone else's convenience

- Not obtaining something we feel should legitimately be ours.[8]

If, before menopause, a woman hasn't learned to identify her anger and what it is telling her (and this describes many women), perimenopause is her best remaining opportunity to do so. At perimenopause, the rewiring of her brain makes her vision clearer and her motivations easier to identify. Using anger as a catalyst for positive change and growth is always liberating.

In the early stages of perimenopause, the irritability you feel may be subtle. Irritability is a low-voltage form of anger that doesn't usually lead to lasting change – or any change. Irritability is like keeping a pan simmering but always adding more water or turning down the heat just before it boils. If we do not attend to the things in our lives that irritate us, nature will turn up the flame on the burner in an attempt to mobilise us.

GLADYS: NEVER BRINGING THE PAN TO A BOIL

Gladys was the perfect example of menopausal irritability. In my office she complained often about her husband, her children, and her job. She had chronic sinusitis, a condition often linked to emotional irritability and anger simmering beneath the surface. Whenever I asked Gladys when she was actually going to take steps to change the aspects of her life that so constantly irritated her, she'd always recover herself immediately, give me a big smile, and say, 'But, dear, my husband is really a wonderful man. And my children are really very loving. I really can't complain about any parts of my life.' Gladys went to her doctor and was put on Prozac, but she never felt as though it, or anything else, ever really helped her. Over the years I cared for her, Gladys's health never improved.

Killing the Messenger: Medicating Our Anger and Irritability to Maintain the Status Quo

In our culture, unfortunately, the usual approach to perimenopausal symptoms such as mood changes and irritability is to prescribe something to soothe us and make us feel better. We seldom ask ourselves – and certainly our doctors rarely ask – 'What is out of balance that needs to be changed?' If we look to hormone replacement therapy for relief without addressing the underlying issues, then even appropriate doses of hormones may not help much.

The women who are most vulnerable to the effects of hormonal swings and have the most difficulty finding relief from hormone replacement regimens and other medication are those who have had problems with mood during menarche, postpartum, and during perimenopause.[9] If the emotional issues in their lives are not attended to, if their midlife losses are not fully grieved and released (if, in other words, they don't listen to their anger and take action), they may end up with full-blown depression – which is sometimes described as anger turned inwards. Depression, in turn, is a very well-documented independent risk factor for heart disease, cancer, and osteoporosis.

Emotional turmoil affects the brain and all its functions. Continuing in the same upsetting situation virtually guarantees that a woman's hormones will stay unbalanced. The longer she allows negative situations to persist, the more out of balance her hormones will become, and the more physically uncomfortable she will feel. A prescription for oestrogen may stop this cycle temporarily, but the body will eventually demand that its message be heard.

DORIS: BYPASSING ANGER

Many women downplay their pain by comparing themselves to someone else who is much worse off. If unresolved, this pattern can be a set-up for health problems, especially at midlife. Here's an example from my practice.

Doris was suffering from high blood pressure and slightly elevated cholesterol, both of which were getting worse as she approached the end of her menopausal transition at the age of fifty-two. Doris told me that her socialite mother had devoted herself to her husband and his career in an unbalanced way that led to rather significant emotional neglect of her children, who were cared for by nannies and household help. Doris had unwittingly created the same pattern with her husband, who was so caught up in his work that he simply wasn't available to her emotionally. But she would not permit herself to express anger at either her husband or her mother. Doris, like so many women whose lives appear relatively privileged, said to me, 'I feel so selfish and foolish for feeling sorry for myself. I really have nothing to complain about. After all, there are all these women who've been raped or been victimised by incest, or whose husbands have left them penniless at midlife. I have so much to be grateful for.'

I call Doris's approach the intellectual bypass – intellectual because the logical part of our brains can always come up with good reasons why we have nothing to complain about. And on the surface this may well be true. However, there's a deeper problem. Comparing our pain to that of someone else invariably takes us away from our own emotions and what we need to do about them. This is because the part of the brain that allows us to feel emotions has far richer and more complex connections with our internal organs, such as the heart and cardiovascular system, than does the area associated with logical, rational thought.[10] Comparisons keep us stuck in our intellect. It's not enough simply to think about our feelings or talk about them. Remember, the word *emotion* contains the word *motion* within it! Our feelings are meant to move us.

Healing doesn't take place until we surrender to our feelings and allow them to wash over us. Doris won't be able to create full cardio-vascular health until she allows herself to feel how painful it is to have a husband who is emotionally unavailable to her, a situation that mirrors so many aspects of her childhood. When she finally surrenders to the grief and rage that have been bottled up for years, first during her child-hood and again during her marriage, she will be on her way to creating not only cardiovascular health, but the gift of a healed life as well.

Emotions, Hormones, and Your Health

Your emotions are your inner guidance system. They alone will let you know whether you are living in an environment of biochemical health or in an environment of biochemical distress. Understanding how your thoughts and your emotions affect every single hormone and cell in your body, and knowing how to change them in a way that is health-enhancing, gives you access to the most powerful and empowering health-creating secret on earth.

Natural foods, supplements, herbs, meditation, acupuncture, and so on are all powerful tools for building and protecting your health. But regardless of what supplements you take and what kind of exercise you do, when all is said and done it is your attitude, your beliefs, and your daily thought patterns that have the most profound effect on your health. How many times have you heard someone say, 'I don't understand it – she always ate well and exercised. How come she, of all people, got ill?' On the other end of the spectrum is the person who smokes cigarettes and drinks too much alcohol, yet lives without any apparent illness well into healthy old age. The answer lies at least in part in the individual's attitudes and emotions. Attitudes and beliefs also influence how well your food is digested and how effective your exercise is. You have, within you, the power to create a life of joy, abundance, and health, or you have the same ability to create a life filled with stress, fatigue, and disease. With very few exceptions, the choice is yours.

Specific Emotional Patterns Are Associated with Specific Illnesses in Specific Parts of the Body

It has now been scientifically documented that specific patterns of emotional vulnerability affect specific organs or systems of the body.

There are dozens of medical studies on breast cancer alone showing that feelings of powerlessness in important relationships and an inability to express the full range of emotions raise the risk of developing breast cancer and lower survival rates from it. Similarly, dozens of studies have suggested that difficulties in handling negative emotions, especially hostility, are linked to sudden death from heart attack.[11] Beyond these are literally hundreds of studies showing that lack of social support, loss of or separation from one's family, or difficulties balancing a feeling of belonging with a sense of independence can affect the immune system and increase susceptibility to infection and autoimmune diseases.

Clinical practitioners have known for hundreds of years that the connection between emotions and states of health is direct and powerful. Amazingly, our outward-focused, cause-and-effect, data-driven culture simply ignored the evidence. Even as late as the 1970s, the pioneering work of scientists such as Walter B. Cannon and Hans Selye, who did groundbreaking research on stress and the mind–body connection, was not accepted in the mainstream. It was scientifically accurate and compelling, but our culture simply wasn't ready for it.

We midlife women *are* ready, and we have the perfect opportunity right now to live this knowledge for ourselves, while also sparking the fire of change in the culture at large.

Our state of health and happiness depends more upon our perception of life events around us than upon the events themselves. This is a truth that our culture does not teach. Instead, we are taught from an early age that our health is largely the result of our genetic heritage, whether or not we've been immunised, how many supplements we take, and how much exercise we get. There is no doubt that these factors can contribute to our state of health. But their influence pales in comparison to the power of our beliefs and attitudes.

How Your Thoughts and Perceptions Become Biochemical Realities in Your Body

Your autonomic nervous system is the system that helps transform your thoughts and emotions into the physical environment that, over time, becomes your actual physical body. This part of the nervous system, which also governs the day-to-day activity of all your internal organs, is divided into two parts: the *parasympathetic* nervous system and the *sympathetic* nervous system. These two systems innervate every organ of your body, including your eyes, tear ducts, salivary glands, blood vessels, sweat glands, heart, larynx, trachea, bronchi, lungs, stomach, adrenals, kidneys, pancreas, intestines, bladder, and external genitalia.

In general terms, the parasympathetic nervous system (PNS) is the brake in your body. It promotes functions associated with growth and restoration, rest and relaxation, and deals primarily with conservation of bodily energy by causing your vital organs to 'rest' when they are not 'on duty'.

In contrast to the PNS, the sympathetic nervous system (SNS) is the accelerator. It revs up your metabolism to deal with challenges from outside the body. Stimulation of the SNS quickly mobilises your body's reserves so that you can protect and defend yourself. This is where the fabled fight-or-flight mechanism kicks in: your pupils dilate, the rate and force of your heart's contractions increase, and your blood vessels constrict, so your blood pressure rises. Blood is borrowed from the intestinal reservoir and shunted to your major muscles, lungs, heart, and brain, preparing you for battle. Bowel and bladder function shut down temporarily, conserving energy needed to power your muscles, whether you choose to stay and fight or run away. (This is the exact opposite of the PNS's function, which is to constrict the pupils, slow the heart, make the bowels move, and relax the bladder and rectal sphincters.)

Since the parasympathetic nervous system deals primarily with restoration and conservation of bodily energy and the resting of vital organs, any activity or thought pattern that engages the PNS puts deposits into your health bank. Conversely, SNS action makes withdrawals from that bank.

It is at this point that perception becomes so important. What is experienced in the body as a challenge from outside – a stressor – will vary from person to person, influenced by each individual's past history, childhood, family background, diet, job, and activities at the moment. Many midlife women live in a state of constant anxiety overload, much of which is a side effect of the culture around us. We want to be good women. We want to do what is right. But the culture around us is changing so fast, and the information overload that it generates is so huge, that we easily become overwhelmed and confused, dancing faster and faster just to keep up. Not knowing what to choose, and what to avoid, we give our bodies mixed signals. We may step on the accelerator and the brake at the same time. Or we may let the accelerator get stuck in the on position, living in a constant state of fight or flight – and making far too many withdrawals from the health bank.

Biologically speaking, we may be undergoing an evolutionary process that will enable our species to handle all this stress more gracefully and healthfully. Frankly, I believe that the multimodal brain of the midlife woman is leading the way. We've always had to be able to do at least three tasks at once. And now, at midlife, when the dictates of our souls make themselves known more fully than ever, we wake up to discover that our brains and bodies are being retooled to facilitate this beautifully.

Stress and Your Temperament

Scientific studies have found a link between temperament, personality, and the ability to deal with stressors. Have you noticed that some people, regardless of what happens to them in their lives, seem to be happy, while some are down even when life seems to be on the upswing? Or that others are anxious or fearful even when they're safe and secure? To a degree, we are born with one of these temperaments, and there is evidence of measurable *biological* differences that go along with each temperament. For example, Stephen Porges MD, has found that each individual has – from birth – his or her own characteristic balance between the PNS and SNS, resulting in what is known as 'vagal tone'.[12] Your individual balance is visible on a type of ECG (electrocardiogram) and illustrates how your heart rate coordinates with your breathing rate, yielding valuable information about your metabolic balance and inherent resilience to stress. Porges has found that, even in premature babies, those who have higher vagal tone, meaning that their parasympathetic nervous system is more activated, are less stressed by external events in the nursery (such as being handled) than are babies with low vagal tone. He has also observed that the personality characteristics that go along with low or high vagal tone (happy, resilient, down, melancholy, anxious, trusting, fearful) appear to follow each individual throughout life.

This explains much about our individual responses to life situations. For instance, it has been clearly shown that one patient may feel great stress while undergoing a relatively simple medical procedure, while a much more difficult procedure might cause little stress in another patient. However, it is also true that the same person may respond minimally to an experience at one time, and then have a massive physiological response to the same experience at another time. This is why attempts to rate stressors are not very useful. A recent study by Dr Charles B. Nemeroff at Emory University School of Medicine in the US found that women who were sexually or physically abused in childhood, compared to those without this history, show very exaggerated physiological responses in later life to stresses like giving a speech or solving arithmetic problems in front of others. They are also at greater risk for depression, anxiety disorders, and other emotional illnesses later in life.[13] Given the large number of women with a history of abuse of some kind, it is not surprising that so many women have mood and other problems during perimenopause.

One of the worst things people can do to themselves is beat themselves up about their inherent temperament or pattern of response to stress. That's why I don't want to suggest that there is some gold standard of emotions that is ideal. This would be no different from telling women they should strive for an ideal weight, height, dress size, and so on. Besides, each temperament appears to predispose people to certain types of genius. If you spent your life wishing you had a 'healthier' kind of temperament, for example, you would not be embracing your full genius or taking full advantage of your natural gifts.

How Menopausal Emotions Affect Our Health

Imbalances between the sympathetic and parasympathetic nervous systems, combined with the changing hormonal milieu of menopause, can increase our body's susceptibility to symptoms or disease. The thymus (which creates your immune system's T cells), the lymph nodes (which create your immune system's B cells), and the bone marrow (which creates your red and white blood cells) are all innervated by the autonomic nervous system. Therefore, each area that creates immune system cells has both an accelerator pedal (sympathetic tone) and a brake pedal (parasympathetic tone).

Why is this important? Because it is via this system that your body records and processes your emotions and the hormones and neuro-chemicals they promote. As I've noted, if you have a backlog of unprocessed emotions, they are going to surface around the time of menopause. As a result, your susceptibility to illness may increase. Over time, if the fear-driven fight-or-flight response is triggered again and again, you can fall victim to diabetes, hypertension, or possibly even an autoimmune disease such as lupus or rheumatoid arthritis. Where you are affected will be determined by the weakest link in your body, the place where your genetic structure has made you most vulnerable.

The bottom line is that what goes on in your mind boosts either parasympathetic or sympathetic nervous system activity. Every thought and every perception you have changes the homeostasis of your body. Will it be the brakes or the accelerator, a health account deposit or a health account withdrawal? This, in a nutshell, is how your autonomic nervous system translates how you view your world into the state of your health.

How Thoughts Affect Hormone Levels at Menopause

The 'language' spoken by your autonomic nervous system is translated to the rest of your body by hormones. The primary messengers of the sympathetic nervous system are hormones called noradrenaline and adrenaline. They are produced in the brain and in the adrenal glands. Every time adrenaline levels go up, levels of another adrenal hormone, cortisol, also go up.

While cortisol provides a much-needed boost in the short term, helping you get through an occasional crisis, it has its dark side. If you live in the SNS's 'fast lane' for a long time, prolonged elevation of cortisol can cause a number of problems. Initially cortisol sparks up your immune system, but if stress keeps the body in a constant state of fight-or-flight readiness, cortisol's effects on the immune system quickly become a liability. White blood cells get dumped into the bloodstream, flooding the system with germ-fighting warriors. Over time, the immune system and the bone marrow become depleted. Long-term overexposure to cortisol causes your skin to become thin, your bones to become weaker, your muscles and connective tissue to break down, your body to develop abnormal insulin metabolism, your tissues to retain fluids, your arms and legs to bruise more easily, and your moods to tend towards depression.

If you persist in the perception that events and demands in your life are stressful and uncontrollable, you are adopting the mind-set that continually whips your adrenals into producing more and more cortisol. Over time, your adrenals may become exhausted, losing their ability to keep up with the demand for increasing amounts of this hormone. This is often coupled with suboptimal nutrition, impaired digestion, and poor assimilation of nutrients, all of which go hand in hand with a stressful life. The resulting immune system incompetence increases susceptibility not only to infectious diseases, but also to autoimmune disorders and all cancers.

The overstimulated sympathetic nervous system also causes an imbalance in a group of hormones known as eicosanoids, resulting in impairment of the cells' ability to metabolise fatty acids. This is associated with weight gain, as the body tends to break down muscle and replace it with stored fat and excess fluid. Imbalanced eicosanoids are also associated with tissue inflammation, which increases the discomfort felt in a host of chronic diseases such as lupus and rheumatoid arthritis. They have also been shown to increase the speed of tumour growth in individuals already harbouring cancer.

In a healthy, normal body, cortisol levels are highest upon waking up in the morning. During the night, the parasympathetic nervous system has done its job of providing rest and renewal to your organs. In other words, a deposit has been made into the 'health bank'. The morning's increased cortisol levels help you get out of bed and get ready for the day ahead. As you wind down in the evening, cortisol levels normally decrease, reaching their lowest at about midnight, easing you into a rejuvenative, restful night. For many stressed-out women, however, the rise-and-fall pattern of cortisol secretion begins to invert itself. Levels are lower in the morning, affording little or no 'fuel in the tank' to start the day, and they're higher at midnight, making it virtually impossible to wind down and rest.

It does not end there. In addition to causing deranged output of cortisol, overstimulation of the sympathetic nervous system also causes decreased production of progesterone, one of your body's natural calming agents. The result is that women who are chronically stressed also tend towards hormonal imbalance between oestrogen, progesterone, and testosterone (which is important in women as well as in men).

Soothing Your Emotions Before They Become Disease

First of all, there is nothing to be gained by categorising emotions as 'good' or 'bad.' Instead, think of them as guidance. The emotions that feel good are guiding you towards health, while the ones that feel bad are trying to get your attention so that you can change either your perception or your behaviour. It really is as simple as that.

Emotions can also become toxic if they are allowed to persist unresolved, rather than being worked through fully and released. Consider, for example, the woman who lost a child and fifteen years later, now well into menopause, still hasn't moved anything in that child's room, keeping it exactly as it was the day the child died. The emotions that drive her to enshrine that room – the unresolved grief, the refusal to move forwards in life, the denial – are toxic. They have not only robbed her of fifteen years of life, but also are setting her up for physical illness, especially given the intensity with which our unresolved baggage from the past arises at menopause.

The ill health and pain you may experience at midlife are not caused by difficult emotions per se, but rather by a willingness to let those emotions persist unresolved – or by a misperception of what they mean in your life. Unresolved, 'stuck' emotions keep setting up the same body biochemistry over and over again. The effect of emotions on our bodies can be likened to water in a river. Our bodies stay clean and fresh as long as our emotions keep flowing, triggering changes in our perception and behaviour. The minute that water stagnates, all manner of decay and germs start to flourish.

One of my menopausal patients arrived at a wonderful insight. She began to realise that whenever she feels happy, she also begins to feel nervous, because it is her perception that whenever good things happen in her life, she has to leave behind past aspects of her life that have supported her. Getting a promotion at work, for example, had always been tainted with pangs of regret, because she knew that moving up changed the dynamics of her old relationships. The people she had been friends with before didn't accept her in the same way any more. I have certainly had the same experience in my own life. The silver lining in that cloud, however, is that by allowing yourself to move continually towards ever-increasing success and joy, you attract new friends and circumstances that support you fully for who you are becoming. The key for this woman is to focus on all the good that has come from allowing herself to become happier and more successful.

Focusing on the positive side of a situation can have a powerful effect on our health. Dr Bernie Siegel tells a story about a patient who overheard doctors say that he had a 'gallop rhythm' in his heart. A gallop rhythm is a dangerous condition, but this patient thought it meant that his heart was as strong as a horse. Because of that perception, the patient's overall status improved dramatically, and he got out of the coronary intensive care unit in record time.

Again, however, beware the oversimplification that 'happiness' is good and 'sadness' is bad. Both emotions are necessary to function as a normal human being. Without sadness, the experience of happiness would lose its sweetness. The healthy way is to strive for a balance of emotional chemicals in your body that support health, and to have those emotions wash in and out like the tides of the sea. Just as the tides are essential for cleansing the ocean, our emotions cleanse our mind and body. At midlife, sadness and regrets from our past may take on a heightened role for a time, helping us to truly clean out the silted-up river bottoms of our emotional lives.

Are We Responsible for Our Health?

Critics of the mind–body connection say that focusing on the emotional dimension of illness makes people feel worse when they are already vulnerable, as though they are guilty of causing their own disease. I agree that there is the potential to carry this philosophy too far and blame ourselves for ill health. However, the value of the mind–body connection is too great to discard. The simple truth is that the people who heal fastest and remain healthiest the longest are those who feel that their lives are fulfilling and joyful. Even when they're ill, they feel that their life has meaning and that they have some locus of control. Those who think, "The world is doing it to me . . . . There's nothing I can do about it . . . . I can't get a break . . . . The world is out to get me . . . . This is just the way the world is', and so on, are disempowered by their thoughts and perceptions. This directly contributes to an imbalance in the autonomic nervous system and associated hormonal systems. Twenty years of medical practice have shown me so clearly that emotions are the primary energy at work, tipping the scales one way or the other, towards illness or towards health, and that the victim mentality is at the root of many illnesses.

Despite what we learn daily about healthy exercise practices, healthy diets, and good medical care, the bottom line is that the most significant way of contributing to our own good health is through the quality of our thought processes. This power is a valuable gift, in light of the absolute lack of control we have over other aspects of life. Think about being on a turbulent flight in bad weather. You have no control over the winds, or the skills or the mental state of the pilot flying the plane. But you do have the power to minimise your dis-comfort. You can decide to read a book, strike up a conversation with the person next to you, take your antioxidants, wrap up in a warm blanket, sleep, listen to music, or watch the film. Alternatively, you can listen to every engine noise and allow yourself to be debilitated by worry for the entire flight. It's your choice.

Ultimately, you are the only one who can make significant deposits into your health bank account. This is not the job of your doctor, your nutritionist, your lover, or your parents. There is no supple-ment, no health care provider, and no exotic herb that can possibly do for you what you can do for yourself.

The key is compassion for yourself. The well-known therapist Gay Hendricks has noted that any area of pain, blame, or shame in our lives is there because we have not loved that part of ourselves enough. No matter what you're feeling, the only way to get a difficult feeling to go away is simply to love yourself for it. If you think you're stupid, then love yourself for feeling that way. It's a paradox, but it works. To heal, you must be the first one to shine the light of compassion on any areas within you that you feel are unacceptable (and we've all got them). The hormonal shifts you experience around the time of menopause can facilitate this.

How Our Midlife Brains and Bodies Are Set Up to Heal Our Past

Though memories are distributed throughout the body and the brain, certain areas of the brain, notably the amygdala and hippo-campus, are especially important for the encoding and retrieving of memories. Interestingly, these areas of the brain are particularly rich in receptors for oestrogen, progesterone, and GnRH, the hormones that fluctuate the most during the perimenopausal years. Given the heightened activity of these hormones in these areas, it makes sense that memory activation and retrieval would be enhanced during the years immediately surrounding menopause.[14] Hurts and losses we've managed to forget or minimise for many years, even decades, may suddenly become overwhelming – even if we think we should be 'over' all that pain from the past.

FIGURE 5: WHY TRAUMATIC MEMORIES MAY BE RELIVED AT MIDLIFE

The brain's memory centres are rich in receptors for the hormones
that fluctuate in perimenopause.
© 2001 by Northrup and Schulz

CHRISTINE: MIDLIFE BRINGS SELF-HEALING

On the tenth anniversary of the day she was raped, Christine wrote, she awoke with a greater rush of energy than ever before. These torrents of feeling had become increasingly powerful as she advanced through perimenopause, like exaggerations of the hormonal crests and troughs of the monthly cycles she described as 'like PMS times ten'. Uncomfortable physical symptoms increasingly accompanied these waves, as her body begged for attention to the wounds left by her sexual assault.

Headaches, body aches, queasiness, insomnia, anxiety attacks, diarrhoea, toothaches, and many other symptoms manifested themselves along the way to my recovery again and again. Over time, I learned to quiet myself and fully experience what I was feeling as each of these 'illnesses' struck me. Each time, strong emotions came up and were eventually released, sometimes within minutes – and the symptoms disappeared.

Christine's openness to the messages being sent by her body helped facilitate her healing.

> The most incredible insight that became clear to me during the process of discharge, release, and healing that occurred time and time again was that I am my own healer. It was amazing to me how interrelated my emotions were with the various symptoms I was experiencing.

SUSAN: STANDING UP FOR HERSELF AT MENOPAUSE

At forty-five, Susan wrote, 'Menopause for me is the courage and push I've needed all of my life.' Both of Susan's parents were alcoholics, and while they 'partied', she and her brother had the responsibility of running the household and taking care of their younger sisters. She left home at eighteen to marry.

> Naturally I married an alcoholic, but I didn't know it until years later. The relationship was very controlling and abusive – mentally, emotionally, and physically. He controlled my every decision, from when I could see my family to where I worked, what furniture to buy, what cars I drove, and the decision to not have children. I convinced myself that we had a wonderful, close relationship. We became my parents, partying and drinking at weekends just like they did – I drank to keep my husband company and to be 'part of' something. I also started smoking up to two packets a day. When I became pregnant at age thirty, he convinced me to get an abortion, saying he was under too much pressure, promising we'd try again the following year. Instead, he had an affair. I hung in there, and eventually he ended it and came back to me. I took this to be proof positive that he truly loved me.

Four years later Susan sought couples therapy, but at the last minute her husband refused to go. Rather than cancel, she went alone. Through her counsellor, she started attending meetings of Alcoholics Anonymous, where she learned that she was not alone. This marked the beginning of a new life for her.

For Susan, the first major milestone was talking about her abortion. Next she gave up smoking. 'That opened up a whole new world for me. I no longer had to stuff my feelings and light up a cigarette. I had a mouthpiece. I had something to say, and oh, I said a *lot* – I had diarrhoea of the mouth. And such honesty!' Then she stopped drinking. 'My husband didn't like this new me at all. I no longer was a party girl, at his beck and call.'

As Susan changed, she felt herself being torn in two, because the life around her, the life her husband had laid out for her, was not changing at all. 'I became a married woman living a single life. We no longer went anywhere or did anything with each other.' There was a series of attempts at marriage counselling, separation, reconciliation, and alcoholism therapy for him, all to no avail. Then came the ultimate boost – menopause! Susan wrote: 'I became perimenopausal at forty-two. I really feel this gave me the courage and the push and the honesty to look at my life with an eye for what I wanted and needed.' She started doing 'so many things I've been wanting to do and never did'. Eventually she filed for divorce and started the life she'd always wanted to have, three thousand miles away from her native New York. 'I had such an easy transition,' she marvelled. 'I walked away from my whole life there – husband, job, friends, and all but the few things I packed when I left – but I suppose I did my grieving while I lived in the marriage. My life is so full today.'

The primary defence against unpleasant memories and emotions is avoidance. This subterfuge often works reasonably well until the perimenopausal transition, when the hormonal shift of focus and accompanying changes in brain activity conspire to bring buried traumas and unresolved issues into the light, expressing them through physical symptoms that cannot be ignored. Whatever causes a woman's lingering wounds, perimenopause can be seen as a built-in support system that sets her up to do deep healing. Although it may not be seen this way at first, it is a gift.

In addition to providing the clarity and courage to face past abuses or pain, menopause can help a woman step back, acknowledge the necessity to change, and do whatever is necessary to separate herself from long-term destructive life patterns. Even the most deeply ingrained patterns can be changed with the support of menopause-induced shifts in the brain, energy, and focus.

Caution: Reinforcing Past Trauma

The disturbing memories and the depression that so often arise at menopause are much less scary and disabling if we see them for what they are. They are evidence that we are now strong enough, deep within, to allow the pain and secrets of the past to rise to the surface and be cleared out once and for all. The midlife investigation and release of the painful patterns from the past is necessary if you are to truly heal. Trust your brain and body to give you the information you need to handle when you're prepared to handle it.

It is valuable to have someone else witness and validate your pain. Many people have found that it was not just the painful experience itself that was so wounding to them as children, but also the fact that there was no one to whom they could safely turn, no one who could understand or validate their reality at the time.

You may choose to work with a therapist, and you may also consider a course of medication to deal with the sleep problems, anxiety, or panic that may arise. However, note that many anti-anxiety drugs are highly addictive. Far too many women have been put on drugs such as Valium during their menopausal transition only to find themselves dependent on them for the rest of their lives. If you're willing to work in therapy and make the requisite changes in your life, you probably won't need to remain on medication for more than six months to two years. (See chapter 10, 'Nurturing Your Brain', for more information on prescription medications and over-the-counter alternatives.)

While I cannot outline the course of recovery in detail here, I do want to caution you about one pitfall: some forms of therapy actually reinforce negative patterns both in your brain and your body. These include 'reliving' the trauma repeatedly and digging for buried memories. Here's why: significant stress of any kind, including the re-experiencing of past painful memories, is associated with high levels of cortisol. This is the very hormonal milieu that increases the likelihood of laying down memories of all kinds, especially traumatic ones, which are mediated through an area of the brain known as the amygdala.[15]

If you are a highly sensitive or suggestible individual, receptive to mental imagery, and you have a lot of cortisol in your bloodstream (as when you're stressed), it is very possible for you to incorporate new traumatic 'memories' into your brain and body that have no basis in your past experiences. Instead, they may be the product of your current environment, combined with the suggestions and imagery you picked up from a well-meaning therapist. For example, if a therapist asks you, 'Did your father rape you when you were three?' and you are in a susceptible biological state, your brain may simply incorporate the question as fact – 'My father raped me when I was three' – whether or not that actually happened. This scenario may then be encoded as a new trauma memory – one that you'll have to cope with on top of the original memories that have arisen on their own.

Ultimately, make it your goal to move on to forgiveness of yourself and those involved in causing you pain in the past. Forgiveness doesn't mean that what happened to you was acceptable. It simply means that you are no longer willing to allow a past injury to keep you from living fully and healthfully in the present.

Finding a Larger Meaning

In some cultures, such as that of Hindu India, midlife is a time associated with the serious pursuit of the spiritual dimensions of life. I see something comparable occurring in the West, where the vast majority of those attending conferences on the connection between the body and soul are midlife women. With our child-rearing years behind us, our creative energies are freed. Our search for life's meaning begins to take on new urgency, and we begin to experience ourselves as potential vessels for Spirit. I've long believed that each of our lives is directed by a force that I think of as God. This force is much bigger than our own intellects, and it always moves us towards our highest possible purpose, working directly through the unique expression that each of us represents. My lifelong interest in metaphysics and astrology has provided me with very clear evidence for this truth.

Barbara Hand Clow, an author who specialises in using astrology to give us more access to our power, explains that all of us must go through several key life passages in order to reach our full wisdom. Each passage is associated with very specific and predictable shifts that, if negotiated consciously, open us to our full potential. In her 1996 book *The Liquid Light of Sex: Kundalini Rising at Mid-Life Crisis,* Clow writes, 'We *form* at 30, we *transform* at 40, and we *transmute* at 50.'[16]

Around the age of forty, the universal energy known as kundalini

THE SEVEN EMOTIONAL-ENERGY CENTRES
The Physical Effect of Mental and Emotional Patterns

Emotional Centre	Organs	Mental, Emotional Issues
7	Can involve any system	Ability to sense or trust in life's purpose Connection to God or universal source of energy Ability to balance responsibility for life events with acceptance of things we cannot control
6	Brain Eyes Ears Nose Pineal gland	Perception: clarity vs ambiguity Thought: left brain vs right brain; rational vs non-rational Morality: conservative vs liberal; social rules vs individual conscience Repression vs lack of inhibition
5	Thyroid Trachea Neck vertebrae Throat, mouth, teeth, and gums	Communication: expression vs comprehension (speaking vs listening) Timing: pushing forward vs waiting Will: wilful vs compliant
4	Heart/lungs Blood vessels Shoulders Ribs/breasts Diaphragm Upper oesophagus	Emotional expression: capacity to feel fully, express and resolve anger, hostility, joy, love, grief, forgiveness Relationships: capacity to form mutual reciprocal partnerships with balance of nurturing of self vs nurturing of others; intimacy with others vs capacity to be alone

Emotional Centre	Organs	Mental, Emotional Issues
3	Abdomen Upper intestines Liver, gall bladder Lower oesophagus Stomach Kidney, pancreas Adrenal gland Spleen Middle spine	Self-esteem, self-confidence, and self-acceptance Personal power: competence and skills in the outer world Over-responsibility vs irresponsibility Addictions to sugar, alcohol, drugs, and tobacco Aggression vs defensiveness Competitiveness vs non-competitiveness; winning vs losing
2	Uterus, ovaries Vagina, cervix Large intestine Lower vertebrae Pelvis Appendix Bladder	Personal power: sex, money, and relationships Fertility and generativity: individual creativity; co-creation with others Boundaries in relationships: dependency vs independence; giving vs taking; assertiveness vs passivity
1	Muscles, bones Spine Blood Immune system	Safety/security in the world; knowing when to trust or mistrust Knowing when to feel fear and when not to Balance between independence and dependence

Sources: C. N. Shealy and C. M. Myss, *The Creation of Health: Merging Traditional Medicine with Intuitive Diagnosis* (Walpole, NH: Stillpoint Publications, 1988). Scientific documentation of the human energy system and updated information from Mona Lisa Schulz, MD, PhD, *Awakening Intuition: Using Your Mind–Body Network for Insight and Healing* (New York: Harmony Books, 1998).

FIGURE 6: EMOTIONAL ANATOMY

The connection between emotions and physical anatomy comes together in the seven emotional centres. These correspond roughly to traditional energy maps of the body that delineate seven energetic centres or chakras.

(which is depicted as a snake in many ancient healing traditions) begins to rise naturally and gradually from the base of our spines, activating each energy centre (or chakra) of our bodies as it does so. Sometimes the resulting sexual energy that is released at this time can be quite intense, driving some women to have affairs or to channel this energy into painting, building a new home, or some other creative pursuit.

This energy activation may also manifest in bodily symptoms. The degree of unfinished business we have in each of these energy centres will determine the type and severity of symptoms we will experience in that area. For example, I personally experienced several bouts of rather severe chest pain in the year when I started to skip periods and have hot flushes, an indication of grief and despair, emotions of which I hadn't been fully conscious. Many other women find themselves feeling heart palpitations, anxiety, pelvic pain, or indigestion at midlife.

When we reframe our symptoms and see them as our inner guidance knocking on the door of each emotional centre, asking us to allow more light and wisdom into that particular area, then we don't feel victimised by our bodies and we have the opportunity to feel empowered by the life energy that is coursing through us at midlife.

For example, my divorce culminated during what is astrologically known as my Chiron return, the peak time for me to transmute and connect more powerfully than ever with my spirit and my life purpose. Simultaneously I've been under the influence of an astrological configuration known as a yod, which means 'the finger of God'. The purpose of this has been to move me out of my old life so that I have the time and motivation to form new, healthier relationships. Though this knowledge has not entirely freed me from the suffering I went through, I take great comfort in knowing that there was a larger purpose and meaning in the events of the last few years – that my experience amounts to something more than a painful divorce and the onset of hot flushes.

THREE

Coming Home to Yourself: From Dependence to Healthy Autonomy

The need and desire to assume more dominion over our lives becomes a burning issue at menopause. Suddenly we find ourselves questioning the meaning and value of many of the relationships that we'd never dared to look at too closely before. Although we all want to maintain the relationships that support us at the deepest levels, we often discover that our old ways of feeling or behaving with those closest to us – whether parents, children, spouses, friends, or bosses – need updating. And any time we update our lives, we have to grieve for the old life that has been lost. Having the courage both to embrace the necessary changes of midlife and to feel the loss that is associated with those changes is a crucial part of creating a firm foundation for health in the second half of our lives.

The Empty-nest Syndrome

You don't have to be a mother to experience the empty nest, that aching sense of personal loss, loneliness, and limbo that so often results when your life undergoes significant change. No matter how secure and settled a woman may feel prior to midlife, the transformative passage into the second half of life almost invariably involves an exodus of some kind. Whether it's the final break up with a husband from whom you have long been estranged, career changes or reversals, the departure of children who have come of age and left home to start lives of their own – lives that no longer include you as an everyday presence or necessity – or all of the above, when your once-bustling home becomes quiet and/or your daily routine suddenly changes and leaves you feeling at a loose end, the experience is not unlike the unexpected death of a loved one. And even if you saw it coming and thought you were prepared for it – even if, in fact, you are the one doing the leaving – it's painful. This is because it's impossible to prepare fully for the kind of upheaval that is so profound it holds the potential to transform you completely from the inside out.

One of my friends, a woman who has managed to maintain a high-powered corporate career while also bringing up two children, recently told me, 'When my youngest left for college this autumn, I was very busy consulting with a wealthy, creative company, which sent me on frequent trips overseas. Though my days were full of excitement, new-ness, and adventure, I nevertheless found myself bursting into tears at red traffic lights while driving. I sometimes feel as though a part of my heart has been ripped out of my chest. After all those years of pur-poseful and fierce mothering, always managing to put my children first in spite of my career, I have been surprised at how very physical and painful this loss feels. And there was no way I saw it coming.'

I can relate completely. As a sneak preview into my own empty-nest scenario, my younger child left home in June of 1999 for a month at camp, just two weeks after my firstborn left for another summer programme in preparation for starting college in the autumn. With my husband gone and the divorce nearly complete, this marked the first time in my life since college and medical school that I had been truly alone in my house. For a while it felt OK. My house was cleaner than it had been in years (not that this was ever a goal of mine), and the freedom from other people's chaos was a pleasant side effect as I began the process of re-creating the house on my terms. I ate whatev-er and whenever I wanted, worked whenever I felt like it, lit candles, and watched films late into the night. I slowly began to enjoy the opportunity to be still and contemplate my life without interruption. After all, I told myself, I wasn't really alone. My daughters would be home soon enough.

But I had a head-on collision with grief and loneliness a month lat-er. I'd picked up my younger daughter from camp, and together we had driven to Dartmouth for a tour, since she was beginning to con-template her college options. As it had been my medical school, not to mention the place where I first met my husband, Dartmouth held many fond memories for me. I remembered vividly the exhilaration

I'd felt on arriving twenty-eight years before, when I was completely smitten by the place. Now I was standing on that same campus, a fifty-year-old newly divorced mum watching the second of her two children make plans for her own life. I was facing not only the loss of my husband and my daughters, but also of all the dreams I'd had for my future. During the three-hour drive home, my daughter slept the whole way, and I realised with surprise that I felt even more lonely than I had when she was gone.

Back at home the next morning, I awoke feeling acutely grief-stricken, and I said to myself, 'Ah, this is the empty-nest feeling I've heard about, the feeling that says, "You're not at home in your new world, and your old world no longer fits you."' I was in limbo, aching for what was and for what might have been. Intellectually I knew this was a growth phase, a kind of labour pain that would yield wonderful things if I could just allow myself to go through it. (It helped to know that I didn't really have a choice.) Rather than smooth it over and find mind-numbing ways to spare myself the anguish, I let myself feel it. I was lonely, disappointed, heartbroken, and scared, and I sat on my bed and cried for everything about my life that was dying.

But there is good news, too. Anyone who has undergone the emotional upheaval of midlife changes can tell you that though the painful feelings associated with the empty nest arise again and again, over time they come less often, their stay is briefer, and their pain penetrates less deeply with each revisit. So our job is simply to be present with them. My own experience, and that of all the women who have shared their empty-nest experiences with me, indicates that the ultimate reward for fully participating in the emotions that wash over us at this time is that the struggle is over sooner than it would be if we tried to resist or deny them. Whether or not a woman realises it going in, that hollow, unsettling, empty-nest experience is a blessing in disguise. Think of it as a kind of labour pain. What you are trying to give birth to is your new life, which your hormones, your brain, and your body have already welcomed and embraced, even though you may not yet be consciously aware of it. To create a renewed life, it is necessary to go into the abyss, into the emptiness you may have spent a lifetime using relationships and busyness to avoid. Having looked into the abyss myself, I can understand why a woman entering it might find the prospect of a positive outcome very difficult to believe in. But now that I have come out on the other side, I know the journey was worth the pain.

PATRICIA: DELAYING THE INEVITABLE

Many women do everything in their power to try to resist change and transformation, often retreating into the kind of nurturing and care-taking they've participated in for their whole life. They spend precious energy trying to keep vital life changes at bay, in essence paddling upstream rather than letting the current carry them into new, uncharted waters. Often their fear of going forwards is so great that it leads to a step backwards instead.

After bringing up five children, Patricia came to a crossroads that took her completely by surprise.

> My husband always ruled the roost, made all the decisions – what groceries to buy, which children helped with which chores, what colour to paint my kitchen – and over the years I learned to deal with it by clamming up and withdrawing into the world I'd created with my kids. When our youngest left home, it hit me like a ton of bricks: it was just me and him. I'd frankly never even thought about that before. We got along OK, but mainly because he did his thing and I did mine. Whenever our purposes crossed, I was submissive and compliant – it had become my habit, and it was easier. Now that the kids were all out of the house, I suddenly realised that this could be my time for *me*. But my husband had never allowed it before; I knew he wouldn't allow it now.

Marriage counselling and divorce were taboo subjects in her husband's family, and Patricia realised that she was unwilling to make further concessions in order to 'colour within the lines' of the way he'd sketched their lives. Instead she decided to avoid the unacceptable future by trying to re-create the past. At the age of forty-seven, she talked him into adopting a baby girl.

> I didn't realise it consciously at the time, but, looking back, I think I knew the baby would spare me from having to put our marriage under the spotlight. I wanted to set the clock back. Going forward was too scary. In some ways it did the trick – it

kept me occupied. But even though bringing up children was my joy in my younger years, I realised – too late – that I'd changed. Devoting my life to children was my past life. Now, in my mid-fifties, I know it's not at all what I want to do at this stage in my life. I'm so tired all the time that I feel sedated, and it's not that it's such hard work physically – it's that my heart isn't in it. I feel tugged, like some force is trying to pull me away from here. I feel like I age ten years for every two. But I'm committed to this little girl now, who deserves all I can give her. I hope I can last until she's grown up.

Boomerang Babies

Variations on Patricia's theme are becoming more and more common, thanks to the higher than ever numbers of adult children who, for one reason or another, boomerang back home – often with children of their own for Grandma to bring up while they try to get their feet under them. If a woman is to claim the second half of her life for herself, to explore her own creative potential and choose the endeavours on to which she focuses her life energy, then she must find a way to stand firm against forces that could induce her to shoulder someone else's long-term responsibilities – forces such as guilt and the compulsion to shield her children from the consequences of their own choices. When decisions and outside circumstances conspire to keep the nest full, there is the strong potential for a woman's new life to become a tired rerun of the old one.

ANITA: FINALLY CUTTING THE CORD

When Anita and Ralph's newly wed (and pregnant) daughter and her husband rented a flat in their block, Anita was thrilled. But over the ensuing months something began to feel wrong.

At first I thought I was in heaven. Jenny was over here all the time, sometimes to do laundry (claiming she was perpetually having trouble with her machine and Jim didn't have time to fix it), sometimes to borrow a cup of sugar, sometimes just to 'hang out'. I thought it was great – it was as if I'd never lost my daughter. Instead of an empty nest, I had the promise of keeping her and having a new little baby around, too. But then, gradually, I started peeling back the layers of what was bothering me. I thought back to when I was a newly-wed, and although I adored my parents, I didn't spend nearly as much time with them as Jenny was spending with me. I began to watch for signs of trouble in her marriage, not realising that I already had recognised a big one – Jenny hadn't really left home yet.

A month later Jim was promoted, which meant a transfer to a town miles away. I felt as though I'd been kicked in the stomach. Jenny is our only child, and she had been my whole life. It was to be a quick move – they had six weeks to tie up loose ends and get settled in their new town – but I noticed that in the midst of all the preparations for moving, Jenny started spending even more time with me.

Two weeks later there was a big row, and the next thing I knew there she was on our doorstep, ready to move 'back home', with a look on her face that was both anguished and maybe a little triumphant at the same time. She told me later that she thought I'd be pleased – she knew how much I was going to miss her. That's partly why my response really surprised her.

It was heart-wrenching for me. I hated to see my daughter hurting, her face blotched from crying and her belly beginning to show evidence of her pregnancy. But somehow, fortunately, I woke up, and none too soon. I told her that moving back was not an option. I told her it was time to move forwards, not back. I realised that I needed to cut the cord and start exploring my own life, and she needed to do the same – otherwise we'd both be stuck in a phase of life that we'd outgrown.

As a woman faces the prospect of an empty nest, daunting though it may be, the bottom line is this: separation is a necessary and, ultimately, blessed thing, clearing the way for her next developmental phase. To block that process can be akin to leaving a pot-bound plant, restricted and stunted, in a too-small container. A woman can choose to facilitate her growth, which may be initially painful, or she can choose to block that growth, a path that results in accelerated ageing and loss of vitality – just as it would for that pot-bound plant. Staying in place, in other words, is not a viable option. Grow – or die.

Powerful Feelings, Powerful Healing

In order to take a new path, you must leave the old path behind. This is one of the most terrifying aspects of the midlife transformation – leaving behind what is familiar and embracing what is unknown. During the first summer after my divorce, for example, I watched my daughter and former husband pull out of the driveway one perfect summer day to go sailing together, a family activity that we had enjoyed for years. I felt left behind, wondering what had happened to my life. In fact, I felt as though, other than my work, I no longer had a real life. When we are standing at a crossroads in our lives, doubts inevitably arise. 'Am I capable of pulling this off? Do I have the talent? The strength? Can I make it out there?' Or, as in my case, 'What's the use of having made it out there if I have no one to come home to?' Plucked from the milieu in which she has already proven herself, and cast adrift in unfamiliar surroundings, a woman would have to be extraordinary not to be afraid. Her self-doubt may be magnified by the fact that as she faces loss, very often the path that will lead to her new life is not clear.

It is vital to a woman's comfort level to understand that the direction of her new path, and her willingness to try it, will come . . . in time. The steps that separate her old life from the new one were not meant to be easy, any more than the birth process is meant to be easy. As difficult as it is to accept, especially in our quick-fix culture, the struggle that accompanies a woman's midlife transformation appears to be an integral part of the learning process, without which she would not have the incentive to set one foot in front of the other. Your empty nest, your altered living space, your disrupted life focus, that directionless feeling – all must first be acknowledged and experienced, with the attendant emotions, in order for the healing process to begin. In the interim, while we experience the upheaval and wait for the new path to become clear, we have to hang out in the 'underworld' for a while, allowing our fears and grief and confusion to be fully experienced. Then, and only then, will the fog begin to lift, revealing hints of new doors, new directions, and a new focus for that shining new life.

All well and good, you might say. But how does one go about fully experiencing powerful emotions without dwelling on them excessively or becoming engulfed in self-pity?

Identifying Your Emotions in Your Writing

There is a writing technique that has been proven effective in helping a woman acknowledge, identify, and express those feelings with focused attention, then release them proactively, on a moment-to-moment basis as they come up, unbidden. It is a skill that requires practice, but the rewards are immediate – and they only get better as your skill level grows. Here's what's involved.

Make a commitment to honour and respect your body by being willing to learn from the emotions that affect it, even if that simply means bringing your loving awareness to it. In other words, be willing to be there for your body and your emotions, just as you would for a child or anyone else you love. If you feel suddenly overwhelmed with sadness or anger, for example, choose to stop and identify that feeling, rather than simply react to it. Acknowledge it. Say to yourself, 'I feel sad' or 'I feel angry'.

Gaze upon your sadness without trying to fix it. The essence of being a good listener – to yourself or to a dear friend – is simply allowing emotion to be expressed freely and honestly. Over time, your caring focus can change pain to compassion. Make the effort to notice your emotions and be with them rather than try to change them, shrug them off, or stuff them into a private corner. Then, once you've focused on them, take the time to write them down.

When I feel strong emotions that stop me in my tracks, I'm almost always helped by writing about the experience as soon as I can find a moment.[1] I sit down, light a candle, put on a tape of some adagio baroque music, take three breaths, and come up writing, recording my thoughts like a good secretary. When a particular thought has a certain buzz or energy associated with it, I urge myself to go deeper, asking what I mean by 'sad', 'angry', 'irritated', or whatever. By the end of one side of the tape, I've generally figured out exactly what the emotion was trying to teach me. And, more than that, I find that the writing moves my energy to a whole new place.

Identifying Your Emotions in Your Body

A related form of awareness involves tuning in to bodily sensations. When you feel the muscles in your temples tighten, for example, simply observe them, and notice how they relax because of your focused attention. Step back and try to recognise the many ways in which each emotion manifests itself in your body – the slump of your shoulders, the lump in your throat, the tension in your jaw muscles, the trembling weakness in your legs, the hollowness in the pit of your stomach, the congestion in your nasal passages as tears flow. Apply the healing power of your awareness to all of these sensations, the emotional and the physical. Your mindfulness first validates the emotions, then eventually clears away any blockage to your ability to be healthy and fully present in your life. The grace and beauty of this approach is that it allows your suffering to have its time, so it can then flow through and out of you, which it will do. In so doing, you are setting the stage for your own healing . . . and for your own ability to move on.

Caring for Ourselves, Caring for Others: Finding the Balance

We are all knit together by continuity of care, which is one of the feminine values that the world needs more of, not less. Yet it is also true that women's lives are sometimes unnecessarily sacrificed to this virtue.

Women of my age are often referred to as the 'sandwich' generation because so many are caught between caring for their still-dependent children while increasingly being called upon to take care of elderly parents or other relatives. This is a time when our programming and our desire to be good daughters, good mothers, and good wives – roles that bring us the love and approval of others – runs headlong into the increasingly urgent need to care for ourselves and the needs of our souls. The resulting competition between those two strong but apparently conflicting desires can wreak havoc with our health if we don't examine these desires carefully and set priorities.

I've watched hundreds of women run themselves ragged at midlife trying to care for a parent with Alzheimer's, hold down a full-time job, and also run a home and family. This three-ring-circus approach to life too often contributes to health problems such as increased blood pressure and cholesterol, anxiety attacks, heart palpitations, severe hot flushes, and insomnia. In fact, research has documented that people who care for parents with chronic disease have more medical conditions requiring treatment than those who don't have this responsibility.[2]

SHARON: TOO GOOD FOR HER OWN GOOD

Sharon first came to see me when she was fifty-one years old, complaining of hot flushes and an inability to fall asleep. When I asked her what her exercise and eating habits were like, she shrugged and said, 'Who has time to exercise or eat well?' Though Sharon was about 2 stone (13.5 kg) overweight and said she wanted to lose weight, she simply couldn't see how she was going to make the time to improve her lifestyle in any way. As I discovered, Sharon was the eldest of five siblings and the only daughter. When her mother died, she was left to care for her father, a man who, at seventy-two, had been somewhat abusive and distant to his children for most of Sharon's life. His health had mildly deteriorated after Sharon's mother died. Though Sharon's father didn't require skilled nursing care, he did need someone to come in and cook his meals, do the laundry, and keep the house clean – tasks that had always been done by his wife.

Sharon automatically added these tasks to her own day even though her father lived about thirty minutes away from her and even though she was holding down a full-time job as a nurse, was married, and had two teenage sons still living at home. The first thing I asked Sharon was, 'Where are your brothers?' She told me that two were living in another part of the country, but two lived in the same town as their father. The obvious next question was, 'Are your brothers assisting with your father's care?' Sharon said that she couldn't really rely on them to help out. After all, they had jobs, wives, and children of their own. 'Besides,' she added, 'they aren't very good at cooking and cleaning. Also, my father really wants me to be the one to come into his house to help out.'

I pointed out to Sharon that if she didn't get some help with caring for her father, chances were she was going to end up with a health problem herself. Then she wouldn't be able to help her dad at all! I've seen this many times in my practice and in my life. I also validated her fear that her brothers might be quite resistant to her need for their help and that they would be likely to resent her for a while. Her willingness to take on the whole job herself had made it quite comfortable for her brothers, a perk they weren't likely to give up easily. And her willingness to sacrifice herself for their approval brought her love, gratitude, and a sense of purpose.

Though Sharon felt victimised by her situation, it had never occurred to her to ask her brothers for help. Nor did she like hearing that suggestion from me. But when I raised the possibility that her weight problem and increased blood pressure were related to her current workload, she could see that something had to give. The first thing I advised was that Sharon take a long, hard look at her beliefs about caregiving.

Sharon, like her mother before her, truly believed that 'if I don't do it, it won't get done'. She had grown up in a household full of boys, none of whom cooked, cleaned, or washed dishes. She and her mother, a woman whom the family described as 'a saint', did all the household work. Not surprisingly, Sharon married a man who didn't share in the household tasks, either. And her brothers all married women who were happy to stay at home, like their mother, and care for their homes and children.

Unfortunately, this sort of martyrdom had already claimed Sharon's mother, who was only sixty-eight when she died of a heart attack. If Sharon wanted to escape the same fate as her mother, she was going to have to revise her beliefs and behaviours about sacrifice and caregiving.

Changing this kind of pattern is rarely easy, however, because when a caregiver like Sharon finally takes a stand, a kind of emotional domino effect gets put into action. When I saw Sharon several months later, she had spoken with her brothers about chipping in towards their father's care. One was so angry with her, he didn't speak to her for a month. But another was a bit more understanding. At the time of writing, Sharon tells me that there has been a split in the family over the stand she has taken. Her brothers have assumed about 40 per cent of their father's care. Their father is learning to do more for himself, and Sharon has lost some weight as well as lowered her blood pressure. Though she feels bad about the rift she 'caused' in her family, she also feels encouraged by the positive changes that have taken place in her health. She knows she is on the right track.

Breaking the Chain of Self-sacrifice

Every one of us makes choices every day. For every choice we make, there will be consequences. The more honest we are with ourselves about the motivation that drives our choices, the healthier we will be. This is as true for caregiving as it is for any other area of our lives, perhaps even more so. The following steps are designed to help you consciously care for yourself while caring for others if and when the need arises.

Step one: Acknowledge that women have inherited a cultural and personal legacy of self-sacrifice that has been passed down to us for generations. If you routinely sacrifice yourself for others, relax. You're normal. We've been socialised to value our contribution to our family or social group – our social worth – more than we value ourselves and our relationship with our soul. For at least the past five thousand years, a woman's worth has been largely determined by how well and how much she serves those who have more power and clout than she has. If you doubt this, remember that women won the right to vote only in 1918, just over eighty years ago. Before that, women's opinions and lives didn't even receive official recognition in the government. We haven't had much time in which to shed the automatic caretaking roles that have won us so much praise for millennia, let alone replace them with new beliefs and behaviours associated with taking our lives as seriously as we take those of others, particularly men.

Step two: Learn the difference between care and overcare. True care of others, from a place of unconditional love, enhances our health. That's part of the reason why volunteering and community service are associated with improved health. But overcare and burnout destroy our health and run our batteries down. Overcare is often motivated by guilt and unfinished business, for which we hope to somehow compensate through the caregiving role. The way to tell the difference between the two is to be aware of how caring for another makes you feel. You must also be 100 per cent honest about what you're getting out of excessive caregiving.

One of my friends told me, 'When I do things to make my family happy, I feel good and loved. The more I do, like baking, cooking, and keeping the house together, the more compliments I get. Though this can be exhausting, and though I keep saying that I need to get a life for myself other than work and cleaning up after everyone, I'm secretly afraid that if I take a stand and delegate responsibility to other family members for some of the caregiving work, they will resent me and not love me as much. So the payoff of doing it all myself is that I get my parents' love and my husband's love.' When I hear something like this, I have to wonder whether it really is pleasure that motivates the caregiving, as she believes, or fear.

Each of us needs to examine what we get from martyring ourselves. One of my patients, a woman whose mother was physically and verbally abusive, learned early on that the only way to avoid being hit was to make all the meals, scrub the floors, and clean the rest of the house. To this day whenever she meets new people, she feels compelled to cook, clean, and bring them gifts to earn their love. She recently told me that she'd had the following insight: 'If you act like a saint, no one ever confronts you. You become a valued part of every group you're in.'

Sainthood of this kind seems mainly an avoidance strategy. On the other hand, the desire to nurture others, including plants and animals, is a positive emotion that seems to be built right in to the biological programming of most women (and many men as well). Studies have shown, for instance, that when volunteers in nursing homes are taught how to give massages to the residents, the health of the volunteers is enhanced as well as that of the recipients. Who hasn't enjoyed the satisfaction gained from making a special school lunch that surprises and delights a child, or helping out a sick friend who needs a meal or someone to look after her children?

It feels good deep inside me to bring comfort to those who are suffering. In fact, my entire career is based on helping others feel better. Often, as I give health assistance to someone, I feel as though I'm in touch with a power that is greater than me but moves through me, helping me as it helps the other person. But many women, including myself, have learned over the years, sometimes through the wisdom of personal illness, that we cannot be available to another in a healthy way unless we're also getting our own needs met.

Step three: Learn the health benefits of benign self-interest. Here's a basic scientific truth: our health is best served by participating in those activities that are in our own highest and best interests. This is not selfish. It is the very basis for a healthy life. There is not a single cell in our bodies that flourishes through sacrificing its own health for the health of the surrounding cells. It simply doesn't make sense. Instead, cells communicate with each other constantly. The health of one affects the health of them all. The more fully you are participating in the work that brings you the most joy, the healthier you and your entire group become.

Step four: Understand that caring for parents or ageing relatives can be an attempt to heal unfinished business from our family past. Claris, one of my menopausal patients whose diabetes was particularly difficult to bring under control while she was caring for her father, told me that the very thought of not caring for her father, who was dying of cancer, caused her to feel overcome with guilt. She said, 'Daddy didn't want any strangers in the house, so I didn't feel as though I could hire a nurse or home help even though the money was available. To tell you the truth, his insistence that I be the only one to help him made me feel special.' When Claris entered therapy after her father's death, she realised that she had never felt her father valued her as much as her brothers, so she tried to prove her worth through caregiving, something she did better than her brothers. She came to see that being constantly available for her father, even though other choices were available, was a way of trying to win the love and approval she had never felt from him in childhood.

Step five: Learn to delegate and ask for help. Caregiving at midlife is yet another opportunity to learn how to have healthy boundaries, set limits, and demand (not ask) that other family members assume some of the burden or pay for your help. If your husband isn't working or is working fewer hours than you are, for example, there's no reason why he can't do his share.

I'm well aware that many women are not in a financial position to pay for outside help to provide care for family members. But in almost every case there is a caregiving solution that needn't fall squarely on only one woman's shoulders. It's time that all men learned the basics of cooking and cleaning. Or, if no one else in the family can or will help out, another tactic would be to work out what your caretaking time is worth, by finding out what it would cost to pay someone to come in and do the work you are doing. Then you could ask your brothers or other family members to pay you directly so that you can cut back on the hours you work elsewhere. That way you would have more time to replenish yourself each day, including time to exercise and eat well.

Like Sharon, you may have to recover from the family programming that leads you to believe your role as a woman must include self-sacrifice. Sharon had to let her father know that he needed to learn how to receive care from someone other than her. And her father also needed to undo a lifetime of conditioning telling him that all his household tasks would automatically be taken care of. It is well documented that older people, including men, can learn and grow until the end of their lives. There's no reason why a man can't learn how to boil an egg, grill a piece of chicken, or stick a load of clothes in a washing machine! Parents who truly love us want what is best for us, even if that means making some adjustments in their behaviour and expectations.

Step six: Plan ahead. Don't wait until a parent or relative is in need of care before discussing a potential plan with your siblings. That way you can avoid the emergency caregiving that seemingly 'just happens' to us but in reality was set in motion by our beliefs and choices years before. One of my friends, an eldest daughter who has just reached forty, has already made it clear to her younger sister, who lives in the same town as their mother, that she has no intention of allowing the mother, a very dependent woman, to come and live with her should something happen to their father. My friend is not being selfish. She's being realistic. She loves her mother but does not intend to sacrifice her life and career for her. Her unblinking approach concerning her mother's possible future care alerts other family members that they can't automatically rely on her to house her mother in the future should the need arise. This breaks the chain of eldest-daughter sacrifice before it even gets welded in the first place.

Getting Clear About Money at Midlife

Whatever the changes that precipitate a woman's empty-nest experience, the only path that will allow the full expression of her creative potential in the second half of her life is the path that establishes her true independence, both financially and emotionally. Even if she currently has a husband who supports her or money coming in from her family, it's important for her to know that if the need arose, she could manage alone. Inability to support themselves financially is the number-one reason why women stay in less than ideal relationships in which they are not treated as autonomous individuals with equal decision-making power.

Though I do not claim to be a financial expert, I do know this: how, what, where, when, and on whom a woman spends money, and where she gets that money, tells you more about her true values, beliefs, and priorities than any other aspect of her life. Our behaviour concerning earning, spending, and saving money lays bare our core beliefs about ourselves and our worth in the world, pure and simple.

The dynamics of money also holds up a mirror to our relationships, telling us how each partner's contribution is valued and whether we are in a truly co-creative partnership. That's why discussing who pays for what and who does what tasks in a relationship is such a loaded and often unpleasant topic.

Cultural Ambivalence About Women and Money

Even though many women now earn more money than their mates, the data suggest that we are still not comfortable, as individuals or as a culture, with that pattern. Consider the following research. Although a study from the University of Missouri in St Louis in the US showed that women now outearn their husbands in one out of five marriages, only 56 per cent of men surveyed in the Virginia Slims Opinion Poll 2000 said that it would be acceptable for their spouses to be the primary wage earners. Many women agree with this. In the same poll, only 61 per cent of women felt that it would be acceptable for them to be the primary wage earners.

When a woman does earn more than her husband, it doesn't wipe out the power differential. If anything, it seems to exacerbate it, due to the ambivalence couples feel about their status reversal. Julie Brines, a sociologist at the University of Washington in the US who studies status-reversal couples, found, for example, that the more women contribute to the family account, the *less* likely their husbands are to contribute to the housework. In fact, when women earned all the money while their husbands stayed at home, these men actually did less housework per week than men who worked outside the home![3] Brines also found that in status-reversal marriages, women cede much of the decision-making power to their spouses. This is the opposite of what happens in traditional marriages, where the husband, who brings home the bacon, tends to call the shots. In other words, when women are the major wage earners, there's not a straightforward relationship between income and power. Instead, there's an effort to achieve balance, even though this so-called balance is anything but.

The implications of this research are clear: no matter how much of the financial burden we shoulder, we still feel responsible for keeping

our husbands happy, for making them feel good about themselves –
especially if they're not earning as much money as we are.

The sad truth is that many of us are still unsure of our worth as
women in relationship to men – which is perfectly understandable
given our history. So we do even more than our share to keep the men
in our lives happy, in case they leave us for someone who appreciates
them more than we do. Secretly we're afraid that if we demand too
much, we'll be left alone.

And then there's that other deeply feminine desire: we want to be
cherished and taken care of. We keep hoping (sometimes despite
ample evidence to the contrary) that to have a husband means that we
will be taken care of. I grew up loving Tarzan movies. Recently I
watched the classic *Tarzan and His Mate*, which I hadn't seen in
years. This time I saw it through a new lens. The programming about
gender roles was very clear: Jane provided the playfulness and the sex,
while Tarzan protected Jane by fighting off wild things and doing a
lot of heavy lifting to make sure she had a secure, comfortable home.
Very compelling. Very appealing.

Evolution is slow in this regard. One of my friends told me that
when she started her final year at university in 1984, none of the ten
women she knew best was in a relationship. But then something
phenomenal happened. In the last term all of her friends suddenly
hooked up with classmates for the graduation party – and later
married them. 'It was almost chemical,' she told me. 'It felt as though
some kind of biological frenzy had hit that was bigger than all of
them. They needed their dates to the party and then they needed
husbands. It was the end of college – time to settle down, find a
husband, and get on with a "normal" life.' She remembered thinking:
'Wow. This is a top college in which women are supposed to be
serious about their careers. How could they suddenly feel so compelled to be part of a couple?'

There's nothing inherently wrong with the desire to get married
and start a family after college or even school. The problem is that
many women move directly from their childhood homes, where they
are cared for, right on to other institutions – either marriage or college
or both – that also provide them with the illusion that they are being
taken care of.

In my own family, as soon as my brothers became eighteen my father
sat them down and told them that they had to start supporting themselves. But he paid for my college years without question. I did put

myself through medical school with student loans and scholarships, but when I got married, during my last month of medical school, I gladly let my husband take care of all the details of buying our first home – a process that mystified and terrified me at the time. He used the last of his educational trust fund as a down payment, and I felt unbelievably lucky to be living this fairy-tale life! We paid off my medical school loans without difficulty.

My husband also made all the decisions about charitable donations and investments, though our incomes were basically equal. Donations went to the educational institutions and charities he favoured. I never questioned this. I found the topic of money burdensome until I was forced to wake up at midlife. I'm not alone; many women find themselves in the same situation. Though we went through women's liberation in college, in the interest of creating a happy home and family life we were always willing to do 'a little more' housework and child care than our husbands. Now our generation has to take the next step.

MARY: IT'S NEVER ENOUGH

Forty-six-year-old Mary had long been convinced her husband was better at finances than she was. He paid all the bills and did the taxes every year. But these activities always upset him. His mantra seemed to be 'There's never enough. There's never enough.' Increasingly Mary felt as though she couldn't ask her husband for money for anything but the barest of essentials, and it seemed the only way she could help the situation was to spend less. Finally, after much soul-searching, Mary decided to get retrained as a nurse, the profession she'd had when she had met and married her husband. Given the nursing shortage and the fact that they lived in a city with several large hospitals, Mary had no difficulty getting a job with a good salary and decent benefits. Within a year or so she began to make substantial contributions to the family income. This made her feel good, even though she hated the on-call part of her job. Despite her contribution, however, her husband continued to exercise iron control over all their financial decisions.

Mary suspected that one reason her husband was reluctant to share the financial decision making, as unhappy as it seemed to make him, was that he was going through his own midlife crisis at work. He seemed depressed about his career and the fact that he hadn't reached the success he thought he should have during his forties – a time he referred to as his 'power years'. He had started talking about retiring early, selling the house, and travelling around the country in a caravan. Mary hoped that her husband was just going through a phase and would recover soon. She suggested that he get some individual counselling, but he became angry with her and said absolutely nothing was wrong with him and that he was not depressed.

Meanwhile, bringing home a salary had allowed Mary to become much more empowered in the world, if not at home. Nevertheless, she began to suffer from a host of health problems, including palpitations, severe hot flushes, and lower back pain. Her periods also became very irregular and very heavy. It was at this point that Mary came to see me, and I asked her what was going on in her life. When she told me, I gave her a series of recommendations to help her physical symptoms. (I will discuss these in later chapters.) I also suggested that she begin to assume a more proactive role in managing the family finances, which she agreed to do.

When she came back three months later, many of her menopausal symptoms were better. She reported that at first her husband had been resistant to her desire to know about their finances and help with spending decisions. However, soon after she initially raised the issue, he started to experience chest pain, which was diagnosed as angina. He realised that if his life continued in the way it had been going, he could die of a heart attack. This was his own midlife wake-up call, and it made him realise that he, too, needed to revamp some of his outmoded beliefs and behaviours.

In the meantime, Mary took steps on her own to increase her financial knowledge. Her new confidence forced changes in her marriage, of course. She told me that she and her husband had to completely rework their agreements about money and household chores. It wasn't easy. But in time, Mary's husband realised that it was in both his and Mary's best interests if both of them knew everything about their mutual finances and agreed upon their spending habits.

Changing Your Cultural Legacy

Middle-class women of my mother's generation were brought up to believe that they would be taken care of by their husbands. With the help of life insurance policies and the unprecedented economic growth that followed the Second World War, many of them were. The majority of my mother's friends, women now in their sixties and seventies, never worked after marriage and never had to return to work after they became widows. The women's movement brought to our collective consciousness the price that our mothers paid for being taken care of in this way, and my generation vowed that we wouldn't become our mothers. (My mother tells me that she is routinely dismayed at the dismissive and abusive ways in which many of her friends' husbands treat them.)

Though we'd like to think that we've come a long way when it comes to earning and handling money, the truth is that far too many women still lack basic money skills and so are overly dependent upon husbands, employers, or family members to do their financial planning for them. It boils down to this: we women are brought up to think that someone else will take care of us financially if we do all the other kinds of caretaking. Our idea of investments is that we invest in the people (usually husbands, but not always) who we believe will provide for us and love us.

How can we women invest in and plan for our own retirement financially if we remain convinced that we don't have the skills or interest to handle money, can't live without people's love and acceptance, and must sacrifice ourselves taking care of others in order to earn that love? No wonder research has found that many women know very little about planning for retirement and old age, investing money rather than just making and spending it, and setting financial goals.

Happily, this situation has now begun to change. Women, particularly midlife women, have now been identified as a lucrative new market for the financial industry. And it turns out that we're good at managing our money. Studies have shown, for example, that women's investment groups do better in the long run than men's. Women tend to focus more on long-term financial goals rather than short-term performance, perhaps because we live longer and know that we are more likely to be supporting children or ageing parents.

The Value of Becoming Financially Astute

Regardless of your current circumstances, it is crucial that you get very clear about your beliefs about money so that you can begin to assume dominion over your money in the same way you are daily assuming dominion over your health. Money is a very concrete form of energy – it is power in our society, allowing you to go where you want to go and stay where you want to stay. Having control over your money gives you a sense of freedom and safety. In study after study, higher socioeconomic status is consistently associated with better health. But I believe it is the sense of empowerment and control, not the absolute number of pounds involved, that makes the real difference.

Many women report that in the early stages of taking financial control, they feel fuelled by both anger and fear. I was no exception. In those first few months after my separation, I found myself possessed by a new sense of purpose, driven by the need to get my life free, clear, and settled. I had to get myself out of debt, pay off the overdrafts, and get the household accounts reorganised. It seemed scary and burdensome at first, but it quickly became exhilarating as I came to the realisation that I *could* do it all by myself. The truth is, I had never actually acknowledged the fact that I had doubted that ability before. I learned I could manage my household finances just as effectively as I had for many years managed my professional and business finances – all without my husband's income, advice, or support. This is not to minimise or disparage his contribution during all the years of our marriage. Rather, it is to acknowledge the personal empowerment that comes from becoming financially independent.

Women who are currently being supported by a husband or other family member can put themselves on the road to financial competence by doing the following exercise for one month. Pretend you are divorced, widowed, or suddenly faced with supporting yourself. Continuously ask yourself questions such as these: 'Where are the insurance documents? The deeds to the house? The mortgage papers? The pension plan? The tax forms from past years? What is the value of the house? What is my net worth? When was the last time I filled out a financial statement?' Having a firm grasp on this type of information can help ensure that you remain in your relationship for all the right reasons – because it fulfils you and makes your life better on many levels – rather than because you believe you would fall apart without it. You simply cannot be available for true partnership and exhilarating co-creation with another until you know how to pull your own weight and have faced your own dependency squarely – and then done something about it.

Coming Home to Yourself

As I write this I am well into perimenopause, a time when I should be in the throes of what many call 'hormone hell'. Yet I feel better now than I have in years. The severe hot flushes I was experiencing in the last few months of my marriage virtually disappeared after my husband left – a phenomenon I've seen repeatedly in other women who've had the courage to leave dead-end relationships. Over and over again I've watched perimenopausal symptoms resolve in women who've had the courage to negotiate the rapids of their midlife transitions consciously and in an empowered way.

But I've also watched something even more profound occurring: the emergence of what can only be described as pure joy, the feeling that arises when a woman is truly coming home to herself. My own experience bears this out, as I marvel at the power of my newfound nesting instinct and at how differently I have chosen to do things now that I have set both feet across the threshold of my new life.

One of the most striking things I discovered after my husband left was an almost physical need to reclaim and redecorate my home, especially the family and spare rooms. One day, with catalogues, telephone, and credit card in hand, within less than an hour I bought a sofa, a rug, tables for the spare bedroom, and even curtains, something that at the age of forty-nine I had never done. My work in combination with my mothering had left no time or inclination to contemplate decor, let alone participate in choosing it. But that was my old life. Now, with my inner landscape rapidly changing, I felt a powerful compulsion to make my outer surroundings reflect the rejuvenation that was going on inside me.

I discovered that feng shui, the Chinese art of placement, helped me enormously in this process. I came to see that our homes reflect our lives, and that by consciously changing them according to the principles of feng shui, we can actually create improvements in our lives on all levels. By using a tool known as the *baqua* map, one can determine which areas of a room or an entire home correspond to specific aspects of life – for example, health and family, wealth and prosperity, helpful people and travel, love and marriage. This information allows you to enhance and change your physical space in order to enhance and change that particular area of your life. And as with all things in life, when you do this, things sometimes get worse before they get better – kind of like taking out the rubbish as part of the process of spring cleaning. When my friend and colleague Terah Kathryn Collins, the author of the 1999 book *The Western Guide to Feng Shui*, did a consultation with me, we both laughed when we realised that my husband had left within four months of the time I had 'enhanced' the love-and-marriage area of our property with a beautiful arbour. She said, 'I see this over and over again. When you enhance an area of your life that isn't working, you first have to let go of the parts that are standing in the way of getting what you really want.' I also put a lighted lamppost in the helpful-people-and-places area of the property. Within two months my life became filled with skilful people who help me on all levels of my life, both at home and at work. (See Resources for feng shui information.)

I wanted my home to be the kind of place where people felt comfortable and welcome. And I wanted to feel at home there, surrounded by colours and textures that drew me in. For the first time in my life, I knew exactly what my personal style was and exactly how I wanted my rooms to look and feel. As the furniture began to come in and the rooms took shape, I felt delighted with the results, going back to look at them over and over again. Slowly it began to dawn on me what I was really doing: I was creating a potential space for all the new energy that was beginning to stream into my life. Whereas before I had been grieving the empty nest, now I was re-creating my old nest into a new place that reflected who I was becoming. It was a nest that would, of course, comfortably accommodate my children, their friends, and the new people who, I felt sure, would be coming into my life.

PAMELA: A HOME OF HER OWN

While for me the process of coming home to myself meant accepting the break up of my marriage, Pamela found a different – and very unconventional – path. She wrote:

I am forty-seven years old and have been in a relationship with Don for eight years, married for five. He's twelve years older, and his philosophy of life is pretty much 'my way or the highway'. Don's unilateral decisions aren't always supportive of me, and last year I decided that I needed to make choices that reflected my beliefs and prepared me for my future. He travels frequently for business and pleasure, and I spent a good deal of time alone in a house that didn't feel like home. I had even created a room of my own, but it wasn't enough.

So I've bought a home of my own. The marriage has had to undergo a transformation now that we are not together on a daily basis, and it could have failed. Don lives where he wants to, and I live where I need to. I cannot describe the joy I feel at living in a place that supports me emotionally and spiritually. I am moved to nurture my home and garden just as it nourishes me. I am delighted by the simplest things. Friends who have visited agree that it is me.

I am grateful that I earn a living and am capable of being financially independent of Don. And perhaps finally succeeding at my career gave me the confidence to create my dream home. After a lifetime of determining my worth through male approval, I am now living from my heart rather than from obligation.

Vocational Awakening at Midlife

For some women, the home – which had been the central focus before midlife – becomes secondary to a new passion, which reveals itself in the form of a vocational calling. Other women leave their previous work 'home' to start their own businesses or change careers. Still others are simply forced by life circumstances into a new path.

The breadth of a woman's interests and contacts outside the home during the childbearing years will have an impact on the ease with which she moves into her new life. Some experimentation may be required before a woman can discover where her passions lie, and it may take longer for some to find their niche than others. Those who continue to define themselves by the roles they no longer have – such as mother or wife – and who have long lived enclosed in those roles may be overwhelmed by fear and lapse into immobility. But the key to finding new passions is getting out and getting moving, even if you don't know where you are going. Sometimes it's simply a matter of stumbling from point A to point B with your eyes wide open to the possibilities.

SYLVIA: DISCOVERING THE ARTIST

Sylvia retired from teaching the same year her youngest son married and moved away. It was difficult for her to relinquish simultaneously her role of mother and mentor to her own children as well as to the students she'd taught for the past twenty-five years. She kept in contact with me through the grieving process, and she admitted there were times she felt she'd never find herself.

'Everything about who I am is wrapped up in kids,' she wrote. 'On one hand, the extra free time made it more difficult, because I didn't know what to do with myself. The days were so long and bleak.' But in retrospect that time was a luxury, because it allowed her to give focused attention to her feelings and let them out – loud and clear. 'My husband continued to go to work, so I was able to cry out loud, wail, even roar in frustration. I made some pretty anguished, animal-like sounds alone in that house – just me and those powerful feelings, bouncing off the walls.'

Then, a few weeks later, Sylvia started looking at her house as though it were a property she was contemplating buying – it had lots of potential but needed adjustments to fit her new life. She knocked down walls and incorporated the kids' rooms into the main living space, creating a great room that could accommodate her monthly meetings with local career women who gathered for the camaraderie and to share new skills, projects, and philosophies. Sylvia did much of the remodelling work herself, despite never having hung wallpaper or laid ceramic tiles before. When it was Sylvia's turn to demonstrate a new skill to the group, she showed them the tilework she'd done in her bathroom. Sylvia started tiling bathrooms for her friends, using handmade tiles and innovative patterns. What started out as a project spanning several weekends has turned into a second profession: two years later, through word of mouth, she has found clients all over the country, and she's recruited and trained two women to help her keep up with the demand. 'I love the travel – I've always been a homebody, and I never went anywhere without my husband. Now I traipse off to visit beautiful homes and work my magic to make those homes even more beautiful, while my husband stays here and runs the household. Several clients asked me to sign my name on a prominent tile in their finished bathroom, like an artist signs paintings. I feel exhilarated and free as a bird. I love this new life.'

JUDITH: FINDING HER TRUE VOCATION

For many women, the key to finding their niche at midlife is in identifying the passions they've always had but never pursued full time. At fifty-four, after more than thirty years in the corporate world, Judith chose to take early retirement. Having looked back over her many years of doing volunteer work, she realised that caring for the elderly was a dream she wanted to pursue. Rather than make excuses for herself because of her age, she undertook a demanding graduate course to prepare for her new work. She wrote:

> I chose to leave my position as a business analyst and embark on a career change. I left with a mission statement: to dedicate my life work to the self-enlightenment, creative development, and joy of being an elderly person, and to provide services to elderly people that enhance their physical, mental, and spiritual growth. I had interviews with managers of elderly people's homes while continuing my volunteer efforts by delivering meals on wheels. This past June I completed the required coursework for a master's degree in gerontological psychology.
>
> I have learned that although it can be extremely painful at times, it is only through the process of transition, with eyes and heart wide open, that an individual can truly succeed in personal growth. Now I feel the excitement and fear of taking my plan to fruition – actually doing what I have been studying and talking about doing! My daughter says, 'Mum, who will employ you at your age?' My husband wishes me to succeed. I know I have *inner resources unlimited* and that new birth is emerging as I enter this new phase of my life.

Many midlife women discover that as they find new direction in life, they themselves become new, and so they attract new friends. One patient put it to me this way: 'I became more interesting. I had more to offer on a personal level – I had more to talk about than kids and soccer practice and my husband's promotion. This new me is someone I really like!'

A Road Map for Navigating
Unknown Territory

Taking those first steps on your journey home to yourself may be one of the hardest things you'll ever do. But as you venture onto this new path you will find that it loses its intimidating aspects and becomes instead a voyage of exploration and discovery. Here are a few signposts to help you along.

Take heart. Though painful, your feelings of loneliness, like all feelings, will gradually lessen and change as time goes on. Be present for your own experience while it's happening. The depth to which you allow yourself to feel pain is the depth to which you will also feel joy. And you have to trust that joy will come again, even though your life will never be exactly the same again. I know that the news is good, because I've been hearing about it for years.

One of my newsletter subscribers wrote:

I haven't felt this good since the whole nonsense started in my early teens. After a hideous perimenopausal epoch in my forties, I look forward to my fifty-second birthday with a big smile! All those years of chasing relationships to make my identity! I now live blissfully alone (except for Harriet the cat) and have an interesting relationship with an unusual man that does not define me. Even though my body will no longer put up with whatever I want to do to it, the aches and pains are treated with acceptance and equanimity. Life is filled with possibilities and delightful friendships, home and garden, dancing the Argentine tango, travel, lots else to do – but great respect for quiet, restful, self-indulgent times.

Embrace the wisdom of routine and discipline. Either start or continue at least one activity that is scheduled regularly. You cannot imagine how healing a regular routine is. In my case, this routine includes daily exercise and a twice-weekly Pilates class. Pilates is a demanding type of exercise that involves moving from and focusing one's attention on what is known as one's 'centre' or 'powerhouse', the muscles of the deep pelvis, buttocks, and abdomen that form a band around the lower body. No matter what else is going on in my life, I make the time to go to the studio and work on the link between my muscles and my brain. The sameness of it and the discipline involved in this activity are very anchoring for me – a part of my life that hasn't changed or gone away. In fact, on the morning my husband left, I went to my class as usual. Though I had no idea what would happen to our marriage at the time, and though my heart was racing and I was scared, getting on the Pilates equipment and going through my usual routine was very calming and reassuring. Though a significant part of my world was falling apart, I could still concentrate on my breathing, the strength of my muscles – and the fact that the planet was going to keep spinning.

Enhance your daily life. In the first few months of my almost-empty nest – my younger daughter was still at home but deeply involved in her own activities – I began the practice of lighting a fire every night and keeping the doors of the woodstove open so that I could enjoy watching the flames as I ate dinner. In all our years of marriage, my husband and I had rarely opened the doors of this stove because it lessens the amount of heat that is produced. But now I was much less interested in thermodynamics, and instead simply wanted to bring the comfort of firelight into my home – especially at dinner-time, when the prospect of facing an evening alone loomed large before me. I also lit candles at dinner each night and played my favourite CDs. Six months later, when my second daughter left for her first term away and I was truly faced with being alone every night, I was determined to use my time to tune in to and deepen my relationship with myself and my spirit. Mostly I wanted to heal the parts of myself that had led to my need to go through a divorce in the first place. And I wanted to get comfortable enough being alone in my home that I didn't need to jump into a new relationship right away just to avoid the pain of my husband's and daughters' absence. I knew that to do so might result in a relationship that simply repeated old, unhealed patterns.

Know that the fear of loss is often worse than the actual loss. I found that my dread of the empty nest was much worse than the actual experience. In fact, I was so busy with work that I enjoyed having only myself to take care of. Besides, I learned that I like reading in bed as late as I wanted, going to as many films as I felt like, taking a bath at any hour of the day or night, and generally discovering what my own needs and desires actually were. Though I had originally planned to have my mother visit and go skiing with me during my first empty-nest winter, the time flew by so quickly that we never got around to it. Nevertheless, it felt good to know that she was willing to come and provide support and recreation if I needed it.

Remember that we're stronger and more resilient than we may think. On the day that would have been my twenty-fifth wedding anniversary, I awoke and just stayed in bed, allowing myself to experience my emotions for a few minutes. I hadn't made it to the quarter-century mark in my marriage, and I felt bad about that. I thought I might spend the whole day feeling sad. But to my surprise, I didn't. Diane, a woman who has worked with me for over twenty years, gave me a funny card. On the cover there was a ridiculous photo of a muscular man dressed up in a tutu with a snake draped over his shoulder. When you opened the card, the greeting read, 'Still looking for Mr Right!' I laughed out loud and put the card in my journal. Later I went out to dinner to celebrate a friend's birthday. The day came and went and I stayed calm and happy. The previous year my heart was breaking on the day of my anniversary, and I dissolved in tears at dinner that night with my two daughters. One year later, I was renewed and at peace.

I won't pretend that going through a divorce and seeing both my daughters leave in the same year was easy. That first empty-nest year was the most difficult time of my life, as I experienced the crumbling of everything I had always thought I could count on. Paradoxically, that year also proved to be one of the most strengthening and exhilarating of my entire life. Looking back, I marvel at how far I've come. By turning my life over to Source energy and being willing to roll up my sleeves and rebuild my life, I've become infused with the energy of hope, relief, and new beginnings. Every day I'm reminded that the energy that supports new life abounds. We just have to believe in it, surrender to it, and ask for help.

FOUR

This Can't Be Menopause, Can It?
The Physical Foundation
of the Change

*M*any women are caught off guard by the first signs of the climacteric. They don't expect symptoms to occur until they've reached the end point – the absolute cessation of periods. But a woman's last period is usually preceded by a long period of transition, which may include symptoms such as hot flushes, mood swings, difficulty sleeping, and night sweats.

Doreen was a vital, youthful-looking woman of forty-six when she had her first hot flush. She'd noticed a certain irritability in the way she related to her husband, who had begun to tease her about being menopausal, but she adamantly denied the possibility. 'I'm still having my periods like clockwork,' she argued. 'My mum was fifty-three when she hit the menopause. I'm not old enough to be going through the change!'

It is true that the age at which a woman's mother had her last period is probably the best predictor of when it will happen to her. But if she doesn't understand that the first symptoms of the climacteric may reveal themselves well before that time – sometimes ten or more years earlier – she is likely to protest, with Doreen, 'This can't be menopause . . . can it?'

The quick answer is this: if you have reason to ask, then it probably is.

What Is Happening in Your Body:
Hormonal Changes

Menopause is officially defined as that point in time when our periods stop permanently. A woman undergoing natural menopause really has no way of knowing whether any given period is truly her last until a year has passed. As menopause approaches, cycles can become quite erratic, and it's not uncommon for several months to go by between periods. By the age of forty some of the initial hormonal changes associated with perimenopause (*peri-* means 'around' or 'near') are well under way. Research has shown, for example, that by the age of forty many women have already undergone changes in bone density, and by forty-four many have begun to experience periods that are either lighter and/or shorter in length than usual, or heavier and/or longer. About 80 per cent of women begin skipping periods altogether.[1] In fact, only about 10 per cent of women cease menstruating altogether with no prolonged period of cycle irregularity beforehand. In an extensive study of more than 2,700 women, most experienced a perimenopausal transition lasting between two and eight years.[2]

Unless you've gone into menopause abruptly because of surgery or medical treatment, perimenopause can be thought of as the other end of a process that began when you first started your periods. That first menstrual period is usually followed by five to seven years of relatively long cycles that are often irregular and frequently anovulatory. Eventually, in the late teens or early twenties, cycle length shortens and becomes more regular as a woman reaches her prime reproductive age, which lasts for the next twenty years or so. In our forties, our cycles begin to lengthen again. Though most of us have been led to believe that twenty-eight days is the normal cycle length, research has shown that only 12.4 per cent of women actually have a twenty-eight-day cycle. The vast majority have cycles that last anywhere between twenty-four and thirty-five days, and 20 per cent of all women experience irregular cycles.[3]

Two to eight years prior to menopause, most women begin skipping ovulations. During these years, the ovarian follicles, which ripen eggs each month, undergo an accelerated rate of loss, until the supply of follicles is finally depleted. Research suggests that, in this culture at least, the acceleration in follicle loss begins at around the age of thirty-seven or thirty-eight. Inhibin, a substance produced by the ovaries, decreases, which results in rising levels of FSH, the follicle-stimulating hormone produced by the pituitary gland.

Contrary to the standard belief, our oestrogen levels often remain relatively stable or even increase during perimenopause. They don't wane until less than a year before the last menstrual period.[4] Until menopause, the primary oestrogen a woman's body produces is oestradiol. However, during perimenopause the body starts making more of a different kind of oestrogen, called oestrone, which is produced both in the ovaries and in body fat.

Testosterone levels usually do not fall appreciably during perimenopause. In fact, the postmenopausal ovaries of many women (but not all) secrete more testosterone than the premenopausal ovaries.

On the other hand, progesterone levels do begin to fall in perimenopause, often long before changes in oestrogen or testosterone. As I will discuss below, this is the most significant perimenopausal issue for the majority of women.

The prevailing message appears to be this: although reproduction is no longer the goal, there continue to be important roles for these so-called reproductive hormones – vital, health-enhancing roles that have nothing to do with making babies. Evidence for this can be seen in the fact that steroid hormone receptors are found in almost every organ of our bodies. Oestrogen and androgens (like testosterone) are important, for example, in maintaining strong and healthy bones as well as resilient vaginal and urethral tissue. And both oestrogen and progesterone are important for maintaining a healthy collagen layer in the skin.

Perimenopause Is a Normal Process, Not a Disease

The main thing to keep in mind about perimenopause is that it's a completely normal process, not a disease to be treated. But in order for her body to continue producing levels of hormones adequate to support health, a woman must be optimally healthy going in – physically, emotionally, spiritually, and situationally. In other words, her future well-being depends not only on the health of her physical body, but also on her non-physical support system, both of which are a reflection of how she cares for herself today and how she has lived up to this point. Because perimenopause occurs at the midpoint of our lives, it is a very good time to take stock and make sure that we are doing everything possible to restore or build our health.

Despite all the media focus on supplemental hormones – which ones to take, what dose, natural versus synthetic, and so on – it is important to bear in mind this often-forgotten fact: a woman's body begins life fully equipped to produce all the hormones she needs throughout life. All of the so-called sex hormones (oestrogen, progesterone, and the androgens) are manufactured from the same ubiquitous precursor molecule – cholesterol. In addition, our bodies also have the ability to convert one type of sex hormone into another. So, for example, oestrogen can be converted into testosterone, and progesterone can be converted into oestrogen. Whether or not these conversions actually take place depends upon our body's minute-to-minute needs, our emotional state, our nutritional state, and so on.

What all this means is that not all women will need or want hormone supplementation. In many cultures hormone supplements are infrequently prescribed, yet women in those cultures rarely have uncomfortable perimenopausal symptoms. How can this be?

First of all, the ovaries only slow down; they do not shut down. Moreover, a woman's body is designed to produce oestrogen, progesterone, and testosterone at other sites besides the ovaries, and it is ready and willing to increase or mediate the output from those auxiliary sites when the need arises at midlife. Research has shown, for example, that oestrogen, progesterone, and androgen are produced in body fat, skin, the brain, the adrenal glands, and even peripheral nerves! But whether or not adequate production occurs depends on what else is going on in a woman's life.

If, for example, a woman is under significant stress – if she is overworked, if her diet fails to meet her body's needs, if she is physically ill, if she smokes and/or drinks, if she is avoiding spiritual issues that are beckoning her, or if she is involved in relationships in which the energy outflow is not matched by the energy coming back – then she may find that her ability to keep up with the demands on her endocrine system is diminished. It will remain so unless and until she is able to implement some changes in those areas of her life that need work. The result may be a tumultuous midlife transition, fraught with her own individual combination of symptoms – from headaches, hot flushes, bloating, and fading libido to mood swings and sleep disturbances.

Given the nature of our current culture, with its ever-accelerating

FIGURE 7: HORMONE-PRODUCING BODY SITES

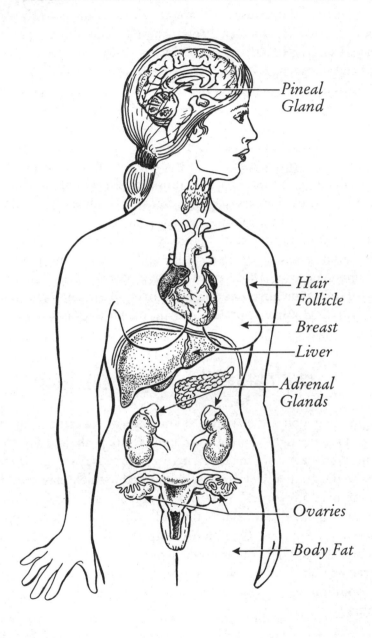

Pineal Gland

Hair Follicle

Breast

Liver

Adrenal Glands

Ovaries

Body Fat

The healthy body is equipped to produce all the hormones a woman needs throughout her life. This natural ability can be supported or thwarted, depending on lifestyle patterns and the state of a woman's health – physically, emotionally, spiritually, and situationally.
© 2001 by Northrup and Schulz

pace of life, about 75 per cent of perimenopausal women have symptoms of menopause that are uncomfortable enough to cause them to seek relief, whether through supplemental hormones, dietary change, exercise, or alternative therapies. If a woman finds that she needs supplemental hormones in order to re-establish a physical and emotional comfort zone, this should not be seen as a personal failure. Rather, it is a wake-up call and an opportunity to implement much-needed change. A woman in this situation might want to consider accepting what I like to call a dusting of supplemental hormones – just enough to provide her with the support she needs for comfort and health, and no more. At the same time she would also be wise to pay attention to the messages her body is sending. It is asking for more than just a prescription or a supplement.

The bottom line is this: before you take something to relieve menopausal symptoms, acknowledge and listen to your body's inner wisdom in creating those outward symptoms. They are uniquely yours. How your hormones behave during perimenopause and how your body and mind respond to hormonal changes is as personalised as your fingerprints.

The Three Types of Menopause

Imagine that you are standing at the foot of a beautiful mountain. You can see the light shining from behind the peak, and you're eager to enjoy the view from the top. There are three ways to get there. You can take the gradually sloping, winding path, which may require you to climb over a few rocks now and then. You can take the short path up, which is much more difficult and will require more equipment and technical support. Or you can skip the climb altogether and get someone else to take you up by helicopter – which sounds easy until you realise that your muscles and organs will not have had the time or the conditioning to cope with the cold and lack of oxygen at the summit.

• *Natural menopause* (the sloping, winding path) occurs gradually, usually between the ages of forty-five and fifty-five, in a woman who has at least one of her ovaries. Duration, in most cases, is five to ten years, though the entire process sometimes takes up to thirteen years.

During this time, periods may stop for several months and then return, and they may increase or decrease in duration, intensity, and flow. All other things being equal, women who are going through a natural menopause may or may not need any treatment for the sake of physical comfort, because their overall health may be strong enough, and their transition may be occurring gradually enough, for their bodies to keep up with the changing demands. It will depend, in other words, on what else is going on in their bodies and in their lives.

• *Premature menopause* (the short path) occurs somewhat faster as well as earlier, in women in their thirties or early forties who have at least one ovary. Approximately one in a hundred women completes the menopausal transition by the age of forty or younger. She may have an illness (such as an autoimmune disease or nutritional deficiency) or some chronic stress (including excessive athletic conditioning) that has adversely affected hormone-related reproductive functions. Duration usually is shorter than natural menopause, at one to three years. Because the transition is quicker, and because the early change is often linked to a pre-existing physical condition, there is a strong likelihood that a woman undergoing premature menopause will need supplemental hormones during the adjustment.[5]

• *Artificial menopause* (the helicopter ride) can occur quite abruptly, induced by surgical removal or disruption of the reproductive tract (including removal of ovaries or surgical disruption of the blood supply to the ovaries), by radiation or chemotherapy, or by administration of certain drugs that induce or mimic menopause for medical reasons (such as to shrink uterine fibroids).

Even tubal ligation has been shown to lower progesterone levels for at least a year following the procedure.[6] And many women who undergo hysterectomy *with* preservation of their ovaries experience symptoms of hormonal change – in addition, of course, to the loss of their periods.

Current estimates in the US are that approximately one in every four American women will enter an abrupt, artificial menopause. Because there's no opportunity for gradual adjustment to the hormonal drop-off, the symptoms of artificial menopause can be severe and debilitating. Almost invariably, supplemental hormone therapy is elected in order to alleviate physical discomfort.

PATTI: ARTIFICIAL MENOPAUSE

Six weeks after vague symptoms (night sweats, weight loss, and a persistent rash in her bikini area) had been misdiagnosed as 'perimenopause and stress', Patti, a forty-one-year-old single mother and owner of a small business, was diagnosed with Hodgkin's disease, a type of lymphoma. Two six-week courses of chemotherapy left her feeling temporarily exhausted and without her curly blonde hair . . . but cured. The one side effect that turned out not to be temporary was the loss of her periods.

She wrote, 'A couple of weeks after the chemo was over, when I was starting to get some of my energy back, I started having night sweats again. This scared me, because I thought it was the cancer coming back, and I thought my mood swings were just due to the constant worry.' Her consultant did some hormone tests and confirmed that Patti had undergone menopause, and she prescribed the appropriate hormone replacement therapy in the form of a skin patch, which gave Patti's body gentle doses of hormone slowly, throughout the day and night. 'I felt much better within just a few days, and I think in my condition – after all I'd been through – it really helped me recover quicker, because my body was pretty traumatised and my mind was frazzled.'

Perimenopause and Hormonal Levels

The conventional view of what happens at perimenopause is that oestrogen levels plummet. This is a gross oversimplification and too often leads to treatment that can make mildly uncomfortable symptoms worse. In natural menopause, the first hormonal change that occurs is a gradual decline in levels of progesterone, while oestrogen levels remain within the normal range or even increase. Because progesterone and oestrogen are meant to counterbalance each other throughout the menstrual cycle, with one falling while the other rises and vice versa, an overall decline in progesterone allows oestrogen levels to go unopposed – that is, without the usual counterbalance. The result is a relative *excess* of oestrogen, a condition that is often called oestrogen dominance – which is precisely the opposite of the conventional view.

If a woman begins to experience uncomfortable symptoms at this stage, it's because her body can sense – and attempts to adjust to – that relative oestrogen excess. Unfortunately, however, there's a great deal of overlap in the symptoms of various hormone imbalances, and it's not uncommon for a woman experiencing symptoms of oestrogen excess to be given a prescription for more oestrogen. Not surprisingly, her mild symptoms worsen as a result.

As the transition continues, progesterone continues to decline, and eventually oestrogen levels may begin to swing widely. The oestrogen highs occur because the ovaries have begun to allow entire groups of follicles to grow and mature during successive menstrual cycles, instead of only one at a time, as though attempting to hurriedly 'spend' those remaining eggs. (This is the reason why the incidence of twin pregnancies increases with age.) The progesterone decline occurs because fewer and fewer of those maturing eggs actually complete the entire ovulation process.

Levels of the hormones FSH and LH, which the pituitary gland in the brain normally releases in precisely metered amounts to stimulate controlled follicular growth and ovulation, become erratic as our ovaries start to skip ovulations. Closer to menopause, hormonal levels start to stabilise. FSH and LH levels smooth out and climb to their new, higher cruising altitude, where they stay for the rest of our lives.

Symptoms of Decreased Progesterone and Oestrogen Dominance

- Decreased sex drive

- Irregular or otherwise abnormal periods (most often, excessive vaginal bleeding)

- Bloating (water retention)

- Breast swelling and tenderness

- Mood swings (most often irritability and depression)

- Weight gain (particularly around the abdomen and hips)

- Cold hands and feet

- Headaches, especially premenstrually

Is There a Test I Can Take?

For years the diagnosis of menopause was simply based on your age and symptoms. Now it's becoming more common to use laboratory confirmation of your hormone levels. Here's why: first, as illustrated by the story of Patti, there are illnesses that mimic perimenopause rather convincingly. (Hypothyroidism is another example; see page 118.) By having your entrance into the climacteric confirmed, you'll simultaneously be ruling out an unexpected medical problem. Second, by determining your levels of the relevant hormones – oestrogen, progesterone, and testosterone, and possibly DHEA and thyroid hormone as well – you and your health care provider can better determine where you stand in the perimenopausal timeline and what approach to take to your symptoms, if any.

If you decide to seek laboratory confirmation, it is important that you understand what tests are available, and what they can (and cannot) reveal about your current status.

Blood Hormone Levels: FSH and LH

The testing method employed by most medical practices is to take a blood sample and send it to a laboratory for analysis of FSH and/or LH levels. This is based on the fact that at menopause and thereafter, a woman's FSH and LH levels rise to their highest ever. But there are problems with this method. First of all, it will tell you nothing about oestrogen levels, because FSH is controlled by inhibin, not by oestrogen. (This is one of the reasons why oestrogen replacement doesn't decrease FSH levels after menopause.[7]) In addition, during the five or ten years of perimenopause – before menstruation ceases for good – FSH and LH levels can fluctuate widely. The ovaries may become inactive for a few days or weeks and then resume production of eggs. It is possible, for example, for a woman's FSH levels to reach postmenopausal levels (greater than 30IU/l) while she is still having normal periods. Her LH levels, meanwhile, will remain in the normal premenopausal range. For that reason, a single high FSH/LH level can't be used to determine whether or not a woman is in menopause. Until a woman has had no periods for a year and has FSH/LH levels well within the postmenopausal range – FSH greater than 30IU/l and LH greater than 40IU/l – it is even possible for her to get pregnant. This is why it's prudent to use contraception for a year after you think your periods have stopped.

Blood Hormone Levels: Oestrogen, Progesterone, and Testosterone

Another common blood test analyses the total amount of oestrogen, progesterone, and/or testosterone in the bloodstream. The largest drawback to this method is that most of the hormone so measured is inactive. The healthy woman's body produces upwards of ten times more of these hormones than she can use, so specialised proteins hook themselves to more than 90 per cent of the hormone molecules produced, inactivate them, and lock the 'doors' that would otherwise allow them to leave the bloodstream and enter the tissues. The biologically active form of the hormone is the part that is unbound or free. This goes quickly into the tissues instead of hanging around in the bloodstream. Thus the standard blood test, which does not distinguish bound from free hormone, will give an irrelevant result, because it measures primarily inactive, unusable, protein-bound hormone.

Preferred Testing Methods

There are two less common but more useful tests, though only the first is available in the UK at present – but do ask (see Resources) as this may change. The costs are equivalent, the ease of taking the samples is the same or better, the laboratory service for the first is readily available, and studies show that the results provide a very accurate picture of where in the perimenopausal transition a woman's body currently stands.

• *Salivary hormone testing* measures the free hormone present in the saliva, which has been shown to be comparable to what is present in other body tissues. Saliva does not contain measurable levels of protein-bound (inactivated) hormone. Used until recently primarily in research, salivary hormone testing is a technology that has proven reliable for roughly thirty years but is still unfamiliar to many medical practitioners.[8] This test can be arranged privately in the UK via the Wisdom Hormone Program in the US (see Resources).

The method also lends itself to samples being taken at a uniform time of day, for more meaningful comparisons. A test kit is sent to your home, with printed instructions. Saliva is collected and placed into provided containers at one or more specific times of the day, then sent in prepaid packages directly to the laboratory, at present in the US. Results are provided to both the patient and the doctor, if desired.

I recommend testing for oestrogen, progesterone, and testosterone levels in your salivary sample, because this will give you a good base-line assessment of your overall hormonal status.

• *Blood tests for free (unbound) hormone levels* are available in the US – only free (unbound) testosterone levels are measured in the UK, with males in mind rather than females, though this may change in the future (see Resources). The main advantage to this method is that the procedure is comfortably similar to that of the standard blood test that most doctors are accustomed to ordering. The main drawback is that the time of day during which your sample is taken is likely to be at the whim of the laboratory's schedule, rather than at a set time of day in the comfort of your own home. Since hormone levels vary throughout the day, your position relative to the normal range may be affected by the hour of your appointment – each individual woman's daily variation can be uniquely hers. Even so, measuring the levels of free oestrogen, progesterone, and testosterone in a woman's blood will be much more meaningful than determining total hormone levels.

Until blood tests are available in the UK, salivary testing is recommended.

LINDSAY: SALIVARY HORMONE LEVELS
VERSUS BLOOD LEVELS

Lindsay, forty-five, had noticed a gradual decline in her libido, despite a solid relationship with her husband and an overall love of life. The next time she saw her doctor, she made a point of mentioning her complaint, and her doctor suggested Lindsay's hormone levels be tested. Lindsay suspected she was entering menopause, and she was excited about the possibility of getting some hormonal support to help rekindle her sexual desire. But the lab results indicated that everything was within normal limits, and her doctor felt that prescribing hormones would be inappropriate under the circumstances.

Unconvinced, Lindsay contacted a laboratory that offered salivary hormone testing and ordered a home test kit to assess her levels of progesterone, oestrogen, and testosterone. As she later wrote to me:

The results showed my progesterone was at the low end of normal range, my oestrogen was right in the middle of normal range, and my testosterone level was way below normal. But my doctor said she didn't have any faith in salivary testing because it was new. I was frustrated, but I like this doctor a lot and didn't want to change. So I let it go for a while. Then I decided to see an endocrinologist, who deals with hormones all the time. He was on the fence about salivary hormone tests, but he was intrigued by the results I had and the way they confirmed my symptoms, which had persisted. So he did another hormone test – a blood test – but this time he specified that my sample be checked for free hormone levels. The results came back showing a pattern similar to what the salivary tests showed – my oestrogen levels were OK, my progesterone was on the low side, and my testosterone was so low it didn't even register. I asked him to call my regular doctor with his findings, and this time she was convinced. She prescribed progesterone and a small amount of testosterone for me (in cream form, for topical use). My libido is back to normal, and I also feel really good about the fact that now my doctor is ordering salivary hormone tests for her other patients. I feel like I've had a hand in helping a lot of women, through her.

Double Testing: If You Test, Test Again

No matter which of the two preferred methods a woman elects to use, I recommend double testing, which acknowledges the fact that hormone levels fluctuate, especially during perimenopause. The best time of day for sample collection is the early morning, and the best time of the month is between days 20 and 23, when progesterone levels are apt to be highest. If your periods are irregular, it is more difficult to accurately assess progesterone levels with just one sample – another reason for double testing. With double testing, the sample is taken or collected and analysed on at least two different occasions *before* treatment. (If symptoms are really severe, you needn't delay treatment. Just get another set of levels about one month after starting treatment so that adjustments can be made.)

Double testing increases the chance that testing will reveal natural biological variations as well as perimenopausal fluctuations. If the results of the second test are vastly different from those of the first, it may be necessary to do one or more additional tests to determine whether the difference is due to laboratory error or to natural fluctuations. Making this distinction can help avoid getting a hormone prescription that at best fails to meet the body's needs or at worst exacerbates the problem.

Menopause and Thyroid Function

The ovaries are the organs that we focus on most commonly at menopause, but the physical foundation of a woman's menopausal experience actually rests on the health of all her endocrine (hormone-producing) organs. Thyroid problems are very common during the perimenopausal and postmenopausal years. While many women with these problems are completely asymptomatic, others may have a wide variety of symptoms. Among the most common symptoms are mood disturbances (most often seen in the form of depression and irritability), low energy levels, weight gain, mental confusion, and sleep disturbances.

Thyroid problems are intimately intertwined with menopause, and not just because of the epidemiological fact that about 26 per cent of women in or near perimenopause are diagnosed with hypothyroidism.[9] According to noted clinician and author John R. Lee MD, there appears to be a cause-and-effect relationship between hypothyroidism, in which there are inadequate levels of thyroid hormone, and oestrogen dominance. When oestrogen is not properly counterbalanced with progesterone, it can block the action of thyroid hormone, so even when the thyroid is producing normal levels of the hormone, the hormone is rendered ineffective and the symptoms of hypothyroidism appear. In this case, laboratory tests may show normal thyroid hormone levels in a woman's system, because the thyroid gland itself is not malfunctioning.

It is no surprise, then, that this problem is compounded when a woman is prescribed supplemental oestrogen, leading to an even greater imbalance. In these circumstances, a prescription for supplemental thyroid hormone will fail to correct the underlying problem: oestrogen dominance.

Even if supplemental thyroid hormone does help alleviate the existing hypothyroidism, in a significant portion of these cases the symptom of depression persists, for a separate and rather surprising reason: depression itself can result in thyroid dysfunction. Treating the hypothyroidism, in other words, may be treating a symptom rather than the underlying cause.

Allow me to explain. In many women thyroid dysfunction develops because of an energy blockage in the throat region, the result of a lifetime of 'swallowing' words she is aching to say. In the name of preserving harmony, or because she has learned to live as a relatively helpless member of her family or social group, she has learned to stifle her self-expression. She may in fact have struggled to have her say, only to discover that it doesn't make any difference – because in her closest relationships she has been defined as insignificant. In order for this complex, entangled state of affairs to be resolved, a woman might need to take not only supplemental progesterone and thyroid hormone, but also an unblinking look at what parts of her life and interpersonal relationships need to change.

Menopause and Adrenal Function

The two thumb-sized adrenal glands secrete three key hormones that help us withstand many of the stresses and burdens of life. However, if a woman has lived for a long time with the perception that her life is inescapably stressful, or if she is chronically ill, the chances are she has asked too much of her adrenal glands and has not given them adequate time to replenish themselves. She may be one of the many today who enter menopause in a state of adrenal exhaustion.

To understand what chronic exhaustion may do to the body and how it affects your menopausal experience, it's important to know what the adrenal glands do for you on a day-to-day basis, through the effects of three distinct but complementary hormones they secrete.

• *Adrenaline* is the fight-or-flight hormone, produced when something is threatening you (or when you think that something is threatening you). It makes your heart pound, your blood rush to your heart and large muscle groups, your pupils dilate, your brain sharpen, and your tolerance to pain increase, so you can be at your best in battle. In modern-day life your battles are likely to consist of daily challenges such as pushing your body to keep going when it's fatigued, dealing with a stressful job, and reacting with quick reflexes to avoid a car crash. Think of these adrenaline surges as withdrawals from a bank, to help you get through life's rough spots. If you have got into the habit of withdrawing adrenaline from your account too often, you'll eventually be overdrawn. Your adrenal glands will be overwhelmed, and you'll have too little adrenaline when you really need it.

• *Cortisol* increases your appetite and energy levels while taming the allergic and inflammatory responses of your immune system. It stimulates the liberation and storage of energy in the body, helps the body resist the stressful effects of infections, trauma, and temperature extremes, and helps you maintain stable emotions. Synthetic versions of cortisol – prednisone and cortisone, for example – are prescribed often in human and veterinary medicine to help the patient perk up and feel better so he or she will eat, drink, and move around more and therefore be better able to fight off illness or recover from an injury. Ideally, cortisol is released into the system only on an occasional basis, rather than in response to chronic stress. Undesirable side effects can occur if cortisol levels become too high for too long. These include loss of bone density, muscle wasting, decreased ability to build protein, kidney damage, fluid retention, fluctuating blood sugar levels, weight gain, and increased vulnerability to bacteria, viruses, fungi, yeasts, allergies, parasites, and even cancer.

• *Dehydroepiandrosterone,* also known as DHEA, is an androgen that is produced by both the adrenal glands and the ovaries. In both women and men, DHEA helps to neutralise cortisol's immune-suppressant effect, thereby improving resistance to disease. (Cortisol and DHEA are inversely proportional to each other. When one is up, the other goes down.) DHEA also helps to protect and increase bone density, guards cardiovascular health by keeping 'bad' cholesterol (LDL) levels under control, provides a general sense of vitality and energy, helps keep the mind sharp, and aids in maintaining normal sleep patterns. Like adrenaline and cortisol, DHEA also improves your ability to recover from episodes of stress and trauma, overwork, temperature extremes, and so forth. And if a woman is experiencing a decline in libido due to falling testosterone levels, often it is declining DHEA levels that are at the root of the testosterone deficiency, as DHEA is the main ingredient from which the body manufactures testosterone.

There is a price to pay for making too many demands on your adrenal glands. Excessive exposure of the body to adrenaline and cortisol can result in mood disorders, sleep disturbances, reduced resistance to disease, and changes in vital circulation, all of which are common complaints in today's living-on-the-edge lifestyle. And because these side effects are not uncomfortable enough to be intolerable, the self-destructive lifestyle often continues. DHEA, which helps the body recover from this sort of chronic abuse, finds itself on duty full time instead of only episodically. Gradually the adrenal glands become seriously exhausted, with the first and most profound effect being their waning ability to produce DHEA. As levels of this restorative hormone fall, cortisol and adrenaline levels begin to fluctuate as well, as the adrenal glands attempt to fill increasingly impossible orders for more support. One of the cardinal signs of adrenal exhaustion – relentless, debilitating fatigue – becomes a prominent complaint. Though this fatigue is often accompanied by depressed mood, irritability, and loss of interest in life, this doesn't mean that the adrenal problem is necessarily the cause of the mood change, any more than similar problems are always caused by thyroid malfunction. That is why these emotional symptoms do not always go away with treatment – the underlying issues remain unresolved.

A woman in a state of adrenal exhaustion is likely to find herself at a distinct disadvantage when entering perimenopause, because in the simplest terms perimenopause is another form of stress. Furthermore, adrenal exhaustion suggests that there are long-standing life problems in need of resolution. These issues will loom all the larger when seen with the no-nonsense mental clarity of perimenopause, but not only will adrenal exhaustion make the transition needlessly unpleasant, it also can deprive a woman of the resources she needs to address those issues and to take full advantage of the creative promise of the second half of her life.

If a woman is feeling chronically tired or depressed, if she begins her day feeling inadequately rested, or if she finds that ordinary stresses are having an impact that is out of proportion to their importance, she may be suffering from adrenal gland dysfunction.

Adrenal Testing

Salivary or serum DHEA and cortisol levels can be easily tested through accredited laboratories. (See Resources.) Conventional blood tests, taken at whatever time your doctor has scheduled your appointment, might indicate that your adrenals are 'normal'. However, a better diagnostic approach will test your levels at different times of the day, which is much more likely to reveal an unbalanced pattern of

Adrenal Stressors

The following stressors can lead to fatigue and, ultimately, adrenal dysfunction – which may, in turn, make some stressors worse:

- Excessive, unremitting worry, anger, guilt, anxiety, or fear

- Depression

- Excessive exercise

- Chronic exposure to industrial or other toxins

- Chronic or severe allergies

- Overwork, both physically and mentally (this applies only if you're doing work that doesn't fulfil you)

- Chronically late hours or insufficient sleep

- Unhealed trauma or injury

- Chronic illness

- Light-cycle disruption: shift work

- Surgery

cortisol and DHEA secretion. If you want to be tested for adrenal function, see a medical practitioner who understands the complexities of adrenal testing.

How to Supplement Your Adrenal Function

If, after testing, you find that you are producing inadequate levels of adrenal hormones, there are several available routes for supplementation of either DHEA, cortisol, or both. But the ultimate goal when it comes to your adrenals is to restore their health and function so that they are eventually able to produce the hormones you need without outside supplements. That is probably going to require making changes in the lifestyle that caused the adrenal depletion. If you supplement your adrenal hormones in dosages that are too high, or if you take supplements for too long, the result can be permanent depression of adrenal function.

DHEA: Supplements are available as tablets, transdermal creams, or sublingual tinctures in the US, although they are only available on a doctor's prescription in the UK. The prescription may be sent to the Nutri Centre (see Resources). It is always best to work with a doctor who can help you monitor your dosage and your blood or salivary levels. Also I recommend making sure you are taking pharmaceutical-grade DHEA (see Resources). Regardless of how you take your DHEA, salivary levels should be retaken every three months. When levels return to the normal range, the dose should be gradually tapered until you're off the supplement completely.

CORTISOL: Some individuals require very small doses of hydro-cortisone, which can be used safely and effectively if prescribed by a doctor knowledgeable about how and when to use it.[10]

DIET: The food plan outlined in chapter 7 is designed to support and recharge your adrenals, among other benefits. Be sure to get enough protein; every meal or snack should contain some protein. And remember that caffeine whips your adrenals into a frenzy; avoid it altogether. Also avoid fasting or cleansing regimes.

SUPPLEMENTS: Supplement your diet at the higher ranges of the nutrients listed in chapter 7 for at least three months for best results. After that, you can reduce them depending upon how you feel.

HERBS: Licorice root is suggested in some cases of adrenal exhaustion. It may help increase cortisol half-life in your body, although more studies are necessary to evaluate this thoroughly.[11] A number of different types of licorice extract are available; I prefer the solid extract. Start with a little dab on the end of a chopstick and mix it with hot water or tea. Gradually work up to 1/4tsp three times per day, if needed. Make sure you monitor your blood pressure, as licorice may increase blood pressure in some individuals. Since low blood pressure is often a symptom of adrenal exhaustion, a small increase in blood pressure to healthy levels is desirable.

What to Expect in Your Transition

Despite the fact that there are stacks of books describing the 'normal' symptoms of perimenopause, many women escape most or all of them. Nonetheless, there are a number of symptoms that women in this culture report frequently, and you may want to review the list on the following pages in order to be informed and prepared. It may also decrease your anxiety about a particular symptom to know that it is related to a normal transition.

Bear in mind the following caveat: it is possible for your expectation of your menopausal experience to become your reality simply because it's what you believe will happen. Remember that in some cultures women rarely report any symptoms from perimenopause, and it is not necessarily written into your biological script that you will have any discomfort either.

Keep in mind also that your mother's menopause experience may have created a powerful unconscious blueprint for you. If your mother's experience was negative, do not assume that you will follow in her footsteps. Focus instead on the ways in which you are different from your mother, and choose a new and improved script for yourself.

The quotations that describe the symptoms below come from patients or newsletter subscribers. I have indicated the chapters in which symptoms and solutions are discussed in more detail.

FIGURE 8: MENOPAUSAL SYMPTOMS TIMELINE

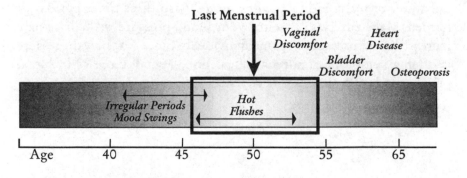

© 2001 by Northrup and Schulz

Hot Flushes

'I've had to give up wearing sweaters because I can suddenly get so hot that I feel the need to open all the windows (even in the winter) and peel off as many layers as I can.'

Hot flushes are the most common perimenopausal symptom in our culture, occurring in about 70 to 85 per cent of all perimenopausal women.[12] They can be very mild or so severe that they result in sleep deprivation and subsequent depression. They begin as a sudden, transient sensation of warmth that can then become intense heat over the face, scalp, and chest area; it may be accompanied by redness and perspiration. They are also sometimes accompanied by an increased heart rate, tingling in the hands, and/or nausea. In some cases the hot flush is followed by a feeling of being chilled. In the majority of women, hot flushes often start just before or during the menstrual periods during perimenopause. Triggered by falling oestrogen and rising FSH, they tend to become more frequent after our periods actually stop. That is the time when oestrogen levels are lowest and FSH levels are highest. Hot flushes usually go away a year or two after actual menopause, although in some (relatively rare) cases they may continue for many years.

Also known as vasomotor flushing, the hot flush occurs when blood vessels in the skin of the head and neck open more widely than usual, allowing more blood to shift into the area, creating heat and redness. Beside hormonal changes, external factors can influence the intensity and duration of a woman's hot flushes. Anxiety and/or tension can magnify them, as can a diet high in simple sugars and refined carbohydrates such as are found in fruit juices, cakes, biscuits, sweets, white bread, wine and beer, and so on.

There are many approaches to cooling hot flushes. Oestrogen replacement is about 95 per cent effective. A 1.5–3 per cent progesterone skin cream also works in about 85 per cent of perimenopausal women; as little as 1/4tsp rubbed into the skin once per day may provide relief.[13] (See chapter 5, 'Hormone Replacement'.) In addition, meditation and relaxation techniques (such as Dr Herbert Benson's famous Relaxation Response) have been successfully used to cool hot flushes in 90 per cent of women, without any hormonal therapy at all.[14]

Many women also find relief when they improve their diets. (See chapter 7, 'The Menopause Food Plan'.) Soya foods (a total of 45–160mg of soya isoflavones per day) provide relief, as do many herbs such as black cohosh, dong quai, or chaste berry. Acupuncture is also very effective. (These approaches are detailed in chapter 6, 'Foods and Supplements to Support the Change'.)

Night Sweats

'I sweat so much at night, I have to get up to change the sheets.'

Night sweats are on a continuum with hot flushes. Traditional Chinese medicine tells us, and many of my patients have confirmed, that 3 to 4am is the most common time for night sweats, which may wake you up drenched with perspiration.

Heart Palpitations

'It's like all of a sudden I'm aware of my heartbeat, whereas before my heart just did its job without me noticing it.'

Like hot flushes, palpitations can range from mild to severe. They are rarely dangerous, though they can sometimes be very frightening. They are the result of imbalances between the sympathetic and parasympathetic nervous systems and are often related to fear and anxiety. If they persist, see your doctor. (See chapter 14, 'Living with Heart, Passion, and Joy'.)

LESLIE: POWER SURGES AT MENOPAUSE

Leslie is an art teacher at a local secondary school and doubles as an unofficial counsellor for her students, who uniformly respect and love her for her obvious devotion. 'I'm one of those art teachers you can spot a mile away,' she wrote. 'I look the part, I guess. I try to do more than just teach kids how to paint or sculpt – I mean, there's art all around us in this world, and much of the joy of life is in appreciating it. I try to demonstrate that in the way I live.'

Leslie likes the image of hot flushes as 'power surges', symbolising a positive, transformative process, and she did not find her hot flushes or any of her other symptoms to be troublesome, nor did she want to mask or muffle them with medication. 'My doctor wasn't surprised when I told her I chose to forgo hormone replacement therapy. She knew I saw this as a way of honouring my body and the natural changes going on within me. At the same time, I did want to provide my body with support and help it adjust, so my symptoms wouldn't be severe.' Leslie chose to provide that support through improved nutrition, herbs, and plant-based hormones (phyto-oestrogens). She takes black cohosh root, which softened her hot flushes within the first week and kept them mild enough that they were merely 'interesting' rather than intrusive. She also drinks a glass of vanilla-flavoured soya milk every morning and evening.

Migraine Headaches

'Ever since I turned forty, I've had a pounding headache the day or two before my period is due. This has never happened before.'

Imbalanced hormone levels contribute to so-called menstrual migraine during perimenopause and menopause. This type of headache usually comes just before your period, when both oestrogen and progesterone levels can fall dramatically. Hundreds of women have been able to recover completely from menstrual and menopausal migraines through the use of 1.5–3 per cent progesterone cream. Apply 1/4–1/2tsp on your skin daily for the two weeks prior to your period, or three weeks out of every month if you're no longer having periods.

Breast Swelling and Tenderness

'My breasts are sometimes so tender, it hurts to hug my children.'

Many women have tender breasts just before their periods. But during perimenopause, you may notice that your breasts feel tender or swollen much more often. This is far more common when a woman is experiencing oestrogen dominance. Relief can often be achieved by following a hormone-balancing diet (see chapter 7, 'The Menopause Food Plan'), ensuring an adequate intake of B vitamins and omega-3 fats such as EPA and DHA (100–200mg once or twice daily), stopping caffeine, and/or using 1.5–3 per cent progesterone cream (1/4tsp twice per day). The addition of whole soya foods to the diet can also be very helpful. (See chapter 13, 'Creating Breast Health.')

Heavy Menstrual Periods

'My periods have become so heavy that I soak through a couple of tampons and an overnight maxi pad in fifteen minutes. Sometimes I even soak through my clothing at work.'

When oestrogen levels are high or even normal but progesterone levels are too low, from lack of ovulation, the monthly oestrogen-driven build-up of the uterine lining (the endometrium) continues unopposed. When it finally breaks down, the result can be erratic, heavy bleeding that can go on for days at a time.

The problem can become so troublesome that some women resort to hysterectomy as a solution, but because heavy bleeding often resolves as a woman approaches menopause, hysterectomy is rarely necessary. The unopposed oestrogen can often be treated with various types of progesterone or contraceptive pills. Since the problem is often worse in women who have too much body fat (fat produces oestrogen), exercise and diet often help. Alternatives such as acupuncture and Traditional Chinese Medicine are also often helpful. In severe cases, the lining of the uterus can be cauterised via laser surgery in a procedure known as endometrial ablation. (See chapter 8, 'Creating Pelvic Health and Power'.)

Irregular or Erratic Periods

'I never know when I'm going to get a period. Sometimes I have a normal period. Then one week later I'll have some spotting. Then I'll go for three months before I have any bleeding again. I have to carry pads with me all the time, just in case.'

When a woman is going through the hormonal changes of perimenopause, just about any kind of uterine bleeding is possible, ranging from periods that become very light and short to periods that space out to every three months or more. And some women have bleeding patterns that are so erratic, they don't seem like periods at all.

If you can live with erratic periods for a while, the problem will go away. It's not really abnormal. But if you also have other symptoms, such as mood swings or headaches, or simply want more regular periods, a very wide variety of treatments are available, ranging from conventional contraceptive pills to effective alternatives like natural progesterone skin cream or the herb chaste berry (*Vitex agnus-castus*), which helps regulate the hypothalamic-pituitary-ovarian axis to produce more progesterone. (See chapter 8, 'Creating Pelvic Health and Power'.)

Fibroids

'I was having irregular bleeding, and when I went to see a gynaecologist, she told me that I had a growth in my uterus that was a fibroid. An ultrasound confirmed the diagnosis. My doctor tells me that we can just watch it.'

About 40 per cent of women develop benign fibroid growths in the uterus during perimenopause. Their growth is stimulated by oestrogen, and they can become quite large. Fibroids shrink dramatically after menopause and, like heavy bleeding, do not usually require surgery or other treatment, especially if they don't produce symptoms. Some fibroids, however, can cause heavy bleeding, depending upon their position in the pelvis. Small ones can be removed through laparoscopic surgery or sometimes by surgical removal through the vagina. Larger ones may require more extensive abdominal surgery. Weight loss, acupuncture, herbs, dietary change, and natural progesterone are all effective alternatives in many cases. (See chapter 8, 'Creating Pelvic Health and Power'.)

Loss of Sexual Desire

'There's nothing wrong with my marriage. I love my husband. But quite frankly, I don't even get turned on by Tom Cruise any more, let alone my husband.'

The first thing that needs to be checked in a woman with loss of sexual desire is her hormone levels. For reasons that aren't clear, some women experience a drop in their testosterone levels during perimenopause; this can result in lack of sexual desire. Adrenal exhaustion can be another factor. If these levels are low, supplementation with small amounts of testosterone or its precursor, DHEA, will restore libido to normal levels. For some women, libido problems are related to lack of oestrogen or thinning of the vaginal tissue. (See chapter 9, 'Sex and Menopause'.) Women who've undergone removal of their ovaries surgically, or whose ovarian function has been compromised by illness, chemotherapy, or radiation, have lost a major source of their normal hormone production. A variety of safe alternatives, such as high-dose soya isoflavones, can often help in situations such as these.

Vaginal Dryness and/or Painful Intercourse

'I just don't seem to be able to get lubricated during sex any more. And when we do have intercourse, it hurts!'

The lining of the outer one-third of the urethra and the lining of the vagina are oestrogen-sensitive. Symptoms may arise from a lack of oestrogen, as well as from decreases in muscle tone and subsequent blood supply in the urogenital area.

For many women, the first sign of perimenopause is a decrease in normal vaginal discharge. This is a direct result of decreasing oestrogen levels. Some may need to use a vaginal lubricant during intercourse because arousal and full lubrication take longer. Topical oestrogen cream, vitamin E suppositories, systemic oestrogen therapy, or increasing intake of phyto-oestrogens such as soya can be very helpful. Some of my patients have been able to increase vaginal lubrication through creative visualisation. (See chapter 9, 'Sex and Menopause'.)

Urinary Symptoms

'I keep getting symptoms that feel as though I have a urinary tract infection. I feel as though I have to urinate all the time, but my urine tests don't show any evidence of infection.'

'I got my first-ever UTI at forty-five – as it turned out, the first of many.'

'Sometimes I lose urine when I cough or sneeze. I'm worried that if this continues, I'm going to end up using adult nappies!'

Recurrent urinary tract infections or urinary stress incontinence (the loss of urine with coughing, sneezing, laughing, etc.) may occur because of the thinning of the oestrogen-dependent lining of the outer urethra. Urinary symptoms often resolve through the use of a small dab of oestrogen cream applied locally. Kegel exercises can also increase blood flow to the area and help with stress incontinence. (See chapter 8, 'Creating Pelvic Health and Power'.)

Skin

'Almost overnight it feels as though my skin has become dry and crepey, especially around my eyes.'

The collagen layer of our skin becomes thinner as our hormone levels fall. A wide variety of highly effective skin treatments is now available that help build collagen, resurface the skin, and prevent wrinkles. Systemic hormones; foods rich in phyto-oestrogens, such as soya; and antioxidant supplements such as vitamin C, vitamin E, glutathione, and proanthocyanidins (from grape seeds or pine bark) also help build collagen and rejuvenate the skin. (See chapter 11, 'From Rosebud to Rose Hip'.)

Bone Loss

'My grandmother gets shorter every year, and more bent over. I don't want that to happen to me.'

For many women, bone loss through the insidious process known as osteoporosis begins as early as the age of thirty – or even earlier. Because of chronic dieting, undereating, overexercising, lack of nutrients, or anorexia, many women do not reach the peak bone density they should when they are in their teens, twenties, and thirties. So when a woman reaches forty and her hormonal levels begin to change, her bone density may already be compromised. When oestrogen, progesterone, and androgen levels start to alter, the collagen matrix that forms the foundation of healthy bone may start to weaken, especially when a woman's nutrition and exercise regimes are lacking. You can maintain the collagen matrix in your bones and also help rebuild healthy bone in a variety of ways, which include getting adequate phytohormones from foods such as soya, from herbs, hormone replacement, and calcium and magnesium supplements, and by doing weight-bearing exercise. (See chapter 12, 'Standing Tall for Life'.)

Mood Swings

'I find myself crying during television advertisements. Then I fly off the handle at my children for no reason.'

As I pointed out in chapter 2, many women experience an intensification of the kind of volatility in their moods that they once felt primarily before their periods, if at all. Part of the reason for this volatility, or for the increase in dark, negative moods, is hormonal. But it may also be a signal from your inner wisdom, trying to get your attention.

Insomnia

'I just don't seem to be able to get to sleep at night. When I do, I often wake up soaking wet and hot. So I throw off the blankets, and then get chilled!'

Many women wouldn't have insomnia if it weren't for their night sweats and hot flushes. For others, anxiety keeps them from sleeping soundly. If your sleep problems are related to hot flushes, they'll often resolve with hot-flush treatment. If they're due to anxiety, you may need to make some changes in your life that the anxiety is bringing to your attention. Other sleep problems may be related to the fact that perimenopause, like adolescence, is a time of transition in sleep patterns. Some of us, like teenagers, will suddenly start requiring much greater amounts of sleep than before. Typically, this changes again after menopause, when we need less sleep than during our twenties and thirties. Some women find daytime naps help during the transition. (See chapter 10, 'Nurturing Your Brain'.)

Fuzzy Thinking

'I keep losing my keys. I walk into a room and forget why I'm there. Sometimes my head feels like it's filled with cotton wool.'

Many women report a feeling of forgetfulness and 'woolly head' during perimenopause. It's not unusual to have trouble concentrating or to do things like putting the mobile phone in the fridge. The same thing often happens postpartum when a woman comes home with a new baby and suddenly feels incapable of understanding her bank statement. The difference between the postpartum period and peri-menopause is that during perimenopause you're giving birth to your-self. It often feels as though the logical side of the brain goes to sleep for a while as a way to force us to become more intuitive and more in tune with our emotions and inner wisdom. Herbs such as ginkgo and St John's wort can help keep your mind clear. Some women find that soya isoflavones or hormones such as progesterone or oestrogen are also helpful. The main thing to remember is that you're not getting Alzheimer's. You're just rewiring your brain for a whole new way of thinking. (See chapter 10, 'Nurturing Your Brain'.)

How Long Will My Symptoms Last?

Many women believe that the symptoms they are experiencing are what menopause – and life – will feel like from this day forward. The truth is that those symptoms, when present, are labour pains, as it were – part of our adaptation to the hormonal changes that take place as our biological focus switches from procreation to personal growth. In other words, the symptoms of the climacteric are temporary. How long they'll last depends on a number of factors, including the type of menopause a woman is experiencing (see page 110), what else is going on in her life at the time, and the ability of her body and soul to support her through this period of transition. In this culture the symptoms of perimenopause, in a natural transition, last anywhere from five to ten years, with a gradual crescendo in the beginning, a peak as the woman approaches the midpoint of the transition, and a gradual decrescendo towards the end as the body learns to live in harmony with its new hormonal support system.

Because all perimenopausal symptoms are interrelated, the treatment of one symptom may alleviate other symptoms as well. Since so many different treatments are effective, an individual woman will want to choose the ones that appeal to her most. Many women select several different treatments at the same time. An example of this would be taking conventional hormone replacement therapy along with a soya product and a good multivitamin, and adding an exercise programme. The bottom line is this: there's no need to suffer through perimenopause. As you read through the chapters that follow, choose the treatments that speak to you. Experiment. Your body is constantly changing. You can't really make a mistake.

FIVE

Hormone Replacement Therapy: An Individual Choice

The science of hormone replacement therapy has evolved very rapidly since the first contraceptive pills were introduced in the 1960s. The pill gave women a magic bullet that enabled them to go about their daily lives without being conscious of their natural hormonal and fertility rhythms. The downside is that these rhythms and the natural wisdom that created them have become pathologised, leading women to believe that synthetic, man-made hormones are safer and better than the 'unpredictable' ones found naturally in our bodies. Conventional hormone replacement therapy is an extension of this thinking: that the female body is deficient and needs to be fixed.

Today, however, there are new options that are much more respectful of the body's wisdom. To understand how they evolved, it helps to know where we're coming from.

A Brief History of Hormone Replacement Therapy

When I was doing my family practice training, I remember going to the library and taking down a book that caught my eye, way up on the top shelf. It was *Feminine Forever*, by Dr Robert Wilson. It described in graphic detail how the lack of oestrogen at menopause led inevitably to the shrivelling of a woman's body, leaving her old and decrepit.

His solution: oestrogen pills to replace what her deficient body no longer produced. This was presented as a sort of magic potion that would leave her 'feminine for ever': youthful, resilient, moist, sexy, and desirable. The way Wilson described oestrogen's benefits, I couldn't imagine a woman who would want to live without it at menopause – a life passage about which my medical training had taught me virtually nothing.

I was still unconscious about how embedded the devaluation of female bodies is within our culture, and how powerfully this devaluation influences the practice of medicine and the science that supports it. (At the time, anyone having her first baby at the age of thirty or older was referred to as an 'elderly primigravida'.) Like many of my peers, my own beliefs were clouded by my cultural legacy: just as male is superior to female, young is superior to old. Salvation would come through denying any differences between male and female, and endeavouring to stay forever young. Our better-living-through-chemistry society was poised to help us control our unruly female physiology through contraceptive pills during our reproductive years and oestrogen during menopause. Not surprisingly, sales of Premarin – the first oestrogen to be marketed – began to soar.

A Shadow Crosses over Premarin

When I was a third-year medical student, one of my mother's close friends confided to me that she had to stop taking her Premarin because she had started to have bleeding. She was later diagnosed with a condition known as adenomatous hyperplasia of the endometrium – indicating that her uterine lining was being overstimulated by the Premarin. Although she never resumed taking Premarin, her bleeding didn't return, and she didn't suddenly shrivel up, either. In fact, she is now eighty-six years old and still climbing mountains and going on long hikes with her friends.

My mother's friend was not alone. In the mid- to late 1970s study after study appeared that proved beyond any doubt that taking oestrogen resulted in an up to fourfold greater risk of developing uterine cancer. At about the same time, contraceptive pills were shown to increase the risk of stroke, pulmonary embolism, and heart attack – deadly complications in young women. Premarin sales plummeted. Women grew afraid of the pill. It would take several years before new studies of lower-dose pills, and major marketing efforts, quelled these fears.

Premarin Sales Revive

Then studies began to appear showing that oestrogen could help prevent osteoporosis. I was intrigued. My husband was doing his training in orthopaedic surgery, and he spent many nights repairing hip fractures in older women, many of whom never walked or lived independently again.

I researched the link between oestrogen and bone health and did a presentation on it for the obstetrics staff at the hospital. Many of my lecturers were dead set against Premarin for any indication – they had been burned too badly by the uterine cancer findings. And although I was convinced that oestrogen replacement could help prevent osteoporosis, I was far more interested in alternatives such as calcium supplementation and exercise. A colleague and I even discussed setting up a long-term study involving diet and exercise, but we were far too busy just trying to complete our courses, and it would take another twenty years for those ideas to be proved and accepted by mainstream doctors.

Meanwhile, other studies showed that endometrial cancer could be prevented if a woman was given progesterone along with her dose of oestrogen. Oestrogen replacement slowly but surely made its way back on to the scene – this time in combination with Prempac-C, a synthetic form of progesterone, which was given to all women on oestrogen unless they had had hysterectomies. (In that case, doctors reasoned, there was no reason to give it.) Progesterone's role was thus reduced to that of a uterine vacuum cleaner – one that prevented excessive build-up of the uterine lining but had no inherent benefits of its own.

Premarin Becomes Synonymous with Hormone Replacement Therapy

Premarin is composed of oestrogenic compounds derived from the urine of pregnant mares. Since its introduction in 1949, it has maintained its place as the queen of the hormone replacement world. In fact, when you say 'hormone replacement', most people, including doctors, still think Premarin – end of discussion.

Its sales hit an all-time high during the 1980s and early 1990s, when study after study (many supported by Wyeth-Ayerst, the maker of Premarin) began to support oestrogen's role in keeping the cardiovascular system healthy. For example, it was shown to lower LDL cholesterol, which the famous Framingham study had identified as a risk for heart attack. Given that cardiovascular disease was also emerging as the number-one killer of women past menopause, doctors everywhere became convinced that all menopausal women needed oestrogen to protect their hearts. Some even refused to care for women who wouldn't take it.

Other benefits were also touted. Premarin seemed to do everything: lift depression, thicken vaginal tissue, stop hot flushes, prevent heart disease, prevent osteoporosis, and even ward off Alzheimer's disease. Premarin was prescribed freely in a one-size-fits-all manner – the same dose for every woman, regardless of her size or her medical history. Prempac-C was added for ten to twelve days of every month to protect the uterus. That was hormone replacement therapy.

Doubts Surface Again

But then a big fly found its way into the ointment. Multiple studies began to support an incontrovertible link between oestrogen supplementation and breast cancer. This link makes biological sense, since oestrogen is well known to stimulate the growth of oestrogen-sensitive tissue, like that in the breast and uterus. Still, the cardiovascular benefits seemed so strong that many women were persuaded to override their fear of breast cancer and continue to take Prempac-C.

At the turn of the millennium, however, several large prospective studies challenged the heart-protection gospel. In a large trial of women who already had heart disease, hormone replacement in the form of Premarin and Prempac-C not only *did not decrease* their risk of subsequent heart attack, it actually *increased* that risk significantly in the first year of use, after which the risk levelled off. As if this weren't disconcerting enough, initial data from the huge Women's Health Initiative, a US government-funded study of thousands of women on Premarin (and often Prempac-C), found that these hormones didn't decrease the statistical risk of heart attack or other heart disease events in healthy women. Other clinical trials also failed to support this link.

Though many experts continue to feel that oestrogen has a cardiovascular benefit, we can no longer assume that this is true for everyone.[1] But whether or not hormone replacement can protect your heart, it has other, very clear benefits. And there are ways to get the benefits and decrease the risks.

Bioidentical Hormones: Nature's Ideal Design

In contrast to Premarin and Prempac-C, the hormones that I recommend are exactly the same as those found in the female body. Though they are synthesised in the lab from hormone precursors found in soya beans or yams, their molecular structure is designed to be an exact match of the hormones found in the human body. Hence we call them *bioidentical* – a term that is far more precise than *natural*, which can be used in confusing and ambiguous ways – eg, Premarin is said by some people to be a 'natural' product because it is made from horse urine. As Dr Joel Hargrove, a pioneer in the use of bioidentical hormones and the medical director of the Menopause Center at Vanderbilt University Medical Center in Tennessee in the US says, 'Premarin is a natural hormone if your native food is hay.'

Because bioidentical hormones are just like the hormones that our bodies were designed to recognise and utilise, their effects are more physiological – consistent with our normal biochemistry – with less chance for unpredictable side effects at low replacement doses than with synthetic, non-bioidentical hormones.

To take advantage of these benefits, you first have to give up the notion that there is an easy, one-size-fits-all answer. There isn't. Some women need or want HRT, some don't. When it comes to hormone replacement therapy, the science we look to for answers is inconsistent, influenced by market forces, and confusing to researchers, doctors, and patients alike. The blessing is that this dilemma forces us to tune in more fully to our inner wisdom, and to make our choices in full partnership with our intuition *and* intellect. This approach is the essence of feminine wisdom.

Moving Beyond Premarin

When Premarin was introduced, the technology to produce other types of oestrogen was not yet available, so it became the gold standard. However, these equine oestrogens aren't normally found in the human female body, and they are often associated with side effects such as headaches, bloating, and sore breasts. In addition, the metabolic breakdown products of Premarin in the human female are biologically stronger and more active than the original equine oestrogens. A host of studies have shown that these breakdown products can produce DNA damage that is carcinogenic in tissue. Given this, it's no wonder that the incidence of breast cancer statistically increases when women are on this drug.[2] In contrast, the metabolic breakdown products of bioidentical oestrogens are biologically weaker, so their effects on tissue do not last as long.

There's reason to believe that bioidentical oestrogen at individualised low doses does not have the same carcinogenic effect on breast tissue as Premarin. But until we have long-term studies on bioidentical oestrogen to compare with the vast amount of data on Premarin, we won't have the scientific verification we need. Unfortunately, Premarin is still the only oestrogen that is being used in all the major studies, such as the Women's Health Initiative in the US.[3] As long as the study uses non-bioidentical hormones at dosages that are not individualised, we won't get the answers we need.

The Balanced Approach:
Individualised Bioidentical Hormone Replacement

It is possible to create a bioidentical hormone replacement regimen using hormone preparations available on prescription from your doctor. Choose any of the bioidentical oestrogen preparations, and if you still have your uterus, ask for Crinone 4 per cent vaginal gel instead of a synthetic progestogen – it is licensed for this use. If your womb has been removed, your doctor will probably only want to prescribe an oestrogen preparation – ask for a bioidentical one and add progesterone cream (1.5–3 per cent by weight) yourself, if you wish. For bioidentical products see the chart on pages 155–6.

These hormones can be taken orally, transdermally, or vaginally, whichever route works best for the patient. Though most women are accustomed to taking pills, the transdermal route is the more physiologically appropriate way to take hormones because they go directly into the bloodstream from the skin. (The body's own hormones are secreted directly into the bloodstream by the endocrine organs.) Oral preparations, on the other hand, first have to be absorbed from the gut and then transported to the liver, where they must undergo further metabolic breakdown before finally getting to the bloodstream.

Research has clearly shown that these bioidentical transdermal hormone replacement regimens provide adequate blood levels of hormone, protect the uterine lining from overstimulation, prevent breakthrough bleeding, and give very effective relief for perimenopausal symptoms.[4]

Why So Many Hormones Are Synthetic

Though it should be intuitively and scientifically obvious that bioidentical hormones in individualised doses would give the best results, many scientists and physicians have turned a blind eye to this concept. The answer is simple: economics.

Bioidentical hormones cannot be patented, so there are no financial incentives for a pharmaceutical company to do the expensive research and development necessary to develop new products containing them. (Unique delivery systems *can* be patented, however, which is why patches such as Evorel, Estraderm, and Femapak, which contain bioidentical oestradiol, can be profitable.)

Synthetic hormones, on the other hand, are made by altering the molecular structure of a hormone enough so that it can be patented. These maintain some of the activity of the natural hormone, but any change in the three-dimensional structure of a hormone, no matter how small, changes its biological effects on the cell in ways that are not completely understood.

Frankly, I trust the wisdom coming from Mother Nature's millions of years of experimentation much more than I trust fifty years of biochemical wizardry from Father Pharmaceutical. But not all women feel this way. Some feel far safer going with what their doctor prescribes. And since beliefs affect biology, what you believe can shape your experience. It's your decision, and my approach is not meant to undermine any individual's positive experience.

What About Contraceptive Pills?

Contraceptive pills are widely prescribed as a convenient way to put the perimenopausal body and its symptoms on autopilot until it's time to move to conventional hormone replacement therapy. There's a currently popular trend to convince women that our menstrual periods themselves are dangerous and that going on the pill as early as our teenage years, and staying on it except to have children, will prevent long-term health problems. Please note, however, that all contraceptive pills consist of synthetics that mask our natural hormonal rhythms and the messages about our health that they convey. Contraceptive pills are also associated with a wide variety of side effects, including blood clots, headaches, and PMS. Although they are appropriate in some cases, I'd rather keep my hormones tuned in to the cycle of the moon and the planets – as opposed to the energy of a pharmaceutical company. You may not be prepared to use other contraceptive methods right now, or you may be using the pill to quell symptoms such as heavy or irregular periods – but just be aware that other options are available.

A Hormone Primer: Essential Information Every Woman Should Know

It's important to keep in mind that hormone replacement therapy involves more than just oestrogen. It also includes the other hormones produced by the ovaries: progesterone and androgens such as testosterone. Some women might be perfectly comfortable with no supplemental hormones; some might need progesterone only; some might need all three. Understanding their original roles in a woman's body, and the kinds of responses some women see when levels drop, can help you make your own very personal HRT decision.

Oestrogen

For generations, oestrogen has been the first (and often the only) hormone to be prescribed for women suffering from symptoms such as hot flushes, vaginal dryness, and mood swings. However, as I noted in chapter 4, oestrogen levels don't fall until late in the menopausal transition, and the majority of perimenopausal symptoms in women with intact ovaries are related more to a lack of progesterone than to a lack of oestrogen.

'Oestrogen' actually encompasses three distinct oestrogenic compounds produced naturally in the body: oestradiol, oestrone, and oestriol. Oestriol reaches its highest level during pregnancy; it has weaker biological effects on breast and uterine tissue than do oestrone and oestradiol. (Women with naturally higher oestriol levels appear to have lower breast cancer rates than others, which has led some practitioners to prescribe oestriol to decrease the risk of breast cancer.[5] Much more research is needed to establish the effectiveness of this approach.)

There is one area in which supplemental oestriol is known to be particularly effective: urogenital symptoms. Applied locally in the vagina, it relieves urinary frequency, vaginal dryness, and other conditions associated with thinning of these tissues.[6]

FIGURE 9: KINDS OF OESTROGEN

17β-Oestradiol
Oestrone
Oestriol

Black Cohosh
Soya Isoflavones
Lignans

Premarin (and others)
Most Contraceptive Pills
Oestrogen agonists
(SERMs)

© 2001 by Northrup and Schulz

As I mentioned in chapter 4, there is reason to believe that oestrogen's role during the childbearing years is quite different from its role after menopause. Before menopause, the primary role of oestradiol is to stimulate growth in the breasts, ovaries, and uterus, and to participate in the growth and maturation of egg-bearing follicles. It also is a major influence in stimulating maternal behaviour. In other words, it promotes childbirth and child care. After menopause, oestrone becomes the predominant oestrogen. No one knows exactly why this happens, but obviously it has nothing to do with procreation. It is likely that oestrogen's ability to protect heart and brain function, as well as bone strength, is part of its purpose in this phase of life.

Remember as well that the ovaries continue to produce small amounts of oestradiol, as do the secondary hormone production sites. As a result, it is biologically possible for a woman to produce enough of her own oestrogen to support optimal health throughout the second half of her life. This is rarely taken into account, perhaps because stress, unmet spiritual needs, and cultural expectations conspire to impair a woman's natural ability to produce adequate levels of the oestrogens.

The most obvious and immediate benefit of oestrogen supplementation is relief from the symptoms of oestrogen deficiency. (See box.) A longer term benefit is oestrogen's ability to help prevent excessive

Symptoms of Oestrogen Deficiency

- Hot flushes

- Night sweats

- Vaginal dryness

- Mood swings (mostly irritability and depression)

- Mental fuzziness

- Headaches, migraines

- Vaginal and/or bladder infections

- Incontinence; recurrent urinary tract infections

- Vaginal wall thinning

- Decreased sexual response

Symptoms of Oestrogen Excess

- Bilateral, pounding headache

- Recurrent vaginal yeast infections

- Breast swelling and tenderness

- Depression

- Nausea, vomiting

- Bloating

- Leg cramps

- Yellow-tinged skin

- Excessive vaginal bleeding

bone mineral loss leading to osteoporosis. It may also help preserve mental function or at least delay the rate of so-called normal, age-related brain changes as well as dementia of the Alzheimer's type. However, there is not enough evidence to support prescribing the hormone for cognitive changes alone.

Oestrogen is available in pills, skin patches, and vaginal creams. In low doses, even synthetic oestrogen in vaginal creams has negligible systemwide absorption and is generally safe for women who need the local effect of oestrogen but don't want any more exposure than necessary.

A NOTE ABOUT 'DESIGNER OESTROGENS'

The oestrogen antagonists are synthetic drugs such as tamoxifen, toremifene, and raloxifene. (These are the ones on the market at present; others are sure to follow.) They get their name from their ability to bind with oestrogen receptors and selectively modulate the effects of oestrogen in different body tissues, hence their name selective oestrogen receptor modulators (SERMs). Tamoxifen (trade name Nolvadex) blocks the oestrogen receptors on breast cells while maintaining some positive oestrogenic effect on bone, uterine tissue, and the cardiovascular system. Raloxifene (trade name Evista) also promotes bone density while decreasing the stimulation of breast tissue by oestrogen. This selective activity is possible because there are two different oestrogen receptors, ER-alpha and ER-beta, each of which predominates in certain tissue. The same oestrogen can produce different effects according to the receptor to which it binds.[7]

Tamoxifen, the most widely used SERM, was first approved by the Medicines Control Agency (MCA) for the treatment of patients with oestrogen-receptor-positive breast cancer in 1973. It is now prescribed for about half of all women diagnosed with breast cancer in the UK. It has been shown to reduce the risk of developing breast cancer in the remaining breast, as well as breast cancer recurrences and deaths. It helps prevent bone loss and also has a beneficial effect on LDL cholesterol. So far, studies have not shown that it decreases the risk of heart attack.

Raloxifene is currently being prescribed to protect women against osteoporosis and heart disease without increasing their risk of breast cancer. However, it doesn't protect bones as well as oestrogen does.

I'm very concerned about SERMs. They are not found anywhere in nature and have not been around long enough for us to truly assess their benefits and risks. Touted for their ability to stimulate the 'good' effects of oestrogen without the 'bad' ones, these drugs are riding the current wave of panic about breast cancer and are being requested by women who really don't need them, or for whom there are far safer alternatives. If a young woman who fears breast cancer begins taking an SERM drug, she will probably be taking it for many years. This long-term blockage of some oestrogen sites with stimulation of others is a double-edged sword. What if we find that these drugs actually increase the risk of Alzheimer's disease by blocking the oestrogen receptors in the brain?

Troubling side effects of tamoxifen have already been documented, including an increased risk of certain visual disturbances, fatal pulmonary embolism, and endometrial cancer. Though studies indicate that raloxifene, unlike tamoxifen, can protect against endometrial cancer, both tamoxifen and raloxifene have been implicated in increasing the risk for colon cancer.[8] They also increase hot flushes in many women, the very symptom for which most perimenopausal women seek treatment in the first place.[9]

Even more disturbing is the recent finding that after five years of use, the anti-oestrogenic effects of tamoxifen on breast cells appear to reverse. The drug now may become breast-cancer-promoting, for reasons that are not clear.[10]

The bottom line is this: unless you have no other alternative, I recommend that you avoid SERMs or limit their use to five years or less. Better yet, stick with bioidentical hormones or the alternatives I outline in chapter 6.

Progesterone

A decline in progesterone is the first hormonal change to cause symptoms in a woman approaching menopause – sometimes years before she suspects she may be nearing the change. Because the body is designed for progesterone and oestrogen to be present in a dynamic counterbalance with each other, the result is oestrogen dominance, with symptoms of both progesterone deficiency and relative oestrogen excess.

Progesterone comes primarily from the ovaries both before and after menopause, but it is also produced in both the brain and the peripheral nerves.[11] Its main job during the childbearing years is to prepare and maintain the uterus for its most important function: pregnancy. It also is a uterine muscle relaxant, preventing premature contractions. Progesterone levels rise in anticipation of pregnancy and stimulate the uterine lining to thicken with rich, well-vascularised tissue to support an embryo, then fall precipitously if pregnancy does not occur. This abrupt drop-off in progesterone is what signals the shedding of the 'nest' (that thickened uterine lining) in the form of menstrual bleeding.

Progesterone also affects brain function. It produces a sense of calmness, and its sedating, anti-anxiety effect helps promote rejuvenating sleep.

Progesterone comes from a temporary yellowish gland in the ovary called the corpus luteum, formed quickly in the small cyst-like structure left behind when a follicle ovulates. The corpus luteum produces increasing amounts of progesterone until the body sends the signal 'We're not pregnant', at which point the corpus luteum is reabsorbed. As a woman reaches her mid-thirties to early forties, the follicle is more likely (at least in this culture) to fail to ovulate, which means the corpus luteum does not form.[12] Over time, this contributes to an increasing deficiency of progesterone.

Note: Our bodies are designed to accommodate very high levels of progesterone during pregnancy. For that reason, symptoms from excessive progesterone are rare. However, depression is a common side effect of some synthetic progestins. And a few women are so

Symptoms of Progesterone Deficiency

- Premenstrual migraine
- PMS-like symptoms
- Irregular or excessively heavy periods
- Anxiety and nervousness

Symptoms of Excess Progesterone

- Sleepiness
- Drowsiness
- Depression

sensitive to progesterone that they become depressed even on very small doses of natural, bioidentical progesterone. Women who have this side effect should try using chaste berry (*Vitex agnus-castus*) to increase their own body's progesterone naturally.

BIOIDENTICAL PROGESTERONE

Bioidentical progesterone supplementation can help alleviate the symptoms of both progesterone deficiency and oestrogen excess, restoring the body's balance.

This provides long-term as well as short-term benefits. As I've noted, a growing body of evidence points to oestrogen dominance as a major factor in promoting breast or uterine cancer in susceptible women. Studies show that when oestrogen replacement therapy (HRT) is taken in concert with an appropriate dose of progesterone, the incidence of uterine cancer does not increase. This is true whether the progesterone is synthetic or bioidentical. We're less sure about HRT's effect on breast cancer. There is evidence that when synthetic progesterone is used, it appears to increase the risk of breast cancer. But we don't yet have long-term studies on the effects of bioidentical progesterone on breast cancer. (See chapter 13, 'Creating Breast Health'.)

FIGURE 10: KINDS OF PROGESTERONE

USP Progesterone
(ProGest,
ProJuven,
Crinone)

Chaste berry
Wild yam

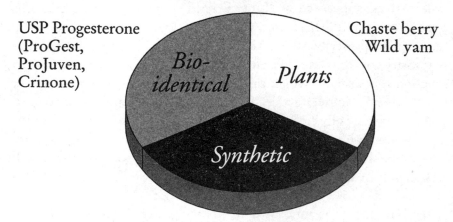

Bio-identical

Plants

Synthetic

Prempac-C
Norethisterone
Norgestrel (and others)

© 2001 by Northrup and Schulz

Another advantage of progesterone supplementation relates to this hormone's relatively unique ability to be converted into other hormones as needed. If progesterone levels are adequate, for example, but testosterone levels are on the low side, supplemental progesterone can actually transform itself into testosterone. Under the right circumstances, supplemental progesterone can even be metabolised into oestrogen. This is one reason so many women enjoy symptomatic relief from using natural progesterone cream in early perimenopause, when there's a great deal of variation in the levels of all three hormones.

Progesterone cream is available by prescription in a 1.5–3 per cent (by weight, ie 950mg–1,800mg) strength, and I've been recommending it for years. You can rub the cream anywhere on your body. One of the best places is right into your hands, because they are very well vascularised. But many women love the way progesterone cream works as a face or body cream.

In most countries natural progesterone cream is available freely, over the counter, but in the UK it is a prescription-only medicine, which means that it can only be obtained by prescription (NHS or private) from a registered doctor. Medicines may be licensed or unlicensed, and this is under the regulation of the Medicines Control Agency. A licensed medicine has passed a lengthy and strict scientific testing, which is also very expensive. Natural progesterone creams are classified as unlicensed and are currently undergoing the tests for application for full licensing, which may mean that your doctor is reluctant to prescribe them. Your doctor's local Prescription Pricing Authority of the Area Health Authority (AHA) may refuse to sanction the costs, in which case the doctor's practice would have to pay the costs – some practices are willing to do this and some are not.

Also, with a fully licensed product the responsibility for prescribing is shared with the manufacturing company, dispensing agency and AHA, whereas for an unlicensed product the doctor takes full responsibility. Unless the doctor is very familiar with the product this may seem like too large a responsibility to take on.

If your doctor is interested in knowing more about prescribing natural (nature-identical) progesterone they can obtain information from the UK importers Higher Nature Ltd (see Resources), but if your doctor refuses to issue a prescription, contact the Natural Progesterone Information Service (see Resources) who can advise you further.

People living outside the UK can obtain ProJuven (natural progesterone cream) from Higher Nature Ltd without a prescription, provided it is legal in their country of residence.

It is illegal to have large quantities of natural progesterone cream sent to the UK from abroad, although you can order one or two tubes yourself for your own use.

The Yam Cream Caveat

Because bioidentical progesterone is often produced from wild Mexican yams, some women try to save money by buying one of a number of wild Mexican yam creams. The problem is, yam contains only a progesterone precursor, which remains inactive when it is absorbed through the skin. Yam creams may offer some beneficial phyto-oestrogens, but they certainly don't provide the documented benefits of progesterone.

Natural progesterone is also available as a 4 per cent or 8 per cent vaginal gel (Crinone), which is fully licensed in the UK – your doctor is likely to be familiar with this product and feel able to prescribe it on the NHS.

THE PROBLEM WITH SYNTHETICS

Synthetic progestogens are an altogether different story. The most commonly prescribed progestogen is norethisterone (Primolut N). Others include medroxyprogesterone acetate (MPA – trade name Provera), norgestrel, and dydrogesterone. Progestogens actually cause or exaggerate many symptoms (see chart on pages 155–6). That's another reason why I don't recommend any of the HRT products that employ synthetic progestogens.

MPA has also been shown to attenuate some of oestrogen's well-documented positive effect on blood vessels. It increases vascular resistance, inhibits blood flow, and increases cerebral artery resistance. A large study of women receiving continuous therapy consisting of oestrogen plus MPA (Premique and Tridestra are examples of this combination) showed a marked increase in myocardial infarction, coronary artery disease death, and venous thrombosis (blood clots in the veins) during the first two years of therapy.[13]

Natural bioidentical progesterone contains no such risk and many benefits. In the famous Postmenopausal Oestrogen/Progestin Intervention trial, oral natural progesterone in micronised form prevented the adverse effects on cholesterol that were seen in those women on Provera (MPA).

Symptoms from Synthetic Progestogens

- Headache

- Depression

- Weight gain and bloating

- Moodiness

- Lack of sexual desire

- Potential narrowing of blood vessels, causing chest pain and lack of oxygen to the heart

---

ELLEN: TOO MUCH OESTROGEN, TOO LITTLE PROGESTERONE

Ellen, a potter and yoga instructor in a university town, noticed a subtle, fuzzy-minded feeling and morning dizziness during the spring of her forty-third year. One day, as she was placing a bottle of aspirin in her shopping trolley, she also realised that though she'd never had headaches before, she'd gradually begun experiencing them regularly – and attributing them to tension, or a weather change, or PMS. On a visit to her doctor, he took a blood sample and tested her FSH level, which was high, convincing him she was menopausal. He told Ellen that her symptoms – the mental fuzziness, dizziness, and headaches – were consistent with menopause and that they'd improve if she took supplemental hormones. He gave her a prescription for Prempac-C to take daily. Within days Ellen was miserable. What previously had felt like a tension headache was now a throbbing, splitting migraine; she felt depressed; she had restless legs that were keeping her awake; and most of her other symptoms persisted.

Same Doll, Different Dress

The latest wrinkle in the hormone replacement scene is prepackaged combinations. The synthetic hormones used in these preparations have been around for years; what is different is the packaging and the ways in which they are prescribed. The most commonly used, Prempac-C, is a combination of Premarin and Norgestrel. Others include Kliofern (a combination of bioidentical oestradiol and synthetic progestogen norethisterone acetate) and Evorel Conti. (synthetic oestradiol plus synthetic norethisterone). The advantage of these last two combinations is that they are convenient and women allegedly don't have any monthly bleeding on them. The problem is that many get spotting and intermittent bleeding for months before their bodies get used to the drug combos, causing many to stop taking them. The biggest drawback is that all of them contain synthetic progestogen and the dosage ratio is fixed.

It's true that the symptoms Ellen experienced were consistent with the climacteric, but in light of her relative youth and the fact that she had not had these symptoms for more than a few months, it was probably early in the course of her perimenopause – which in many women is associated with low progesterone levels and a relative excess of oestrogen. The blood test for FSH levels, upon which her doctor based his diagnosis of menopause, is an inaccurate way to assess the big picture. It's like looking at a single frame in a very long film. In fact, the symptoms Ellen experienced after taking the prescribed oestrogen were consistent with oestrogen overdose.

Even without knowing this, Ellen did the intuitive thing: she stopped taking her oestrogen. Within twenty-four hours she started feeling better, and she vowed to 'tough it out' without going back to the doctor. But her original symptoms persisted, and eventually a friend referred her to another doctor, who ordered salivary hormone tests for oestrogen, progesterone, and testosterone. The results confirmed that Ellen was in an early stage of perimenopause, with her primary hormonal change being low progesterone. Now using a natural progesterone cream to gently supplement her body's own dwindling supply, Ellen feels much better, and she understands a lot more about the transitional process. 'I'm a work in progress,' she wrote. 'My hormonal status is changing, and I know that what works for me now might need to be tweaked a little in six months.'

Testosterone

Testosterone is produced in both the ovaries and adrenal glands. Its primary job is to provide vital assertive energy and sexual drive. Testosterone and other androgens can increase the ease with which a woman becomes sexually aroused, as well as the frequency with which she follows through by initiating sexual activity. Testosterone also increases sensitivity of the erogenous zones, frequency of orgasm, intensity of sexual fantasies, and incidence of orgasmic dreams.

Not all women's testosterone levels drop perimenopausally – in fact, androgen levels actually increase in some. But if a woman is suffering from adrenal depletion due to chronic stress (see chapter 4), a precipitous drop in testosterone may occur, with symptoms of declining libido and overall energy depletion. Surgical removal of the ovaries, uterus, or both, as well as chemotherapy, radiation, or autoimmune disease, can also contribute to a drop in testosterone levels severe enough to cause symptoms.

For reasons that have yet to be clarified, some women experience a gradual decline in testosterone from early adulthood to old age, while other women continue to produce plenty of testosterone throughout life. The adrenals surely play a role, but whether there are other factors remains to be seen. Before you decide to try testosterone supplementation, it is essential to have laboratory confirmation of a deficiency via saliva or blood testing for free (unbound) testosterone (see Resources). As with other menopause-related symptoms, there is considerable overlap among the three hormones. In many women, for example, a decline in libido is due to an oestrogen deficiency, while testosterone may be normal. There is no benefit from taking supplemental testosterone if there is no deficiency to begin with.

This bears emphasis because testosterone supplementation has become a popular topic on the chat show circuit, and doctors report a rush of requests for testosterone from women who think it will jump-start a flagging sex life. If there is a deficiency, the benefits include heightened sex drive and sexual function, higher levels of energy overall, better muscle tone, and improved mood and outlook. There also is evidence that restoring normal testosterone levels can help improve

Symptoms of Testosterone Deficiency

- Decreased libido

- Impaired sexual function

- Decreased energy overall

- Decreased sense of well-being

- Thinning pubic hair

Symptoms of Testosterone Overdose

- Mood disturbances

- Acne, particularly on the face and scalp

- Increased facial hair growth

- Deepened voice

bone mineral density. Incorporated into a vaginal cream, testosterone can also help restore normal vaginal wall thickness and lubrication. However, if there is no deficiency, supplementation will probably lead to overdose, which can produce symptoms most women find objectionable.

Bioidentical testosterone is available from formulary pharmacies (Boots the Chemist) and can be used as a skin or vaginal cream by those women who require it. Testosterone is also available in a patch. (Andropatch, though this is only licensed for male use in the UK). (See Resources.)

How to Decide Whether or Not to Take Hormones

Whether you should or should not take supplemental hormones at menopause depends on a number of factors, including your overall physical health, emotional and spiritual well-being, nutritional status, lifestyle, and so forth. All these factors can influence how well your secondary hormone-production sites are able to keep up with your body's new needs. For some women, just learning that the symptoms of perimenopause are temporary is enough reassurance; they become willing to experience those symptoms without masking them with medicine. And once we relax and allow our fears and resistance to fade, the symptoms themselves may lessen. This is the 'placebo effect' in action, and it is a significant factor in menopausal treatments, as well. Knowing that we can ask for and receive help creates its own healing energy.

Taking Stock Before Making the Decision

Before deciding on hormone replacement, it is important to take an honest look at yourself and at your medical history – including that of your family members – so you can draw an accurate picture of your own goals and needs. Some women choose HRT primarily to relieve symptoms during the climacteric, then discontinue the hormones once the menopausal transition is complete. Others have known risk factors for certain health problems such as heart disease or osteoporosis, in which case they're likely to decide to take HRT on a long-term basis. Still others feel caught in the middle: they'd like to try HRT, but there's an aspect of their personal or family health history that they worry will place them in a higher risk category if they take supplemental oestrogen. Therefore, the first step you need to take in making the HRT decision is to identify your risk factors and decide how much weight you intend to give them.

When I say 'how much weight you intend to give them', I mean that only you have the power to decide how much influence your cultural and family script will have on your reality. Perimenopausal discomfort is a reality for most Western women, while women in some other cultures have a different experience. Studies show that while 70–85 per cent of North American women are affected by hot flushes, only 18 per cent of Chinese factory workers in Hong Kong experience them.[14] I can assure you that the basic biology of the ovaries in China is not different to that in the West. This speaks to the strength of expectations and how an entire culture can come to dictate what each individual will experience. Notwithstanding, each of us has the power to acknowledge this influence and then change our response to it.

Selected Hormone Options

TYPE	PRODUCT	ROUTE OF ADMINISTRATION	OESTROGEN	PROGESTERONE
SEQUENTIAL COMBINED THERAPY	Adgyn Combi	Tablets	Oestradiol (S)*	Norethisterone (S)
	Climagest	Tablets	Oestradiol (S)	Norethisterone (S)
	Cyclo-Progynova	Tablets	Oestradiol (B)	Levo/norgestrel (S)
	Elleste Duet	Tablets	Oestradiol (B)	Norethisterone (S)
	Estracombi	Patches	Oestradiol (B)	Norethisterone (S)
	Estrapak	Patches and tablets	Oestradiol (B)	Norethisterone (S)
	Evorel-Pak	Patches and tablets	Oestradiol (B)	Norethisterone (S)
	Evorel-Sequi	Patches	Oestradiol (B)	Norethisterone (S)
	Femapak	Patches and tablets	Oestradiol (B)	Dydrogesterone (S)
	Femoston	Tablets	Oestradiol (B)	Dydrogesterone (S)
	Femoston 2/20	Tablets	Oestradiol (B)	Dydrogesterone (S)
	Nuvelle	Tablets	Oestradiol (S)	Levonorgestrel (S)
	Nuvelle TS	Patches	Oestradiol (S)	Levonorgestrel (S)
	Premique Cycle	Tablets	Conjugated oestrogens (S)	Medroxyprogesterone (S)
	Prempak-C	Tablets	Conjugated oestrogens (S)	Norgestrel (S)
	Tridestra	Tablets	Oestradiol (S)	Medroxyprogesterone (S)
	Trisequens	Tablets	Oestradiol (B)	Norethisterone (S)
CONTINUOUS COMBINED THERAPY	Climesse	Tablets	Oestradiol (S)	Norethisterone (S)
	Elleste Duet Conti	Tablets	Oestradiol (B)	Norethisterone (S)
	Evorel Conti	Patches	Oestradiol (B)	Norethisterone (S)
	Femoston Conti	Tablets	Oestradiol (B)	Dydrogesterone (S)
	Kliofem	Tablets	Oestradiol (B)	Norethisterone (S)
	Kliovance	Tablets	Oestradiol (B)	Norethisterone (S)
	Nuvelle Continuous	Tablets	Oestradiol (S)	Norethisterone (S)
	Premique	Tablets	Conjugated oestrogens (S)	Medroxyprogesterone (S)
GONADOMIMETIC	Livial	Tablets	Tibolone (S)	
UNOPPOSED OESTROGEN (if uterus is intact an adjunctive progestogen must be used)	Adgyn Estro	Tablets	Oestradiol (S)	none
	Climaval	Tablets	Oestradiol (S)	none
	Dermestril	Skin patches	Oestradiol (B)	none

Selected Hormone Options

TYPE	PRODUCT	ROUTE OF ADMINISTRATION	OESTROGEN	PROGESTERONE
UNOPPOSED OESTROGEN (if uterus is intact an adjunctive progestogen must be used)	Elleste Solo	Tablets	Oestradiol (B)	none
	Elleste Solo MX	Skin patches	Oestradiol (B)	none
	Estraderm MX	Skin patches	Oestradiol (B)	none
	Estraderm TTS	Skin patches	Oestradiol (B)	none
	Evorel	Skin patches	Oestradiol (B)	none
	Fematrix	Skin patches	Oestradiol (B)	none
	FemSeven	Skin patches	Oestradiol (B)	none
	Harmogen	Tablets	Oestrone (S)	none
	Hormonin	Tablets	Oestriol/oestradiol/ Oestrone (S)	none
	Menorest	Skin patches	Oestradiol (B)	none
	Oestrogel	Gel	Oestradiol (B)	none
	Premarin	Tablets	Conjugated oestrogens (S)	none
	Progynova	Tablets	Oestradiol (B)	none
	Progynova TS	Skin patches	Oestradiol (B)	none
	Sandrena	Gel	Oestradiol (B)	none
	Zumenon	Tablets	Oestradiol (B)	none
ADJUNCTIVE PROGESTOGEN	Adgyn Medro	Tablets	none	Medroxyprogesterone (S)
	Crinone	Vaginal gel	none	Progesterone (B)
	Duphaston HRT	Tablets	none	Dydrogesterone (S)
	Micronor HRT	Tablets	none	Norethisterone (S)
OESTROGEN ONLY (local application)	Estring	Vaginal ring	Oestradiol (B)	none
	Ortho Dienoestrol	Vaginal cream	Dienoestrol (S)	none
	Ortho-Gynest Pessary	Pessary	Oestriol (B)	none
	Ortho-Gynest Cream	Vaginal cream	Oestriol (B)	none
	Ovestin	Vaginal cream	Oestriol (B)	none
	Premarin	Pessary	Conjugated oestrogens (S)	none
	Tampovagan	Pessary	Stilboestrol (S)	none
	Vagifem	Vaginal cream	Oestradiol (B)	none
	Vagifem	Vaginal tablets	Oestradiol (B)	none

*(B) = bioidentical; (S) = synthetic

Statistics predict what will happen to groups in general, not to specific individuals. Studies have shown that a woman's faith in (or rejection of) her cultural and genetic/familial script can play a significant role in how her reality plays out. People who are known in their families as 'black sheep' are the least likely to fall victim to diseases that run in the family, perhaps because it is their own personal attitude and style to reject rules and colour outside the lines. Since most health care providers are trained to look at statistics when making decisions and predictions about our health, it is crucial that each of us emphasise our innate ability to become 'black sheep' when and if this stance can improve our health and outlook.

Although scientific studies may change how we think about something intellectually, our behaviour and what we actually do with scientific information is shaped far more by our day-to-day relationships with friends and family than by any other factor. If, for example, you've watched your mother, sister, or best friend come alive again after going on some form of HRT, you're apt to feel very positive about the benefits of this approach. If, on the other hand, you've watched a family member suffer from headaches, sore breasts, and weight gain from taking too high a dose of oestrogen, you're not going to be very eager to try it yourself. And if you are surrounded by aunts, grandmothers, or other older female role models who are vibrantly healthy, live well into their nineties in good health, and have never taken HRT of any kind, your inner blueprint for what is apt to happen after you go through menopause without medication will be quite positive.

My own personal legacy includes cardiovascular disease. My mother lost both her parents to heart disease, and my beloved father collapsed and died on the tennis court at the age of sixty-eight, a victim of a ruptured cerebral aneurysm, when my mother was only fifty-two and perimenopausal. She finished the climacteric as a widow, during an era when women were expected to fade physically and socially after menopause. Though my mother tends to avoid conventional wisdom in general and visits to the doctor in particular, her sister and her friends were told again and again that without supplemental Premarin they would become little old ladies with fragile skeletons and weak hearts. But my mother greeted that prediction with a dismissive wave of her hand. Now well into her seventies, she climbs mountains wearing a heavy backpack and can ski rings around me on the slopes. She has an active social calendar, her mind is razor sharp, her blood pressure is 120/60, and no form of oestrogen medication has ever entered her vibrant body. (She does occasionally use a splash of natural progesterone skin cream, because it helps the 'creakiness' in some of her joints.)

Which of my family's medical legacies will I inherit? I firmly believe that through the physical and emotional choices I make – and the expectations and beliefs with which I live my life – I shape my own future. I believe that my daughters and grandchildren will do the same. Would I like to have the same level of health when I'm in my seventies that my mother now enjoys? Of course I would, but I believe it will happen because I have chosen it, not because I have inherited it.

What Are Your Goals?

Too many women (and doctors) see the HRT decision as an either/or, yes/no decision. I'd like to reframe it as a process. As a first step, it is important to define the goals you hope to achieve with HRT. Contrary to the message conveyed by pharmaceutical marketing efforts, HRT will not give you a means of moving backwards, of denying the ageing process and keeping you young for ever. In fact, to do so would be counterproductive to your physical, emotional, and spiritual health. If you are determined to deny that you have passed middle age, HRT cannot put you at peace with that fact. However, a personally tailored programme – with or without supplemental hormones – can help reduce physical symptoms and health worries so that you can focus your energies on finding your creative passions, which in and of themselves can stoke the flames of your life force. HRT can help mask the heart palpitations and irritability often associated with perimenopause. But it cannot resolve the underlying relationship problems that might be utilising those symptoms to get your attention.

Every day more and more studies are showing how effective modalities such as dietary change, food supplements, exercise, and herbs can be in supporting a woman through her menopausal transition. Though some doctors still don't know about these approaches and may not mention them to you, they often work as well or better than HRT. They can also be used in addition to HRT, to reduce dosage levels, side effects, and potential risk. In other words, you don't necessarily have to choose between HRT and alternatives. Think of your perimenopausal support as a smorgasbord. You get to choose what appeals to you at the moment and leave what doesn't.

Becoming an Active Partner in the Decision

For our mothers and grandmothers, the decision to take HRT (or not) was very often a passive one, made by their doctors (or husband or best friend!) with their own involvement limited to 'being good patients'. Or they decided by not deciding and simply let time go by. In those days there were very few HRT preparations available, so the choices were only two: yes or no. And until very recently, the potential benefits were too often clouded by side effects from the wrong type of medications or fear of long-term consequences. And in the late 1990s, less than 20 per cent of US women used hormone replacement therapy, and those who did often discontinued it within six months.[15] The figures are similar for British women.

This trend is now changing. More women know their options and know that they can change their regimens if they are not working. They have access to a wealth of new information about menopausal physiology and medicine. Above all, their HRT options have increased dramatically just over the last five years. Today the question 'Do I need or want HRT?' is, in fact, a series of questions, including 'What kind?' 'What strength?' 'In what combination?' 'For what reason?' 'For how long?' and 'At what risk?'.

The number of options can be intimidating at first, but in the end there is a great deal more satisfaction among women who are choosing HRT today. And although I discourage using HRT as a means of numbing oneself to what is happening in body and mind during perimenopause, there is nothing to be gained from suffering. Given the range of formulations and dosages now available – as well as the many alternatives to HRT – you can create an individual treatment programme that supports you through the change, rather than helping you deny that it is happening.

EVIE: BRITTLE DIABETES, BRITTLE HORMONES

Evie is an energetic, upbeat insurance saleswoman who steadfastly refuses to allow her diabetes – which she's had since the age of thirteen – to dominate her life. She checks her blood glucose levels regularly and gives herself two injections of insulin each day, but she's considered a 'brittle' diabetic and still suffers at least one diabetic crisis each year.

Evie takes these episodes in her stride, sometimes exasperating her friends and loved ones who wish she'd take her condition 'more seriously', but she admits that she gets 'prickly' when they dote on her. She has also begun to make the connection between the state of her diabetes and the state of her emotions. When she is upset with one of her children, her boss, or her husband, her insulin and dietary needs can change dramatically and quickly. It also came as no surprise to Evie's doctor that because of her metabolic problems, her blood sugar levels went wild as she bumped and jolted through her menopausal transition. She wrote, 'There's an amusement park nearby, with a really scary roller coaster. Oestrogen, glucose, FSH – everything was bouncing all over the place.'

Because her levels were so erratic and sensitive, it was hard getting her regulated, but with trial and error Evie and her doctor managed to arrive at a hormone replacement programme that gently alleviated her discomfort, stabilised her metabolism (and therefore her glucose levels), and supported her body through the transition. 'It was a pretty tough trip for a while, but I noticed a difference within weeks of getting the right levels of hormones.'

Clarifying Your Needs

In order to make the best choice for you, you need to clarify your needs, then become an active partner in getting them met. This may mean consulting more than one health care provider – a herbalist in addition to your obstetrician or gynaecologist, for instance. It may also mean asking your doctor to try an approach he or she is unfamiliar with – and sharing the responsibility for the results.

To begin, review the following eight health factors and determine which, if any, apply to you. This will help you focus your thinking about which replacement regimen to use, if any, and for how long.

Factor 1: You want relief from discomfort, particularly hot flushes that disrupt sleep. This is the most common reason why women choose HRT, especially oestrogen. However, discomfort is also the most common reason for women to stop taking HRT – the formulation and/or the dosage prescribed may not be right for their particular metabolism, resulting in persistent medication side effects and/or symptoms of overdose.

If relief from symptoms is your sole reason for seeking treatment, treatment will probably be needed only until the perimenopausal transition is complete, which can be confirmed either by a lack of menstrual periods for at least a year or by the laboratory tests outlined in chapter 4. There might be a brief perimenopause-like adjustment when coming off hormone treatment, but if you are weaned off the hormones over a period of several months, the symptoms generally are mild. Many women come off HRT once they've become well established on regimens that include herbs, soya, exercise, or dietary supplements. This approach often smoothes the adjustment.

If you want symptomatic relief but your personal preference is to stay away from supplemental hormones, there are many non-hormonal treatments available over the counter or from health care practitioners such as naturopaths and acupuncturists. (See chapter 6.)

Factor 2: You are suffering from urogenital symptoms. The health of the vaginal lining and urethral tissues is highly influenced by the hormonal milieu in our bodies. Women may seek relief from stress incontinence (they leak urine when coughing, sneezing, laughing, or lifting heavy objects), urge incontinence (they have difficulty making it to the lavatory without leaking), recurrent vaginal yeast infections, vaginal dryness and/or discomfort during intercourse, recurrent bladder infections, or urinary frequency (they need to urinate more than eight times during the day, or one or more times during the night).

Taking oestrogen (by mouth or applied locally) and/or androgen hormones (applied as a skin patch or as a cream formulated for vaginal application) helps maintain healthy vaginal and urethral tissue, even when relatively small doses are used. As little as 1 to 2mg of natural testosterone in a cream base, applied to the vagina two to three times per week, for example, is often all that is necessary. And sometimes the phyto-oestrogens found in herbs, soya, or flaxseed (linseed) can restore vaginal tissue to its premenopausal moistness and resilience. (See chapter 6.)

Some women find that systemic oestrogen (taken by mouth) doesn't help vaginal and urethral tissue. No one knows why this is the case, but local application is the answer.

Factor 3: You currently have a healthy heart but are at increased risk of cardiovascular disease. A woman's increased risk of heart disease is usually related to (1) a positive family history (heart disease or stroke in father younger than the age of fifty-five, or in mother or other first-degree female relative at the age of sixty-five or younger) and all the emotions that go with it, (2) lifestyle factors such as smoking or lack of exercise, or (3) a predisposing factor such as low HDL cholesterol, high LDL cholesterol, or high triglycerides.

Oestrogen replacement decreases LDL cholesterol and increases HDL cholesterol.[16] It also has been shown to have a positive effect on blood vessel walls that seems to involve nitric oxide, a chemical produced in the body that helps keep blood vessels dilated. (Viagra, the drug for male impotence, also exerts its effect through the nitric oxide pathways.)

Some studies, but not others, have shown that conventional oestrogen replacement can increase the risk of blood clots, including pulmonary embolism.[17] Oestrogen has also been shown to increase the level of triglycerides in some women.

Nonetheless, the consensus among many women's health experts is that the benefits of oestrogen on the cardiovascular system outweigh the risks. This beneficial effect is partially obliterated when a woman takes norethisterone or another synthetic progestogen along with her oestrogen. Virtually all the currently available combination hormone therapies contain synthetic progestogens, and I don't recommend them.

I feel strongly that oestrogen would show a far greater potential benefit if women used individualised regimens consisting of natural, bioidentical hormones. Because of their deleterious effect on blood vessels, I believe that synthetic progestogens (especially Provera (MPA)) are more dangerous than taking no hormones at all. Tried and tested methods to decrease heart disease risk also include avoiding smoking, regular vigorous exercise, taking supplements such as vitamin E, following a diet rich in fruits and vegetables, consuming soya foods, and keeping weight normal. (See chapter 14 for my heart health programme.)

Factor 4: You have already been diagnosed with heart disease. You may have seen headlines about the recent epidemiological studies suggesting that women who already have significant heart disease when they start taking HRT are at slightly *increased* risk of having a life-threatening cardiovascular event, such as heart attack or stroke, during the first year of starting their hormone supplementation. This risk abates after the first year, however.

Many scientists feel that this is due to a hormone-stimulated increase in chemicals called 'inflammation factors', such as C-reactive protein, which was found in the bloodstream in amounts that were 85 per cent higher in women taking HRT. However, this is once again a case where you need to read the small print. Nearly all the women in the study were taking Premarin and synthetic progestogen. As I've said above, I believe that the increased risk boils down mainly to the adverse effects of medroxyprogesterone acetate (trade name Provera). It is also true that oestrogens at high enough doses have long been associated with increased risk of blood clots that predispose to heart attack, especially in smokers.

Here's the bottom line: women with or without heart disease should avoid synthetic progestogens and keep their oestrogen doses as natural and as low as possible.

Factor 5: You are at increased risk of osteoporosis or already have been diagnosed with bone loss. A woman whose mother or grandmother has osteoporosis is at increased risk of this potentially disabling condition, though it is unknown whether this is because of a genetic inheritance or because we tend to 'inherit' habits, lifestyle choices, and life expectations, which may predispose us to less-than-optimal bone strength. (See chapter 12 for additional risk factors, many of which are under our control.) Oestrogen replacement definitely helps prevent bone loss associated with menopause, and continuous use of oestrogen decreases the risk of fracture by 50 per cent or more. The bone-preserving effects of oestrogen are maintained only as long as a woman stays on it.

Androgens such as testosterone also play a role in preserving bone health. Those women with naturally high testosterone levels have a decreased risk for osteoporotic fractures. Low-dose testosterone supplementation has been found to help maintain bone mass.

A number of drugs – calcitonin, the bisphosphonates such as alendronate (trade name Fosamax), and SERMs such as tamoxifen (Nolvadex) and raloxifene (Evista) – have also been shown to help prevent loss of bone and decrease fracture risk. As with hormone replacement, they are effective only as long as a woman is on them.

High doses of soya protein, regular weight-bearing exercise, and vitamin D are also very effective ways of maintaining bone density and decreasing fracture risk, both at perimenopause and beyond.

Factor 6: You are at increased risk of Alzheimer's disease. At this point in our limited understanding of this organic brain disorder, a positive family history is the strongest predisposing factor, although most individuals who get it don't have any genetic predisposition. There is less consensus regarding some studies' suggestion that high levels of aluminium intake (from using aluminium cookware or consuming food from aluminium cans) might also contribute to an individual's risk of Alzheimer's disease.

Despite our lack of understanding about underlying causes, preliminary research suggests that even among women with a strong family history of Alzheimer's, taking supplemental oestrogen results in a lower incidence of the disease or delays its onset. Unfortunately we don't have the kind of long-term prospective studies on large numbers of women that could give us the definitive answers we're seeking. In other words, when it comes to oestrogen and Alzheimer's, we're at the same place as we were back in the early 1990s with oestrogen and heart disease – lots of evidence but no definitive proof.

In the meantime, it is clear that all hormones can affect brain function – androgens and progesterone as well as oestrogen – and that many women continue making enough of these throughout life to protect their brains. In fact, a recent British study of postmenopausal women not on HRT found that those with the highest levels of endogenous oestradiol were the least likely to have Alzheimer's disease.[18] And there are many additional things a woman can do now to protect her mental functions in later life. (See chapter 10, 'Nurturing Your Brain'.)

Factor 7: You are at increased risk of breast, uterine, ovarian, or bowel cancer. A positive personal or family history for one or more of these hormone-related cancers makes the hormone replacement therapy decision very anxiety-provoking for many women. Here are the facts: recent research has suggested that the dose and formulation of HRT are important factors in the cancer issue. Though all types of oestrogen at high enough doses over a long enough period of time can potentially stimulate breast cancer growth, I feel that Premarin, because of its association with DNA damage and because it has a stronger biological effect than bioidentical oestrogens, may be more carcinogenic than bioidentical oestrogens. In other words, the increased risk of breast and uterine cancer shown by past studies may have been related to oestrogen overdose or the wrong kind of oestrogen, rather than oestrogen per se.

If oestrogen is taken in a way that more closely mimics the way it is produced in the body – in physiological doses calibrated to the body's needs, in bioidentical formulation, and partnered with bioidentical, not synthetic, progesterone – it begins to lose its sinister profile. (See chapter 13.)

For the woman who is in the highest risk category for breast, uterine, or ovarian cancer but who desires support through the symptomatic phase of perimenopause, there are two options that are unlikely to adversely affect that risk. First, she can take bioidentical hormones at the lowest possible levels during the five years or fewer when her symptoms are the most troubling. This will involve fine-tuning her doses with the aid of salivary testing, so she takes no more than the amounts necessary to achieve physiological balance and symptomatic relief. Second, she can opt for non-hormonal, herbal treatments. (See chapter 6.)

With regard to colorectal cancer, the picture is clearer. Colorectal cancer accounts for 11.2 per cent of all cancers among US women – third after breast and lung. In both prevalence and mortality it out-ranks endometrial, ovarian, and cervical cancers. A summary of ten studies with information on the timing of oestrogen use indicates a 34 per cent reduced risk of colorectal cancer in current users. This pro-tection is nearly lost within a few years of stopping hormone therapy. Though no one knows why for sure, it appears that oestrogen causes a decrease in bile acids, substances manufactured in the liver that are associated with the promotion of colorectal cancer.[19]

Factor 8: You reached menopause prematurely (prior to the age of forty) or artificially and abruptly (due to surgery, illness, chemo-therapy, or radiation). Women with this history are more likely to need systemic HRT, a programme that provides physiologically appropriate hormone levels throughout the body, rather than more locally acting products, and rather than relying solely on herbal treatments and dietary approaches. There are several reasons for this. First, the physical and mental symptoms associated with a premature or abrupt cessation of natural hormone production are usually more severe than with a more gradual perimenopausal decline. Second, both premature and artificial menopause appear to create an increased need for the cardiovascular, bone, and brain support provided by HRT. With premature menopause, the woman's body is left without endogenous hormone support for more years than if menopause had occurred later in life. I recommend using a combination of bio-identical hormones, with the dosage based on your blood or salivary hormone levels.

SANDY: SURGICAL MENOPAUSE

Sandy had an 'instant' menopause at thirty-five, when her ovaries were removed because of severe endometriosis. This created the abrupt hormonal withdrawal characteristic of artificial menopause. Her symptoms were quite pronounced. Until her surgery, Sandy had believed that she would not take HRT when she reached her natural menopause. Now, to say the least, her discomfort was intrusive. And the fact that she would be without her normal complement of hormones for approximately fifteen extra years meant that her bone density, heart health, and mental functioning might suffer in the future. As a result, Sandy felt she had no choice but to start HRT. 'Frankly,' she wrote, 'I was so miserable I couldn't give my full attention to the decision beyond that point.' She and her doctor decided on a skin patch that delivered bioidentical oestrogen (17-β-oestradiol), along with natural progesterone oral capsules. With minimal tweaking, they arrived at the optimal dose for her, and her level of comfort vastly improved.

'At that point,' Sandy wrote, 'I could start applying myself to decisions that would affect my future. I really had not wanted to take HRT after menopause, but I didn't want to increase my chance of osteoporosis or heart disease, so it felt right to take HRT under the circumstances. Then it hit me: I can have the best of both worlds! I decided I'll take these hormones until I'm fifty-five, when I'd proba-bly have completed my menopausal transition naturally, and then I'll wean myself off the hormones and sail through my menopausal years au naturel. I feel much happier about this plan. I feel like the idea was a thank-you gift from my body for bending the "rules" and providing it with hormones during these extra fifteen years of menopause.'

When to Start HRT

Over the years I've watched scores of women left to 'tough it out' during their stormy perimenopausal years because their doctors didn't want to prescribe hormones until they were definitely past menopause. There's no need for this. You should feel free to start what you need when you need it – and that includes hormones, herbs, foods, lifestyle changes, or a combination of all these. Because menopause is really a retrospective diagnosis, you won't know you're there until you're there!

For the woman who wants help with perimenopausal symptoms and finds that a non-hormonal approach does not provide sufficient relief but who is afraid that supplemental oestrogen might increase her risk of breast or uterine cancer, HRT is not necessarily out of the question. (See chapters 8 and 13.) As I've said above, I'm not convinced that there is any significant risk from taking bioidentical oestrogen at a low dose only during the five years or less that menopausal symptoms are likely to be the most intrusive. After that, she can wean herself off some or all of the hormones or replace them with other alternatives. Astoundingly, there are no studies that prove that taking oestrogen is contraindicated even in women with breast cancer, though many doctors and their patients are justifiably nervous about taking this hormone in such cases.

So far, I've been able to quell my own hot flushes with a daily serving of soya protein powder that contains 160mg of soya isoflavones. I also use natural progesterone skin cream, dong quai, and a Chinese herbal combination. (See chapter 6.) I may eventually take some form of low-dose bioidentical oestrogen. Currently, however, my salivary oestrogen levels are still in the normal range. I also follow a diet that keeps insulin levels normal, exercise regularly, and get acupuncture treatments from time to time. My blood pressure and cholesterol levels are low, and my bone density is fine.

RENÉE: LOSING CONTROL, FINDING COMPASSION

Though many of us have fixed ideas about how we will negotiate menopause and what we will and won't do, we need to be willing to let go of all our preconceptions once we actually begin going through the experience. Renée's story is a beautiful example of this.

> I'd decided a long time ago that I wasn't going to colour my hair when it went grey and I wasn't going to take supplemental hormones when I hit menopause. Menopause for me was going to be a beautiful thing. I had it all worked out.

Principles of HRT

- Establish your natural hormonal levels by getting a baseline test in your late thirties or early perimenopause.

- Replace only those hormones that need replacing.

- Use the lowest dose that does the job.

- Use bioidentical hormones that are an exact molecular match to those naturally occurring in your body.

- Support your HRT regimen with a healthy diet, the right nutritional supplements, and exercise.

- Be realistic. The goal is not to turn back the clock. Rather, the goal is to optimise your comfort and overall health so you can live the second half of your life with maximal vitality and mental clarity.

Then on my forty-seventh birthday my father died without warning, of a massive heart attack. My mother, confused and scared and in need of support, moved in with us. Then my husband, David, lost his funding and suddenly was faced with the prospect of being unemployed by the end of the year. And I was practically blindsided one week later with my first hot flush, which was so powerful it actually steamed up my glasses. Emotionally, financially, hormonally, and in terms of my overall sense of security, it felt like the proverbial rug was being pulled out from under my feet. My hot flushes became increasingly bothersome, particularly when they happened in the middle of the night and interrupted my sleep. I was feeling short-tempered with my mum and with David, and the house felt claustrophobic – I suppose I just couldn't handle all the unexpected stresses that came up at what felt like the worst possible time in my biology. When my gynaecologist suggested that I needed a little hormonal support, I sighed with relief and accepted it, and I feel much better now. In fact, just making the decision to accept help made a big difference in the way I felt, right away.

The lesson I learned from all this applies to more than just menopause: you can't control everything. I've always been a big control freak, but now I understand that in some ways we're all just along for the ride, and we need to be compassionate with ourselves and willing to change direction once in a while, in order to adjust and accommodate to what life throws our way, no matter what stage of life we're in at the time.

A Dusting of Hormones

So, let's say that you've decided that you may want to try hormone replacement therapy. You are still having periods, but you're getting hot flushes before they start. You also have occasional night sweats. I'd recommend that at this point you get your hormone levels tested. The ideal time is about a week before your period is due, because you'll be able to see what your peak progesterone level is at that time, and it will also give you an idea of how much oestrogen and testosterone is normally circulating in your system. These levels will also give you an idea of what level you want to replace to once you start hormones.

The next thing you do, depending upon your hormone levels, is to start replacing the hormone that is lowest. In most cases, this will be progesterone, and maybe oestrogen. Increasingly we're finding that many perimenopausal women also have an androgen deficiency. As already mentioned, natural progesterone in the form of a 1.5–3 per cent skin cream has been shown to give good blood levels. This alone may be all you need. Try it for two weeks before your period, then take two weeks off after your period starts. You can also use it for three weeks on and one week off. Most women notice a reduction of their symptoms within a month of starting this cream. Continue with this as long as you're getting good results.

If your oestrogen level is too low, you'll want to start with the lowest level of oestrogen available. Oestrogen is available by prescription only, so you'll need to work with a doctor to get the right dose and blood levels for you. Many women like the convenience of the oestrogen patch, which comes in many different strengths and can be left on the skin for several days. Others prefer to take a pill. If you're taking oestrogen, you have to be sure that you have enough progesterone to prevent excessive build-up of your uterine lining. This can be accomplished in some women with 1.5–3 per cent progesterone skin cream. Others may need a higher amount of progesterone, I recommend Crinone vaginal gel.

If your doctor doesn't know about this approach, either educate him or her or find someone who does. (See Resources.)

How Long Should You Stay on Hormones?

The length of time you continue to take hormones depends entirely on why you are taking hormones and what other things you are doing to achieve the same benefit. For example, if you originally started oestrogen to maintain bone health but have since incorporated regular weight training into your lifestyle, you can probably taper off the oestrogen and still maintain your bone density. If, on the other hand, you are a confirmed couch potato and you know you are at risk of osteoporosis, then you'd better keep taking your oestrogen, or one of the other drugs to maintain bone density, for the rest of your life.

With bioidentical hormones at low levels, the benefits of HRT may far outweigh any risks – especially if you feel good on them, have risk factors that HRT is known to ameliorate, or have a health history that doesn't include a lot of healthy ninety-year-old relatives! The vast majority of women start taking hormones, herbs, or both for immediate relief of menopausal symptoms such as hot flushes or vaginal dryness. Others are far more concerned about Alzheimer's, osteoporosis, or possible heart disease prevention. Taking hormones for short-term symptom relief is very different from taking hormones for long-term disease prevention. Most women experience most of their menopausal symptoms during a five- to ten-year period, after which the symptoms abate naturally.

Not Carved in Stone

Because every woman's body is a work in progress, your hormonal status – and your need for a particular type of support programme – may well change. If you elect to take supplemental hormones, it is wise to have your hormone levels checked every three to six months during the first year of hormone use. Compare the results to how you're feeling. This can help indicate if, and where, your prescription needs fine-tuning. After you have reached a comfortable level, you only need to test every year or so.

Remember that formulations that work well for one woman do not necessarily provide optimal results for another. You may want to try a different formulation, a different delivery system, or a different dosage, or switch from hormone supplementation to non-hormonal herbal support or vice versa. Be calm and at peace about this decision process – you can always change your mind if what you've chosen falls short of your expectations.

SIX

Foods and Supplements to Support the Change

*F*or thousands of years, long before our culture placed its trust in pharmaceuticals, women relied upon their intuition and Mother Nature to keep themselves and their families healthy. Guided by their inner wisdom, our ancestors plucked healing plants from nature's colourful pharmacy – fragrant chamomile for calming teas, fresh ginger to prevent nausea and calm the stomach, and foxglove to regulate the heartbeat.

It is remarkable that our herbalist ancestors, though separated by thousands of miles, often drew upon the same herbs to treat the same conditions. Native American Indian women and their Chinese counterparts, for example, both used angelica (dong quai) to treat menopausal symptoms.

Today this ancient, intuitive wisdom is being augmented by objective scientific studies confirming what wise women have always known: plants contain a wide range of ingredients, such as essential fatty acids, phyto-oestrogens, and antioxidants, that can heal and help keep us healthy at all stages of our lives, including perimenopause.

To use herbs and foods optimally requires an adjustment in thinking. Plant medicine and food do not work in the body the way drugs, or even bioidentical hormones, do. Modern pharmaceuticals and hormones usually consist of one purified active ingredient (often derived from a plant source and then altered biochemically) that is carefully standardised and measured for its biological effect.

Whole herbs and foods, on the other hand, contain many different active ingredients that act synergistically in the body. There is good reason to believe that to get the full range of benefits, you need to consume the whole plant – or a product made from part of the whole plant such as leaves or roots – rather than a single ingredient. This is why some studies show that whole soya foods give better results than capsules or pills containing isolated soya isoflavones.

In allopathic Western medicine, we try to target a symptom or illness with a single drug – we give contraceptive pills, for example, to stop heavy bleeding or to regulate irregular periods. Contraceptive pills control symptoms, but they do nothing to treat the underlying imbalance.

Herbs and foods, on the other hand, with their exquisite combinations of interactive ingredients, work to balance the body at a number of different levels simultaneously. Accordingly, there are many different herbs or foods that one might use to regulate the menstrual cycle or as overall perimenopausal tonics, including soya foods, ground flaxseed (linseed), dong quai, or chaste berry, to name just a few. All contain substances that help balance the endocrine system in slightly different but synergistic ways.[1]

Herbs also work best when considered as part of an overall plan that includes a good diet, exercise, and improved relationships. In other words, we need to approach herbs and foods with a holistic mind-set that asks, 'What foods or herbs will best help me balance my body so that it can heal itself?', rather than the more dualistic 'What pill do I need to take to remove this symptom?'

Who Should Consider Herbs?

- Your symptoms are mild but you'd like a little support.

- You believe that herbs are simply more natural and beneficial than prescribed hormones.

- You'd like to avoid HRT because of fear of breast cancer or another health concern.

- You're on HRT of some sort but would like the added benefits of herbs.

- You cannot tolerate HRT.

Basic Principles of Herbal Therapy at Menopause

In order to use menopausal herbs well and wisely, you need to understand the following basic principles.

• All plant foods contain what are known as phytonutrients. *(Phyto-* means 'plant'.) These are unique substances produced during the natural course of growth and are specific to a particular plant's genes and environment. In addition to providing taste and nutritional value, phytonutrients can play therapeutic roles by modifying physiological processes in our bodies. This is the basis for botanical medicine. An example of this is the phytochemical indole-3-carbinol, found in cruciferous vegetables such as broccoli. This substance appears to convert the most potent oestrogens in the body into weaker, less carcinogenic forms. High consumption of cruciferous vegetables is associated with a decreased risk of breast cancer, breast tenderness, and bloating, all of which are related to oestrogen levels that are too high.

• The line between using herbs as foods and using them as drugs can be blurry. For example, ephedra (ma huang) can be an effective treatment for asthma and sinusitis, but it should be avoided as a daily supplement. In general, the greater your intake of an herb, the greater the potential for druglike effects. For safety, keep doses moderately low, and follow the directions on the packet or a herbalist's recommendation. It is also best to let your doctor know what herbs you take regularly, because some herbs interact with some drugs in a way that either decreases the drug's potency or changes its effect.

• Recent advances in the standardisation of herbal supplements has led to more consistent quality and potency. The most effective products are those that combine the whole plant (or plant part, such as the root) with a standardised percentage of the primary active ingredient.

• The common menopausal herbs mentioned in this chapter have been used safely and effectively for thousands of years and rarely have side effects. However, a few people may react to some of them, some of the time – just as with any food or drug. There are also many herbs with known toxicity that shouldn't be used except under the care of an experienced herbalist. Examples include belladonna, blue cohosh, lobelia, and poke root.

• Phyto-oestrogens, the natural hormones found in plants, are not the same as the hormones found in the female body, although they may have somewhat similar beneficial effects. Phyto-oestrogens are found in more than three hundred plants, including some that we routinely eat in the UK, such as apples, carrots, oats, plums, olives, potatoes, tea, coffee, and sunflower seeds. Soya and linseed are particularly rich in these substances.[2] Phyto-oestrogens can be divided into two main families: the *isoflavones,* which include substances such as genistein, daidzein, equol, and coumestrol, and the *lignans,* which include matairesinol, enterolactone, and enterodiol.

The oestrogenic activity of phyto-oestrogens is lower than that of human oestrogens – in the range of a hundredth to a thousandth that of oestradiol. They also have antioxidant and antiproliferative activity that is still being elucidated. This means that they have the ability to prevent free-radical damage to cells, the number-one cause of premature ageing of tissue, and they also help prevent abnormal cell growth.

Like other oestrogens, phyto-oestrogens bind to oestrogen receptors throughout our systems. (Research has shown that oestrogen receptors are found on the surface of nearly every cell of our bodies, not just those of the vagina, uterus, and breast tissue.) When they bind, they exert a balancing, or 'adaptogenic', effect.[3] This means that if your oestrogen levels are low, the herbs will have an oestrogenic effect, but if your oestrogen levels are too high, they will block the stronger oestrogens. That's why the same herb – dong quai, for example – can be used both for conditions in which there is too much oestrogen (such as PMS) and for those in which there is too little (hot flushes).

Phyto-oestrogens do not stimulate the growth of oestrogen-sensitive tissue such as in the breast and uterus; in fact, they have been shown to inhibit breast tumours in some animal studies, probably because they occupy oestrogen receptor sites and prevent overstimulation of the cells.[4] Menopausal herbs have never been implicated in promoting cancer in humans, either, and indeed, some herbs are noted for their anti-cancer properties.[5] For this reason, menopausal herbs are an excellent choice for those who are concerned about cancer.

• Many plant extracts exert a tonic effect on the female pelvic organs, and other organs as well. What this means is that they stimulate blood flow and sometimes even increase the weight of these organs.[6] Herbs such as black cohosh and chaste berry have also been shown to reduce menopausal symptoms by acting on the pituitary gland.

• In general, herbs exert their influence in a much slower, more gradual way than drugs or even the bioidentical hormones that I often recommend. So be prepared to wait three or four weeks before noticing an effect from an herbal supplement.

• Finally, menopausal herbs are often given in combination, since experienced herbalists have found that their actions are synergistic and produce better results when used this way. Chinese herbal formulations set the standard for this synergy.

Key Menopausal Herbs

The following are some of the best-studied herbs used for menopausal symptoms. They can be used singly or in combination. Please note that this list is far from comprehensive. Many others, such as peony, hops, motherwort, and false unicorn root, are also effective.

DONG QUAI (*Angelica sinensis*): Dong quai (also known as angelica, dang gui, and tang kuei) has excellent phyto-oestrogen activity and has been called female ginseng because of its ability to enhance energy and a sense of well-being. It is used for amenorrhoea, irregular periods, and excessive uterine bleeding. My acupuncturist, who is from Taiwan, tells me that dong quai is one of the most widely used herbs in China and that many women take it throughout their repro- ductive and perimenopausal years.

Dong quai also has analgesic and anti-allergy effects, is anti- bacterial, is a smooth muscle relaxant, and can stabilise blood vessels.[7]

Dong quai is widely available over the counter. It is the foundation of almost all menopausal formulations and can be taken indefinitely. In Asia, women simmer the raw dried herb with chicken to make a soup or stew. Angelica root can be found in many herb shops or health food stores. It is also processed into capsules, tablets, and tinc- tures. (It is best to avoid alcohol-based tinctures.) The recommended dosages for most over-the-counter dong quai preparations are probably too low to be helpful (the usual dose is 4.5g per day). Increasing the dosage on your own is unlikely to cause any problems, but it's always best to be under the supervision of a certified herbalist or practitioner of Traditional Chinese Medicine.

Note: Do not take dong quai if there's a chance you're pregnant.

CHASTE BERRY (*Vitex agnus-castus*):   Chaste berry comes from the chaste tree, which is native to the Mediterranean. It is widely available at natural food stores, often under the name vitex or agnus castus. It has been shown to have a profound effect on pituitary function, increasing the secretion of LH (luteinizing hormone) and decreasing the production of FSH (follicle-stimulating hormone), which in turn shifts the production of hormones towards more progesterone and less oestrogen.[8] This is thought to be the main reason why it helps balance the irregular periods that result from the hormonal swings of perimenopause. It also acts somewhat like the neurotransmitter dopamine. Chaste berry is particularly beneficial for women who are having PMS-like symptoms or are experiencing scanty, irregular periods. It has been shown to suppress appetite, relieve depression, and improve sleep. It can take several months to work.

The usual dose is 1tsp of crushed fruit per cup of water one to four times per day, or 20–75 drops of the 1:3 liquid extract one to four times per day (or as directed on the bottle).

Note: Chaste berry can cause rashes in susceptible individuals. Don't take it with neuroleptic medicines such as haloperidol (Haldol) or thioridazine (Melleril), or when pregnant or nursing.

BLACK COHOSH (*Cimicifuga racemosa*):   Black cohosh has been used in the US for hundreds of years. Native Americans called it cramp bark. It is also a popular Chinese herb and is often used in formulations for perimenopausal symptoms. It binds to oestrogen receptors, where it selectively represses the elevation of LH that occurs at menopause.[9] Its oestrogenic effect decreases hot flushes, night sweats, and emotional instability. It is also helpful for PMS symptoms. A standardised extract of black cohosh sold under the trade name Remifemin is one of the most widely used herbs in Europe, where it is a well-documented alternative to HRT. Clinical studies show that it relieves menopausal symptoms such as depression, vaginal dryness, hot flushes, and menstrual cramps. Many women take Remifemin alone for good relief of menopausal symptoms.

The usual dose for Remifemin is 2 tablets (60 or 120mg per tablet) twice per day. Or take black cohosh in any of the following forms, three times per day: powdered root or as a tea, 1–2g; solid, dry 4:1 powdered extract, 250–500mg; fluid extract, 1:1 tincture, 4mg (1tsp, or about 5ml).

Note: Black cohosh can interact with medicines for high blood pressure and may result in excessively low blood pressure in some women.

LICORICE ROOT (*Glycyrrhiza glabra*): Licorice is a perennial, temperate-zone herb that grows 3 to 7ft high. The parts used are the dried runners and roots. Licorice root is one of the most extensively used and scientifically investigated herbal medicines. The active constituents of licorice include both isoflavones and lignans. Licorice has many pharmacological actions, including oestrogenic, anti-inflammatory, anti-allergy, antibacterial, and anti-cancer effects. It helps regulate oestrogen/progesterone ratios. It also helps replenish adrenal function, so it is very good for fatigue.

The usual dose is 1/4tsp of solid extract once or twice per day.

Note: Blood pressure should be monitored to be sure that it stays stable. The cortisol-like activity of this herb may cause a problem in those who are prone to hypertension. In those with low blood pressure, this herb can help correct and balance the problem.

Any of the key menopausal herbs above, either alone or in combination, often help to relieve a wide variety of symptoms including vaginal dryness, hot flushes, and mood swings. My advice is to try one or more for at least a month. If you are still troubled by your symptoms, add another of the key herbs, or choose from the more specific remedies listed in other chapters.

Menopausal Healing Foods

Though many common foods contain vitamins, minerals, and phyto-oestrogens that are healthful for the perimenopausal transition, a few stand out as particularly helpful: soya, fresh ground linseed, and foods containing bioflavonoids. No matter what type of perimenopausal treatment you choose, if any, I'd suggest supplementing your diet with at least one of these 'superfoods'.

Soya

Soya, like menopausal herbs, can be used as a safe alternative to hormone replacement, offering most of the benefits of HRT without any of the risks or side effects. On the other hand, if you are taking hormones and are happy with your regimen, you can still enjoy the benefits of soya. In fact, a diet rich in soya and other phyto-oestrogens may allow you to decrease the total dose of hormones you are on and still maintain all the benefits.

Mainstream medical research is confirming that soya protein, as a regular component of the diet, can lessen both the frequency and the intensity of hot flushes and other perimenopausal symptoms. Soya protein appears to benefit just about every system in the body. Many perimenopausal women report that it helps their skin, hair, and nails, and after about two to three months on high doses of soya, many report a return of vaginal moisture to premenopausal levels. It also helps women with mood swings, PMS symptoms, migraine headaches, irregular periods, and weight gain, and has been shown to decrease calcium loss through the kidneys.[10] Studies also show that soya protein helps decrease fat and increase lean tissue in menopausal women.[11] It has also been shown to decrease the risk of breast and endometrial cancer because of its anti-proliferative effects.[12]

Hundreds of studies are documenting the other benefits of soya. For example, a recent study followed fifty postmenopausal women who consumed three servings of soya milk (7.5oz each) or three handfuls of roasted soya nuts per day for twelve weeks, for a total daily dose of 60–70mg of isoflavones.[13] The following benefits were reported:

Heart. Researchers measured a 5.5 per cent increase in 'good' HDL cholesterol and a 9 per cent reduction in 'bad' LDL cholesterol. Many other studies have also documented soya's ability to lower choles-terol. In fact, on 26 October 1999, the US FDA approved the health claim that soya protein reduces the risk of coronary artery disease.[14] It has also been shown to have a beneficial effect on blood vessel reactivity, which may be why it helps migraine headaches.[15]

Bones. The study noted a 13 per cent increase in osteocalcin, a marker of bone formation, and a 14.5 per cent decrease in markers for osteoclasts, cells that cause bone loss. Soya protein revealed a bone-forming benefit that oestrogen does not provide.

These same benefits have not been found with isolated isoflavones in tablet form, though a type of artificial isoflavone known as ipriflavone has been shown to increase bone density.[16] There are a number of different brands of plant-based oestrogen-mimicking pills on the market, but no controlled studies have been done that show the effects of the various doses. Nor are there any studies showing that the body can absorb isoflavones from the pill versions as well as from whole soya foods. This is probably because whole soya contains other known and unknown ingredients in addition to the isoflavones.

Colon cancer and bowel problems. Preliminary results of another study showed that a diet enhanced with soya protein may help reduce colon cancer incidence in people who have a history of the disease or who have had precancerous polyps removed. Based on these preliminary results, Dr Maurice Bennink of Michigan State University in the US suggests that there could be both a 50 per cent reduction in risk in cancer incidence and an additional delay in onset of ten to fifteen years in patients taking soya.[17] Numerous animal studies also show that soya protein (not isoflavone pills) can reverse precancerous colon conditions. Animal studies show, too, that soya has an inhibitory effect on inflammatory bowel conditions such as Crohn's disease and ulcerative colitis.

SERMs. Many women on tamoxifen have reported relief of symptoms such as hot flushes and depression when they increase their intake of soya.

IS THERE A SOYA–THYROID CONNECTION?
One of my newsletter subscribers wrote to me about her recently diagnosed thyroid disease and asked a question I hear frequently: does soya intake interfere with thyroid function?

> Based on a standard blood test, I have been told I am developing Hashimoto's thyroiditis. My doctor says it is not related to perimenopause, but I am a forty-five-year-old woman and you said in your newsletter that perimenopause and thyroid problems often occur together. I'd like to increase my intake of soya to help with my perimenopause symptoms and protect my heart and bones. But I've read that eating a lot of soya causes hypothyroidism. I'm confused. What should I do?

My reader may have seen a report on some studies done on animal cells in vitro, or on infants using soya-based formulas, that have suggested the possible anti-thyroid effect of soya. However, a randomised, double-blind, placebo-controlled study was done recently at the Health Research and Studies Center in Los Altos, California, on thirty-eight menopausal women between the ages of sixty-four and eighty-three who weren't on hormone replacement therapy. Over the six-month period during which these women took 90mg of soya isoflavones per day, no anti-thyroid effect was shown.[18] This correlates with the epidemiological evidence in Japan, a country whose inhabitants show no increased risk for hypothyroidism, even though the Japanese consume an average of 100–200mg of soya isoflavones per day.[19]

Here's the bottom line: there is no convincing evidence that soya intake increases the risk of hypothyroidism during perimenopause. However, women often begin increasing their intake of soya during perimenopause, a time when they often get their thyroid function checked for the first time as well. And given that fully 25 per cent of perimenopausal women have a thyroid problem, many believe that soya is responsible. If you have any doubt about your thyroid function, get it tested. It's a simple blood test, and it will put your mind at ease.

SOYA BENEFITS ARE DOSE-DEPENDENT

It is not always easy to compare soya foods, gram for gram, in terms of effectiveness, because some soya foods contain more isoflavones than others. A lot depends upon where the crop is grown and how it is processed. One serving of a typical soya food contains 20g of protein and about 30mg of soya isoflavones (genistein, daidzein, etc). In contrast, some supplements made from whole soya are much more concentrated.

Most US research studies have been done with only 40–60g of soya protein per day (two to three small servings) because that is the most US volunteers will eat! It is also the minimum amount you'll need to eat to get any noticeable effect. At this level of consumption, it takes about four to six weeks of consistent use to notice an effect. This is consistent with research that shows that when women ate 60g of soya protein per day in the form of a powdered drink mix, they had a 45 per cent reduction in hot flushes after twelve weeks.[20] Research and my clinical and personal experience suggest that most women need about 100–160mg of soya isoflavones per day to get significant relief from other menopausal symptoms, such as vaginal dryness, as well as to protect their heart and bones.

Each of the following servings contains approximately 35–50mg of soya isoflavones:

- 1 cup soya milk

- 1/2 cup tofu

- 1/2 cup tempeh

- 1/2 cup green soya beans, available fresh or frozen

- 3 handfuls of roasted soya nuts

Powdered soya protein can be mixed with water, milk, or juice. Various brands are available. This is a particularly convenient way to get the benefits of soya. Some brands, such as Revival, contain the equivalent of four to six servings of soya in one drink. (See Resources.)

Add soya foods to your diet gradually; otherwise you might experience flatulence, since your intestinal bacteria have to adjust to this new food. You can use digestive enzymes to help (See Resources).

SUE: DEPRESSION LIFTED, BREASTS HEALED

I've heard many inspiring stories about how soya foods have changed women's lives. Here's a letter from a woman named Sue.

About a year ago my mum got me started on Revival, and I will be forever grateful. She herself had started taking Revival after she was diagnosed with breast cancer. She went through rigorous chemotherapy, radiation, and tamoxifen treatment. She is now doing well and is cancer-free.

I was on Prozac and Prempac-C for years and had not been able to eliminate either of them. Cutting back on Prozac or Prempac left me unfit to live with. Two weeks after starting Revival, I began cutting back the prescription medications and was off all the drugs and hormones within six weeks – with no ill effects. Now for the real surprise.

For years I have feared my regularly scheduled mammogram. I would usually get called back at least once for repeat views because I have severe fibrocystic breast disease and I've had two densities in my left breast that they've been watching closely. Yesterday I went for my regular mammogram and was absolutely shocked with the result. The left breast densities are almost totally gone – if you try really hard, you can see them. And the fibrocystic density has greatly diminished. On the old films the density could be seen throughout the breasts. Now there's about 30 per cent normal breast tissue. I was told I no longer have to go for a mammogram every six months. I'm down to just once per year.

WHAT TO EXPECT WHEN YOU ADD SOYA TO YOUR DIET

Depending on the amount you're eating, you may notice a decrease in hot flushes within a few days of adding soya to your diet. The average woman in Japan (where hot flushes are relatively rare) eats four to six servings of soya per day, or the equivalent of 100–200mg soya isoflavones.

Some perimenopausal women have found that their periods returned when they began taking soya or one of any number of menopausal herbal mixtures on the market. A patient came to me for a consultation after this happened, because her regular gynaecologist was very worried that the herbs were having a dangerous adverse effect. However, the phyto-oestrogens in soya or menopausal herbs do not cause periods in women who are completely through the menopause.

Irregular periods during the menopausal years are due, instead, to fluctuating hormonal levels. It is very common for a menopausal woman to go for months without having a period and then start menstruating regularly again for several months or even years. Soya intake won't prevent this. And the same is true of women who've reported that their fibroids began to grow when they started taking high doses of soya. Soya doesn't promote fibroid growth, though the highly fluctuating oestrogen levels associated with perimenopause often cause very rapid fibroid growth. In fact, some women report a reduction in the size of their fibroids when on soya compared to when they take conventional hormones.

A woman taking Revival wrote: 'I have been taking Revival for many months with great success (it reduced the size of my fibroid and slowed the bleeding). I started HRT and within a month my fibroid was growing again and I was bleeding again. I stopped. I am now back on Revival and here to stay.'

Another of my patients told me that when she started to take a soya drink from her health food shop, her hot flushes and hypoglycaemia (low blood sugar) symptoms went away completely. Later, she said, 'I began to doubt that something as simple as a soya drink could eliminate hot flushes. So I stopped it. Sure enough, my hot flushes returned within a week. So I started taking my soya again. I wish I hadn't stopped it, because it took another two weeks for it to kick in again.'

SOYA CAN BE USED BY THE WHOLE FAMILY

Making soya part of family meals can benefit everyone in your family. In men, soya protein has been found to help maintain healthy prostate tissue. In fact, many have found that they no longer need to get up at night to urinate once they start taking supplemental soya. Ongoing research is studying the effects of soya on prostate cancer.

USE ORGANIC, NON-GMO SOYA PRODUCTS

It is estimated that about 20 per cent of the American soya crop has undergone genetic modification to enhance drought resistance and other desirable traits. Such genetic engineering raises some disturbing ethical and health questions, and in Europe, unease about this development has led to the banning of genetically modified organisms (GMOs). The same movement is now becoming active in the US. Until we know more about the possible health or environmental risks, stick with soya that has been organically grown and that is labelled non-GMO.

Flaxseed (Linseed): Super Source of Lignans, Fibre, and Omega-3 Fats

Flaxseed (linseed) is the best available source of anti-cancer and phyto-oestrogenic compounds known as lignans – with a concentration more than a hundred times greater than other lignan-containing foods such as grains, fruits, and vegetables. Lignans are plant substances that get broken down by intestinal bacteria into two chemicals, enterodiol and enterolactone. These substances then circulate through the liver and are later excreted in the urine.[21] Linseed is also an excellent source of fibre and of omega-3 fats.

There are a number of reasons why we all should be interested in incorporating more lignans into our diet. The following are some of the most compelling.

LIGNANS

Lignans have potent anti-cancer effects. An impressive number of studies have shown that linseed lignans help in both prevention and treatment of breast and colon cancer because of their ability to modulate the production, availability, and action of the hormones produced in our bodies.[22]

Lignans are potent phyto-oestrogens. In women who consume linseed, studies have shown significant hormonal changes, including alterations in oestradiol levels, similar to those seen with soya isoflavones. This makes linseed oil or ground linseed a great choice for women who can't use soya or who simply want another source of phytohormones.[23]

Lignans are good antioxidants. Like soya and many herbs, lignans have antiviral, antibacterial, and antioxidant properties, which means they help prevent free-radical damage to tissues – the cellular-level injury associated with ageing and disease.

Lignans help protect the cardiovascular system. Studies have also found that lignans in the form of linseed significantly lower LDL cholesterol (the 'bad' cholesterol), raise HDL cholesterol (the 'good' cholesterol), and reduce the incidence of atherosclerosis.[24]

FIBRE

Linseed is an excellent source of fibre. In addition to its phyto-oestrogenic properties, linseed is rich in both soluble and insoluble fibre. Adding a daily serving of ground linseed to your diet may eliminate any problems you have with constipation. (Just be sure you take it with enough liquid.) While the fibre in wheat bran is quite hard and can irritate the bowel, the fibre in linseed is much softer. When combined with fluid, linseed fibre forms a mucilage in the body that can significantly help reduce the risk of diabetes and cardiovascular disease. Fibre has been shown to reduce both total cholesterol and triglyceride levels in the bloodstream.

The total dietary fibre content in 45g of linseed (about 1/4 cup) is 11.7g. This is nearly four times greater than the fibre contained in a 1/2-cup serving of oatmeal.

OMEGA-3 FATS

Linseed is an excellent source of omega-3 fats. These fats are essential for the health of every cell in our bodies, including the cells in our brains and hearts. A deficiency of omega-3 fatty acids, which is quite common, can result in fatigue, dry skin, cracked nails, thin and breakable hair, constipation, immune system malfunction, aching joints, depression, arthritis, and hormone imbalances.

Omega-3 fats are found not just in linseed, but in fatty fish (especially salmon, mackerel, sardines, and anchovies), fish oil, liver, kidneys, egg yolk, and algae. Linseed meal is an excellent source of omega-3 fats if it's freshly ground. (Linseed oil also provides omega-3s, but it does not provide fibre. In addition, the oil must be kept refrigerated, or it will turn rancid.)

Remember, however, that you can't rely on linseed products alone to meet all your needs for essential fatty acids. While it contains EPA (eicosapentaenoic acid), linseed doesn't have DHA (docosahexaenoic acid), a brain tissue building block that your body can't manufacture. Fish, especially the cold-water fatty kinds, remains a good source of DHA. That may be why studies show that individuals who consume fish exhibit a lower incidence of depression. If you can't or don't want to consume fish regularly, I think DHA (100–400mg per day) is one of the best supplements you can take. (See Resources.)

HOW TO TAKE LINSEED: Not all linseed is created equal. I recommend buying golden linseed grown in the northern Great Plains regions of North America (Manitoba and the Dakotas), where the rich soil and climate support linseed that is high in omega-3 fats and flavour. (See Resources.) Avoid the brown linseed found in most health food stores. It doesn't taste very good and its nutritional value pales in comparision to golden linseed. Grind your daily serving (1/4 cup) in a coffee grinder (I bought one especially for linseed) and then stir the meal into soups and beverages, or sprinkle it on cereal or salad. I add half my daily dose to my morning soya drink and eat the other half with plain yoghurt at the same meal. This combination makes a wonderfully fibre-full, phyto-oestrogen-rich, perimenopausal power breakfast. And it takes less than three minutes to prepare!

Bioflavonoids

Another rich food source for phyto-oestrogens are the bioflavonoids contained in many herbs and fruits. Bioflavonoids compete with excess oestrogen for receptor sites and are therefore also helpful for balancing menopausal hormones and tonifying the pelvic organs. The white, spongy inner peel of citrus fruits is a very rich source, so eat some of it along with your orange or grapefruit. (I usually just take the orange peel and eat the inner white part directly – the same as I would an artichoke leaf.) Other rich sources of bioflavonoids include cherries, cranberries, blueberries, bilberries, many whole grains, grape skins, and red clover. In supplement form, 1,000mg of bioflavonoids with vitamin C daily has been shown to relieve hot flushes.[25]

Traditional Chinese Medicine and Acupuncture for Menopause

Over the years I've referred hundreds of women for acupuncture and Traditional Chinese Medicine (TCM), a system of medicine that is over two thousand years old, for the relief of a wide variety of gynaecological problems, including those related to menopause. I have personally used elements of Traditional Chinese Medicine, including various herbal formulas and acupuncture, to relieve menstrual cramps and hot flushes.

Traditional Chinese Medicine is by its very nature holistic, tailoring treatment to the individual's body, mind, spirit, and emotions. This system of medicine views our health as a balance between the two contrasting states of yin and yang. The following is a very simple explanation, courtesy of my own personal mother–daughter acupuncture team, of the most common pattern that occurs during menopause.[26]

According to Chinese medicine, the part of us that is referred to as yin – our vital fluids – begins to diminish as we grow older. This leads to an excess of yang – vital energy and heat – and/or stagnation of *chi* (life energy). Ideally, when our yin, yang, and *chi* are in balance, our body acts something like a kettle containing liquid (yin) heated by fire (yang). The resulting steam (the enhanced *chi* flow) circulates throughout the body, warming and nourishing it.

How much and to what degree yin becomes depleted depends upon our lifestyle, diet, and genes. Depletion of yin causes the vital liquid in the kettle to burn off, so that the fire burns without producing the steam necessary to moisten and nourish.

Excess heat leads to hot flushes, the most obvious symptom, as well as to dryness of the skin, eyes, and vagina. Excess heat can dislodge the *shen* (spirit) from the heart, causing restlessness and insomnia. If excess heat enters the blood, it can cause heavy menstrual periods. *Chi* stagnation can cause pain anywhere in the body, as well as moodiness and emotional instability. A combination of excess heat and *chi* stagnation can lead to restlessness and anxiety.

Diet

According to Chinese medicine, diet is the most effective way to relieve many symptoms, and my experience bears this out. All heat-producing foods and substances should be eliminated. Caffeine, alcohol, refined sugar, food colouring, preservatives, and additives (including antibiotics and hormones fed to animals during the production of most meat, chicken, and eggs) will cause excess heat and yin depletion. Red meat should be consumed in small quantities, but being a complete vegetarian (vegan) is not recommended. You should eat at least 2–4oz of meat or fish every week or two, depending upon your size and lifestyle. It is also helpful to limit spicy, pungent foods, such as curries or chillies, and greasy, fried, or oily foods.

Foods should be lightly cooked, not raw or cold. (These days I microwave my salad greens for about thirty seconds with a little lemon juice on them.) The body has to work much harder to digest raw food, which creates heat and *chi* stagnation. Cold food, contrary to popular belief, doesn't cool the body in a balanced way. Instead, cold and ice create blockages in the *chi* channel, which creates *chi* stagnation. The following foods are especially cooling and helpful: melons, bean sprouts, tofu, white ocean fish, celery, apples, asparagus, and grapes.

Smoking obviously makes everything worse. When you smoke you are quite literally breathing in fire and toxins that enter the brain and bloodstream directly. It is also well documented that smoking poisons the ovaries, decreasing our oestrogen levels about two years sooner than would normally occur.

Practitioners of traditional Chinese medicine also discourage the regular use of ginger and Asian ginseng (*Panax ginseng*) and Siberian ginseng during perimenopause because both are considered heat-producing.

Chinese Herbs for Menopause

An incredible variety of Chinese herbs and herbal combinations are available to treat every condition known to humanity – and the symptoms of perimenopause are no exception. While many individual Chinese herbs have Western counterparts, the most effective Chinese herbal combinations are unique to this system of medicine. Many of these so-called patent formulations have been tested and refined for thousands of years.

A full discussion of Traditional Chinese Medicine and Chinese herbs is beyond the scope of this book. The preparations mentioned below don't even begin to scratch the surface of what is available and safe for almost all people to take. Since most herbal prescriptions are based on an individual's unique constitution, it is best to work directly with a practitioner trained in this system.

If you are buying herbal formulations from a health food shop, make sure that the ingredients are listed on the label.

The following are particularly useful for perimenopausal symptoms:

JOYFUL CHANGE is a safe, general perimenopausal herbal tonic. It consists of over twenty-five different herbs, including dong quai, black cohosh, and peony. It was especially created for the complex menopausal symptoms of women in our culture by knowledgeable practitioners of Chinese medicine. It is effective for symptoms such as hot flushes, insomnia, and dryness. It also addresses the cause of the symptoms by draining heat and nourishing yin. Joyful Change is helpful for balancing the menstrual cycle in those women whose periods have become irregular and scant because of skipping ovulations.

YUNNAN BAI YAO (also known as Yunna Pai Yao) is very helpful in controlling the heavy bleeding that is so common in perimenopausal women. It should not be used on a long-term basis (more than a month) because it is not a cure. In other words, you should also take measures to address and treat the underlying cause of your bleeding, such as oestrogen dominance or a fibroid.

TIAN WANG BU XIN WANG is said to nourish the heart yin and anchor the spirit. It is helpful for anxiety, restlessness, and insomnia. This herbal combination can be taken indefinitely; it is widely used by the general population in China, not just menopausal women.

CHAI HU LONG GU MULI WANG moves the liver *chi* and sedates the spirit. It is helpful for moodiness, emotional instability, and outbursts of anger and feelings of frustration. It is also used to treat insomnia.

Acupuncture

Acupuncture is an essential part of Traditional Chinese Medicine. Because it works to normalise the flow of life energy or *chi* in the body, it is particularly appropriate for perimenopause, a time when our energy is completely renewing itself. It is extremely effective for relieving hot flushes, insomnia, night sweats, anxiety, restlessness, emotional instability, moodiness, menstrual cramps, and excess bleeding.

Though most people resort to acupuncture only after conventional Western drugs and surgery have failed, and though it is often effective even in these difficult situations, acupuncture is best used as preventive health care or at the onset of symptoms. It can unblock stuck *chi* long before the problem manifests in actual illness.

When I was in my thirties, I was able to eliminate my menstrual cramps with acupuncture treatment. They have never returned. I have also referred patients for acupuncture who have had illnesses ranging from migraine headaches to chronic urinary tract infections. Acupuncture can help regulate menstrual periods, control heavy menstrual bleeding, stop seizures, and even in some cases help shrink fibroids. Research has shown that acupuncture improves cortisol balance in the body, enhances immune function, and helps quell addictions to cigarettes and alcohol.

Acupuncture works by redirecting the flow of *chi* along energy pathways in the body known as meridians. Because the meridians have no known anatomical counterparts, allopathic medicine dismissed acupuncture's effectiveness for years, until the presence of meridians was definitively demonstrated in a French study. Researchers injected a radioactive tracer into both traditional acupuncture points and into random sham points. The tracer that was injected into the genuine acupuncture points could easily be tracked as it ran up the meridians.[27] The clinical evidence of acupuncture's effectiveness has also become too compelling to ignore.

Start Somewhere

Don't let all these choices overwhelm you or become another heavy list of 'shoulds'. The wisdom in nature is user-friendly, and you have a lot of it within you already. To tap in to it, just pick the herb, the formula, or the foods that seem to jump out at you and say 'Try me'. Because all of the herbs and foods I've mentioned contain phytohormones of some kind and have virtually no side effects, feel free to experiment.

SEVEN

The Menopause Food Plan:
A Programme to Balance Your Hormones and Prevent Middle-age Spread

*O*ver the years, countless women in their late thirties or forties have come to me with one or more of the following complaints: 'Where did this spare tyre around my middle come from?' 'Why can't I lose that last 5 to 10lb I used to be able to shed within a few weeks?' 'Why is it that although I weigh the same as I did at college, my body seems different?'

Some women find themselves gaining weight at midlife even if they are eating no more than before. Others simply change shape: their waistlines thicken, and fat accumulates on their abdomen, flanks, and shoulders. Most of us have to make changes in our diets and exercise regimens if we expect to negotiate menopause without 10 to 20lb or so of extra baggage, weight that, in addition to wreaking havoc with our appearance, is also a well-documented health risk.[1]

The underlying reason for these changes is that midlife women experience a slowdown in metabolic rate of about 10–15 per cent compared to earlier in life. Our bodies also become more efficient at taking energy into our cells and storing it in the form of fat.[2] In addition, as oestrogen levels fall, our appetite increases.[3] Nature designed this for two reasons: to allow us to survive on less food as we get older and, in some cases, less able to fend for ourselves; and to assist us in putting on a supply of body fat that can produce the oestrogen and androgens our ovaries are no longer producing at the same rate.

If we were still living the hunter–gatherer lifestyle that our genes evolved to support, these midlife metabolic changes wouldn't be a problem. But in a culture where we are constantly told, 'You can't be too rich or too thin', nature's midlife metabolic slowdown is simply not welcome.

Thankfully, there are ways to negotiate these metabolic shifts and rebalance your hormones without any significant weight or fat gain. I know this path from the inside out, not only professionally but also personally.

Making Peace (Once Again) with My Weight

My weight has been an issue for me since I was twelve years old, when I went on my first diet. In my teens and early twenties I was always trying to weigh 10 to 20lb less than I should have, given my rather sturdy frame and large muscles. (No one understood at that time that weight could be a very misleading measure of health.) Throughout my teens, I struggled to weigh 8 stone (52kg), a weight I achieved only for a month or so when I starved myself in college. In my twenties, I ran regularly and was able to maintain my weight at around 9 stone (56kg) with a great deal of effort, which included fighting constant cravings for sweets.

After my pregnancies I, like so many other women, was never able to get my weight back to 9 stone (56kg) no matter what I did. I had run headlong into another aspect of Mother Nature's wisdom, which has set up postpartum weight gain so that we new mothers will be likely to stay alive during lean times to nurse and care for our children.

In my thirties, after I had breast-fed my two daughters for a total of nearly four years, my weight stabilised at around 10 stone (63kg). During these years I added weight training to my fitness regimen, and I figured that my weight gain was as much muscle as fat. (Muscle weighs more than fat, but it also burns calories far more efficiently.)

Finally, in my early forties, I came to a place of peace with my weight and size, even though my skeleton will never be a size 8! Through careful attention to my diet – which has consisted mostly of whole foods, healthy fats, lots of fruits and vegetables, and lean protein – and consistent exercise including weight training, I managed to maintain my body fat percentage at a healthy 25 per cent and my weight at about 10 stone (63kg), plus or minus (mostly plus) a few pounds. Yes, it still would have been nice to lose 5 to 10lb, but I wasn't willing to change my lifestyle further – or give up my regular, though modest, servings of chocolate brownies or pie – to lose them.

My Metabolism Takes On a Life of Its Own

A month or so after becoming fifty – about the time my periods became irregular – I began, inexplicably, to gain weight. Every day the scales showed another pound, even though I wasn't eating or exercising any differently. I was horrified. Yes, horrified. Lest you think that this is too strong a word, let me explain. I have the kind of body shape and metabolic rate that could very easily lead to obesity if I were not so disciplined about my diet and exercise routine. There was an upper limit on the scale beyond which I would not allow myself to go, and that number was 10 stone 4lb (65kg). But now I stood by helplessly and – in the space of a few weeks – watched the scales climb to 10 stone 9lb (67kg), 1lb less than I had weighed at the end of my pregnancy with my first daughter!

I knew that a new plan of action was called for. But what should it be? I'd been so sure I'd finally won the battle of the bulge and found a comfortable way to eat that would work for me for life.

Ketosis and Me

For the last seven or eight years I have recommended and followed the low-carbohydrate, relatively high-protein dietary approach advocated by Drs Mary Dan Eades and Michael Eades in their book *Protein Power.* But this time I decided to try a more extreme form of carbohydrate restriction. I went out and bought a copy of *Dr Atkins' New Diet Revolution.* The cover said two million copies had been sold; could that many people be completely wrong?[4] In any case, given the connection between carbohydrates, insulin, and weight gain (which I will discuss in more detail below), Atkins's research and clinical expertise made sense to me.[5]

I had also researched ketosis, the metabolic state that results when you cut down carbohydrates enough to begin burning body fat for fuel. Although critics cite ketosis as a danger of high-protein diets, I knew that this metabolic state was safe for people with no kidney problems, at least for the limited amount of time recommended by Atkins and quite probably for much longer periods. More than that, it appeared to be associated with consistent and relatively fast weight loss.

I decided to follow the Atkins 'induction' diet to the letter for at least fourteen days. I bought some urine testing strips at the chemist to test for ketosis. (Ketone bodies, which result from the breakdown of body fat, are excreted in the urine and can be easily tested for at home.) According to Atkins, the presence of ketones in the urine is a virtual guarantee that you're burning fat for energy. Then I cut my carbohydrate intake to less than 20g per day, a level of restriction I'd never tried before.

According to Atkins, the vast majority of people reach a state of ketosis within forty-eight hours. That is how long it takes their liver's glycogen stores to be depleted so that the body begins to use its fat for energy. So I cut the carbohydrates, waited forty-eight hours, and then began to test my urine two to three times every day. Nothing. The strips didn't turn purple. Though I actually felt good and had a lot of energy, I didn't go into ketosis until I began to add relatively high doses of the supplement L-carnitine.

After a full ten days of carbohydrate restriction, I managed to produce just a little bit of ketosis – the urine strips measured 'trace'. But even then I failed to lose weight or inches. In fact, I put on 3lb on the induction part of the Atkins diet. I had now plateaued to a new high. Talk about frustration! Here I was, exercising regularly, eating a very limited amount of carbohydrates, keeping the rest of my food portions normal, and following a diet that has helped millions lose weight. But it didn't work for me. Like many other perimenopausal women, I had hit a metabolic wall; our midlife bodies hold on to fat for dear life.

As a result of my experience, I did more research, talked to more experts, and continued on my quest to solve my weight dilemma. Within four months, I got back down to 10 stone (63kg) again.

The following programme is based on my own experience, reports from thousands of my newsletter subscribers, and many of my patients. It is designed to help you tame your midlife fat cells, balance your hormones, and safeguard your health on all levels.

Five Steps to Midlife Weight Control

Step One: Measure for Health – Waist/Hip Ratio, Body Mass Index, and Body Fat Percentage

Midlife weight gain is not necessarily a health risk. In fact, those extra pounds we gain at perimenopause often go away once we get past menopause, when our metabolism restabilises.

However, the hormone shifts of menopause also predispose us to central obesity (excess belly fat), which *is* a problem. Abdominal fat cells are more metabolically active – and potentially more dangerous – than the fat cells on your hips and thighs. They can contribute to insulin resistance, a metabolic condition in which your body has to secrete more and more insulin to clear the sugar out of the blood.

And they can pump out too much androgens and oestrogen. The classic apple-shaped figure is associated with an increased risk for heart disease, breast cancer, uterine cancer, diabetes, kidney stones, hypertension, arthritis, incontinence, polycystic ovary disease, urinary stress incontinence, gallstones, stroke, and sleep apnea.[6]

Your waist/hip ratio is a quick way to gauge your risk. Measure around the fullest part of your buttocks. Then measure your waist at the narrowest part of your torso. Divide your waist measurement by your hip measurement. A healthy ratio is less than 0.8. The ideal is 0.74. A ratio greater than 0.85 is associated with all the health risks listed above.[7]

The body mass index (BMI) is another way to measure your health risk. To determine your BMI, simply find your weight and your height on the table on the following page. A BMI of 24 or below is ideal. Higher BMIs are associated with an increased risk of diseases of all kinds. The jury is still out about how much additional risk is associated with a slightly elevated BMI, in the range of 25–29.

Percentage of body fat is the final number you'll need. This can be measured by your doctor or at a health club. Though it's possible to purchase over-the-counter devices that measure body fat, I have not found them to be very accurate. It is possible to have a healthy body fat percentage (between 20 and 28 per cent for women) and have a BMI that is higher than 24. This is especially true in athletes who have a great deal of muscle mass.

If your waist/hip ratio, BMI, and body fat percentage are all in the healthy range, then you simply have to fine-tune what you are already doing to maintain your weight and balance your hormones. If not, then do whatever you can to lower your risk. A 1999 study from Harvard Medical School in the US found that women who put on approximately 20lb in adulthood experience a decline in physical function and vitality even greater than that associated with smoking. Weight gain was also associated with an increase in bodily pain, regardless of a woman's baseline weight. Happily, this is all reversible. Once the overweight women lost weight, all characteristics of health and vitality improved.[8] This is very good news. You don't have to reach your ideal weight; even a modest 5 or 10lb fat loss – or achieving

FIGURE 11: BODY MASS INDEX CHART

Weight in Stone and Pounds

Height (Feet and Inches)

	5'0"	5'1"	5'2"	5'3"	5'4"	5'5"	5'6"	5'7"	5'8"	5'9"	5'10"	5'11"	6'0"	6'1"	6'2"	6'3"	6'4"
7 2	20	19	18	18	17	17	16	16	15	15	14	14	14	13	13	12	12
7 7	21	20	19	19	18	17	17	16	16	16	15	15	14	14	13	13	13
7 12	21	21	20	19	19	18	18	17	17	16	16	15	15	15	14	14	13
8 3	22	22	21	20	20	19	19	18	17	17	17	16	16	15	15	14	14
8 8	23	23	22	21	21	20	19	19	18	18	17	17	16	16	15	15	15
8 13	24	24	23	22	21	21	20	20	19	18	18	17	17	16	16	16	15
9 4	25	25	24	23	22	22	21	20	20	19	19	18	18	17	17	16	16
9 9	26	26	25	24	23	22	22	21	21	20	19	19	18	18	17	17	16
10 –	27	26	26	25	24	23	23	22	21	21	20	20	19	18	18	17	17
10 5	28	27	27	26	25	24	23	23	22	21	21	20	20	19	19	18	18
10 10	29	28	27	27	26	25	24	23	23	22	22	21	20	20	19	19	18
11 1	30	29	28	27	27	26	25	24	24	23	22	22	21	20	20	19	19
11 6	31	30	29	28	27	27	26	25	24	24	23	22	22	21	21	20	19
11 11	32	31	30	29	28	27	27	26	25	24	24	23	22	22	21	21	20
12 2	33	32	31	30	29	28	27	27	26	25	24	24	23	22	22	21	21
12 7	34	33	32	31	30	29	28	27	27	26	25	24	24	23	22	22	21
12 12	35	34	33	32	31	30	29	28	27	27	26	25	24	24	23	22	22
13 3	36	35	34	33	32	31	30	29	28	27	27	26	25	24	24	23	23
13 8	37	36	35	34	33	32	31	30	29	28	27	26	26	25	24	24	23
13 13	38	37	36	35	33	32	31	31	30	29	28	27	26	26	25	24	24
14 4	39	38	37	35	34	33	32	31	30	30	29	28	27	26	26	25	24
14 9	40	39	37	36	35	34	33	32	31	30	29	29	28	27	26	26	25
15 –	41	40	38	37	36	35	34	33	32	31	30	29	28	28	27	26	26
15 5	42	41	39	38	37	36	35	34	33	32	31	30	29	28	28	27	26
15 10	43	42	40	39	38	37	36	34	33	32	32	31	30	29	28	27	27
16 1	44	43	41	40	39	37	36	35	34	33	32	31	31	30	29	28	27
16 6	45	43	42	41	39	38	37	36	35	34	33	32	31	30	30	29	28
16 11	46	44	43	42	40	39	38	37	36	35	34	33	32	31	30	29	29
17 2	47	45	44	43	41	40	39	38	36	35	34	33	33	32	31	30	29
17 7	48	46	45	43	42	41	40	38	37	36	35	34	33	32	31	31	30
17 12	49	47	46	44	43	42	40	39	38	37	36	35	34	33	32	31	30

☐ Underweight ▧ Weight Appropriate ☐ Overweight ■ Obese

a BMI that is one number lower than your current number – can dramatically improve your health, lower blood pressure, and balance your hormone levels.

Step Two: Test Your Metabolic Stressors

In her book *Fight Fat After Forty* (Piatkus), Dr Pamela Peek, a researcher with the US National Institutes of Health, documents the connection between toxic stress and toxic weight gain – the kind of weight that accumulates in the abdomen and puts women at risk of premature death. Toxic stress can come from any daily challenge, but a number of circumstances make it especially common in women over forty: the resurfacing of childhood trauma, perfectionism, relationship changes such as divorce and caregiving, job stress, acute or chronic illness, dieting, and the effects of menopause.

This explanation clicked with me because initial perimenopausal weight gain coincided with new stresses in my life. The scales started to climb just before the Christmas holidays, when my older daughter arrived home for her first holiday from college and we officially launched our first Christmas season as a 'broken' family. My daughters were scheduled to split their holiday time between my house and their father's, a situation I had always been sure would never happen to us.

I was also caring full time for my best friend, who was recovering from major spine surgery. I was preparing her meals, trying to anticipate her needs, watching her go through excruciating pain unrelieved by narcotics, and generally trying to provide a safe place where she could heal. For well over a month I was basically on call twenty-four hours per day, with only an occasional break. In retrospect, no wonder the pounds piled on.

Get out your calendar, do some detective work, and see if you, too, have a stress pattern that could be leading to weight gain. Be particularly aware of the danger of the late afternoon hours when the main hormones that allow us to mount a response against stress – serotonin and cortisol – tend to fall, leaving us feeling more vulnerable to our underlying emotions. In particular, when serotonin, the 'feel-good' neurotransmitter, is depleted, we are apt to eat anything in sight – particularly refined carbohydrates – to bring it back to normal.

The effect of stress on weight also works in the opposite direction. One of my perimenopausal physician colleagues recently went on a trip with one of her grown-up children, who is at medical school. They went to a stimulating medical meeting and then explored the Grand Canyon together. Though she paid no attention to her diet and ate whatever she wanted, she arrived home 6lb lighter! She told me, 'I think that my cortisol levels returned to normal because for ten days I got to sleep through the night and not worry about being called in for an emergency. And besides that, my serotonin was up from all the exciting conversation and healthy sunshine I was getting!'

Step Three: Exercise

If you don't already exercise, there is no time like the present to start. Your muscles are loaded with insulin receptors. The more muscle mass you have and the more heat you generate from your muscles on a regular basis, the more efficiently you'll burn carbohydrates and body fat. You'll also be protecting your bones and your heart. In fact, of all the lifestyle changes that best predict permanent weight loss, regular exercise is number one. I recommend at least thirty minutes of sustained exercise at least five times per week.

If you already exercise, change your routine. Perhaps you've found yourself, like me, stuck at a metabolic roadblock, even though you've already cut back on carbohydrates and are exercising regularly. When this happens, it is usually because your body has adjusted to your current level of activity – just as it's possible to maintain your weight on as little as 1,000 calories per day – the body's metabolic rate simply decreases to accommodate its perception of starvation.

In order to get your stubborn fat cells to release their load, you have to confuse them a little. Try a different exercise routine that recruits other muscles. If you've been walking, try a stair-stepper, an elliptical trainer, weight training, or a cross-country ski machine. The idea is to get your body out of its metabolic rut.

I personally had to increase the intensity and length of my weight-training sessions while cutting back on my walking – something that had become so easy I barely even broke a sweat. The weight workouts were much harder. Over time this switch worked.

Step Four: Get Your Thyroid Checked

About 25 per cent of women develop or have pre-existing thyroid problems by the time they reach perimenopause. Low thyroid function is associated with a decreased metabolic rate. If you have any symptoms of thyroid problems (fatigue, weight gain, cold hands and feet, thinning hair, or constipation), get your thyroid checked. I finally did this during my own metabolic slowdown and found out that my thyroid hormone levels were consistent with what is known as subclinical hypothyroidism. I had no symptoms other than the weight gain. I started on a very low dose of thyroid hormones – levothyroxine (T_4) and triiodothyronine (T_3) – which I may or may not have to continue. (Though most doctors prescribe only levothyroxine, many women do better on a combination of T_3 and T_4.) Like any medication decision, I'm taking this month by month. My blood tests are back to normal. It's difficult to say whether the thyroid hormone replacement is what finally turned my weight gain around, because I also changed my exercise routine and cut down on all refined carbohydrates. In addition, the stress I was under decreased dramatically when the holidays ended and my friend recovered fully.

Step Five: Eat Foods That Normalise Insulin and Blood Sugar Levels and Balance Hormones

All perimenopausal women should follow a diet, supplement, and exercise programme aimed at modulating excess oestrogen. This is crucial for those with symptoms of oestrogen dominance such as fibroids, painful breasts, or heavy bleeding.

The standard Western diet almost guarantees some kind of oestrogen dominance or hormone imbalance because it is high in simple (or refined) sugars and starches, the wrong kinds of fats, and low-fibre, nutrient-poor fast foods.

The dietary approach I'll outline below addresses three interlinked hormonal conditions that are very common during perimenopause: 1) too much insulin, leading to insulin resistance; 2) too much oestrogen and not enough progesterone; and 3) an imbalance of the regulatory substances known as eicosanoids.

The Elements of Imbalance

Before I get to the specifics of my programme, I'd like to give you a quick overview of the basic science underlying this approach, so you see how all the elements fit together.

Insulin Resistance

Insulin is produced in the pancreas and is responsible for ferrying glucose from the bloodstream into our cells, where it is used for fuel.

Good health depends upon our body's ability to make and utilise just the right amount of insulin to keep our blood sugar at optimal levels and our metabolism working normally. Consumption of refined carbohydrates results in an immediate surge in blood sugar. This triggers the pancreas to secrete large amounts of insulin to process the blood sugar. Every cell in the body has insulin receptors on the surface. These allow insulin to 'open the door', so that glucose can enter the cell.[9] But over time, when blood sugar levels continue to be too high, the insulin receptors lose their ability to respond to this abnormal metabolic burden. They become insensitive, and a condition known as insulin resistance develops, in which more and more insulin is poured out, to less and less effect. Eventually neither the body tissues nor the pancreas can keep up with the blood sugar load. Virtually every cell in our bodies is adversely affected by this abnormal metabolic state. In severe cases, an individual with this condition may be diagnosed with type 2 diabetes and require insulin injections to meet the demand.

Obesity contributes to this problem. Body fat is loaded with insulin receptors, and the fatter you get, the more insulin it takes to get blood sugar into the cells. Type 2 diabetes will often disappear simply with weight loss alone.

About 25 per cent of the population appears to be genetically resistant to the adverse effects of overproduction of insulin and insulin resistance. These individuals usually manage to stay very slim no matter what they eat. But 75 per cent of the population is not so lucky, especially during perimenopause. As women age, they tend towards decreased total muscle mass and increased body fat – regardless of body weight. This is a set-up for insulin resistance and for the myriad health and hormonal problems associated with it. Any woman who experienced gestational diabetes when pregnant is also at greater risk for insulin resistance and syndrome X (see box) during perimenopause.

Most perimenopausal symptoms, such as heavy bleeding, cramps, fibroids, and PMS, will respond to a diet that keeps your blood sugar and insulin levels stable – a diet that will also keep your eicosanoids balanced. In general, insulin and blood sugar levels stay normal on a diet of unrefined whole foods that include carbohydrates with a low to moderate glycaemic index, such as fruits, vegetables, and whole grains. The glycaemic index is simply a measurement of the rate and degree to which a given carbohydrate-containing food raises blood sugar levels. High-glycaemic-index carbohydrates – including

Syndrome X

The medical conditions associated with insulin resistance are collectively known as syndrome X, a term first coined by Dr Gerald Reaven, a world-renowned endocrinologist at the Stanford University School of Medicine in the US.[10] They include:

- Increased risk for type 2 diabetes[11]

- Abnormal cholesterol levels[12]

- Hypertension

- Heart disease: coronary artery disease and peripheral vascular disease[13]

- Obesity

- Anovulation[14]

- Overstimulation of ovarian testosterone[15]

- Polycystic ovary disease

- Excess hair on the face, hair loss, or male pattern baldness in women

- Adult acne

- Increased risk for breast cancer and endometrial cancer[16]

alcohol, starchy and sugary foods such as biscuits, sweets, fizzy drinks, and white bread, and almost all refined, processed foods – are quickly metabolised into sugar, triggering a rush of insulin into the blood.

On the other hand, carbohydrates with a low glycaemic index break down slowly, raising blood sugar to relatively low levels over a longer period of time. This allows them to be metabolised with only a small amount of insulin.

Evolutionarily speaking, most of the high-glycaemic-index carbohydrates are 'new' foods that have been rapidly increasing in our diets only over the last century. Up until then, for millennia, our food supply and metabolism evolved side by side along with the active lifestyles that also keep insulin levels normal.

Oestrogen Dominance

A diet high in refined carbohydrates makes all perimenopausal problems worse because of its adverse effect on hormone balance. It reinforces the tendency toward central obesity (see page 194), which in turn favours production of oestrogen and androgens. Central obesity and high insulin levels – which can occur even in women of normal weight and BMI – are also associated with higher blood triglyceride levels. This, of course, has a negative effect on heart health, but it also interferes with the normal mechanism by which the body deactivates free oestradiol. A relative increase in the amount of metabolically active oestradiol in the bloodstream can target oestrogen-sensitive breast and endometrial tissue, resulting in possible excessive growth of these tissues. This is one of the reasons why hyperinsulinaemia with insulin resistance is a significant risk factor for breast cancer as well as polycystic ovary disease.[17] High insulin levels also increase tissue sensitivity to a protein known as insulin-like growth factor (IGF-1), which is known to stimulate the growth of breast and other tissues.[18]

Eicosanoid Imbalance

The typical Western diet can result in imbalances in a large, powerful group of cellular messengers known as eicosanoids. These hormone-like substances control virtually all the biochemical processes in your body, and your health depends on their balance. For example, too much of certain kinds – known as series 2 eicosanoids – and not enough of series 1 and 3 eicosanoids can result in inflammation, decreased oxygen availability in cells, and excessive blood clotting.

One of the best-known eicosanoids, prostaglandin F2-alpha, is implicated in menstrual cramps. Every medication for menstrual cramps on the market, from Ponstan to Fenopron, works by blocking the body's synthesis of excess amounts of prostaglandin F2-alpha. Another eicosanoid, interleukin-1, is also partly responsible for the inflammation in arthritis, which is blocked by aspirin and other NSAIDs.

Prostaglandins and other related eicosanoids, such as the prosta-cyclins, thromboxanes, and leukotrienes, regulate such diverse functions as blood pressure, blood clotting, inflammation of all kinds, the immune system, the sleep/wake cycle, uterine contractions during birth and during the menstrual cycle, the release of gastric acid in the stomach, and the dilation and constriction of blood vessels and of the airways in the lungs.

Although eicosanoids act very much like hormones, they are produced not in glands, which discharge their contents into the bloodstream, but instead inside the cells themselves, where they act and then vanish very quickly. Until the early 1980s scientists didn't have the sophisticated equipment necessary to measure them. This is why some doctors even today may not understand that imbalanced eicosanoids are the final common pathway for many disease processes. If you've ever had a headache, menstrual cramp, rash, or joint swelling and pain, you've felt the effect of imbalanced eicosanoids.

Fortunately, you usually do not need drugs to balance eicosanoids. Although eicosanoid levels are affected by virtually every aspect of our lives, including our emotions, the most powerful and practical way to achieve healthy eicosanoid balance is through your daily diet.

The number-one reason for imbalanced eicosanoids – and all the diseases and symptoms associated with them – is the standard Western diet, which has the following characteristics:

- Too many refined carbohydrates, resulting in the overproduction of insulin. Too much insulin favours the production of the pro-inflammatory eicosanoids, like prostaglandin F2-alpha and the cytokines.

- Deficiencies in the polyunsaturated fats known as omega-3 fats. Omega-3 fats are necessary for the function of nearly every cell in the body, particularly those of the nervous system, brain, eyes, and immune system. Omega-3 fats also favour the production of series 1 and 3 anti-inflammatory eicosanoids, which are necessary to balance the 'bad' series 2 eicosanoids. Currently levels of the especially important omega-3 fat DHA (docosahexaenoic acid) are 40 per cent lower, on average, in American women than in European women.

- Too many trans fats, usually from margarine. (See pages 213–14.) These block production of series 1 and 3 eicosanoids and favour the pro-inflammatory series 2 eicosanoids.

- Deficiencies in the micronutrients that are necessary for optimal eicosanoid metabolism. Too little vitamin C, vitamin B_6, and magnesium, for example, favour the overproduction of pro-inflammatory eicosanoids.

Unremitting stress is also a factor in eicosanoid imbalance. It results in the overproduction of adrenaline and cortisol, stress hormones that also favour the pro-inflammatory eicosanoids. Caffeine, which is often used to alleviate the effects of stress and fatigue, has the same effect.

FIGURE 12: THE HORMONAL BERMUDA TRIANGLE

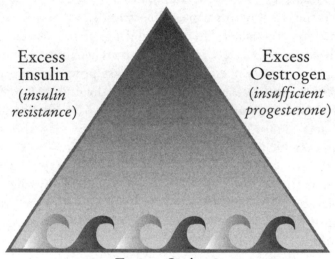

Excess
Insulin
(*insulin
resistance*)

Excess
Oestrogen
(*insufficient
progesterone*)

Excess Series 2
Eicosanoids
(*insufficient Series 1 and 3*)

During perimenopause, dietary factors and hormonal shifts can
produce three interlocking conditions as dangerous to our health as the
proverbial Bermuda Triangle is to planes and ships.
© 2001 by Northrup and Schulz

The Hormone-balancing Food Plan

Given the average lifestyle of today's perimenopausal women, it's not difficult to see why insulin, oestrogen, and the eicosanoids become unbalanced, putting us at increased risk for everything from heart disease and high blood pressure to arthritis and breast cancer. Fortunately, when you follow the food plan I suggest here, you won't have to wait long to feel better. In a matter of days, you'll probably notice that your sleep improves, you begin to lose excess fat, various troublesome symptoms begin to disappear, and your skin takes on a healthy glow. At the same time you'll be reducing your risk of the diseases of ageing.

To keep your blood sugar, eicosanoids, and hormones balanced, do the following:

Eat at Least Three Meals a Day

Many women skip both breakfast and lunch, saving up their calories until dinner. The problem with this approach is that the metabolic rate naturally peaks at noon and decreases after that. So the food you eat at night is far more likely to be stored as excess fat compared to the food eaten earlier in the day. Here's another reason why you can't afford to skip meals for weight control: it is well known that yo-yo dieting and periodic starvation lower your overall metabolic rate over time, resulting in a body that is so metabolically efficient that it is possible to remain at the same weight despite a very low calorie diet. That's why, when I faced my own midlife weight gain, severe calorie restriction was not an option. I had starved myself too many times in my teens and twenties, including fasting. I've always had a relatively slow metabolic rate, and now midlife was lowering it further. I couldn't risk another slowdown. It is also clear that severe food restriction often results in a decrease in beneficial lean body mass but not necessarily a decrease in body fat. That means that after severe food restriction, you might end up with a higher percentage of body fat than when you started.

Most perimenopausal women do best when they keep their blood sugar stable throughout the day by eating frequent, smaller meals. I highly recommend a snack at around 4 pm, right during the time when blood sugar, mood, and serotonin tend to plummet. This snack can keep you from overeating at night when you get home. (If you don't, you're apt to begin your evening meal the minute you get home and then end it when you go to bed, in a desperate attempt to make up for a full day's worth of deprivation.)

To negotiate the metabolic challenges of midlife successfully, you need to be patient. And you also need to rethink your 'diet' mentality. In other words, you need to think of your new metabolism as something that will require a new way of living and eating, not another quick-fix diet. (I certainly learned that when I tried the Atkins induction programme.)

Focus on Portion Size, Not Calories

Instead of calorie counting, concentrate on eating the highest-quality food available, in smaller portions. Cup your two hands in front of you. That's how big your stomach capacity is. Limit your intake to no more than that at each meal or snack. Overeating in general – regardless of the food – is associated with overproduction of insulin. Note that, in general, the food portions in US restaurants are much bigger than in Europe, which is one of the reasons Americans are so overweight compared to Europeans.

In order to keep my weight stable, I've had to cut down on my total food intake, eliminate grain products most of the time (see below), reduce my consumption of desserts to no more than once per week, make lunch the biggest meal of my day, eat very lightly at dinner, and increase my exercise time.

Eat Protein at Each Meal

That means eggs, fish, lean meat, dairy food, or a vegetarian alternative to animal protein, such as soya protein powder, whey protein powder, whole soya beans, tofu, or tempeh. Beans contain protein, but they also contain a considerable amount of carbohydrate. Though the carbohydrate in beans tends to be on the low end of the glycaemic index, beans can be too high in carbohydrate for some perimenopausal women. They work very well for others. You have to judge this for yourself.

Protein needs vary depending upon your size and physical activity. The bigger and the more active you are, the more you need. In general, if you have any tendency towards weight gain at midlife, your diet should be about 40 per cent protein, 35 per cent low-glycaemic-index carbohydrates, and 25 per cent fat. You don't have to adhere to this rigidly at every meal and snack, but it's an average to aim for over about a week's time.[19]

If you are at risk of any condition, including cancer, stimulated by excess oestrogen, you might want to increase your protein even more. Protein can actually decrease your risk. Here's how it works. When the liver, body fat, and ovaries metabolise oestrogen, they use an enzyme system known as cytochrome P450. A diet rich in protein increases the activity of the entire P450 system, thus helping to protect your body from overstimulation by oestrogen. In one study, for example, individuals who were fed a diet that contained 44 per cent protein, 35 per cent carbohydrates, and 21 per cent fat experienced a profound shift in their body's ability to deactivate excess oestrogen.[20]

Cut Down on Refined and High-Glycaemic-Index Carbohydrates, Including Alcohol

Remember, not all carbohydrates are created equal. One gram of carbohydrate from table sugar has a different metabolic effect than the same amount of carbohydrate from blueberries. This difference is measured, as explained earlier, by the glycaemic index, a number that indicates how high and how fast a given food will raise your blood sugar. White bread tops the scale with a glycaemic index of 100. Certain foods with a high glycaemic index, such as baked potatoes or bananas, can still be part of a healthy diet for some people, depending upon your unique metabolism.

Eliminate as many refined carbohydrates from your diet as possible. That means cutting out white rice and foods made with white flour, such as muffins, rolls, bagels, biscuits, French bread, bread sticks, crackers, snack foods, pretzels, and pasta. You also need to eliminate fizzy drinks, which are nothing but sugar water. An occasional diet drink is OK if you're not sensitive to aspartame. (See chapter 10.)

It also means eliminating or cutting back heavily on alcohol in every and any form, including wine spritzers, wine, beer, and spirits. Alcohol is nothing but sugar in a form that is so absorbable that its effects are felt within minutes in the brain. One of the first things women notice when they eliminate the empty calories found in alcohol is that they lose weight very quickly. Many also notice that their hot flushes go away as well. That's because alcohol significantly interferes with oestrogen metabolism and causes an almost immediate

If You Are a True Carbohydrate Addict

Women who grew up in alcoholic or chaotic family systems may have brain and body chemistry that is overly sensitive to the effects of food, and particularly to the neurochemical known as serotonin. Serotonin is released in the brain quite rapidly when you eat refined-carbohydrate-rich foods such as most breakfast cereals or biscuits. True carbohydrate addicts cannot stop after eating a few biscuits or potato crisps. They don't seem to have a normal satiety mechanism in place. If this describes you, I recommend consulting one of the following books:

The Carbohydrate Addict's Lifespan Program: A Personalized Plan for Becoming Slim, Fit, and Healthy in your 40s, 50s, and 60s and Beyond, Richard F. Heller and Rachael F. Heller (Plume Books, 1998)

Potatoes, Not Prozac, Kathleen DesMaisons (Simon & Schuster, 1999)

The Sugar Addict's Total Recovery Program, Kathleen DesMaisons (Ballantine Books, 2000)

hormonal imbalance, with too much oestrogen in the blood relative to progesterone.

You also need to eliminate or cut back strongly on sweet things: sweets, biscuits, cakes, pastries, and ice cream. You may still want to have them on special occasions, but as your blood sugar and eicosanoids become balanced, you'll find that your craving for these foods will decrease dramatically and you won't like the way you feel after eating them.

Remember, your body will be able to burn stored fat and keep your insulin and blood sugar levels normal only when you don't eat or drink excessive amounts of the wrong kinds of carbohydrates. Otherwise excess blood sugar will be stored as fat, which will accumulate not just on your hips but also in other places, like your arteries and in your heart and brain.

The challenge here is to find the amount and type of carbohydrate intake that allows you to either maintain or lose weight. Some individuals can eat as many as 300g of carbohydrates a day and not put on weight. Others, myself included, have to keep that number much lower. This is an individual matter and also varies with stress levels. The type of carbohydrate consumed also matters. You may be able to consume up to 200g of carbohydrates per day from beans, rice, vegetables, and fruits, for example, and either maintain or lose weight. But if you consume those same 200g in the form of biscuits and cake and alcohol, you'll gain weight.

Consume Grain Products with Caution

Even if you have eliminated refined grains in all forms, you can still get into trouble with whole wheat, whole rye, whole oat, or millet flour. A fascinating line of research now suggests that the degenerative diseases that currently plague the human race didn't arrive on the scene until agriculture became widespread. Paleoarchaeological studies show that many of the ancient Egyptians were fat and had dental caries – diseases associated with a grain-based diet and virtually absent in hunter-gatherers.

Many carbohydrate-sensitive individuals find that eating grain products triggers binge eating. I've certainly seen this happen with brown rice – a 'health food' that I used to consume regularly but have had to virtually eliminate. I've also had to eliminate nearly all whole-grain bread products, even the unleavened ones. (One line of thinking suggests that yeast bread is difficult to digest because of the potential for yeast overgrowth in the intestines. Unleavened bread is better tolerated by many, but not everyone. Even a whole-wheat unleavened tortilla wrap sandwich at lunch makes me feel groggy and bloated these days.) Looking back, I can see that eating too much bread has been a problem with me for years. But at perimenopause, my body finally said 'Enough!'

Eat a Wide Variety of Fresh Fruits and Vegetables Daily

You need to aim for at least five servings a day, but it's easy, at least in the summer, to get in more. Remember that a serving is small, as little as 100g in many cases. The healthiest fruits and vegetables are the ones that are the most colourful. That's because the pigments in these foods, such as the carotenes or carotenoids, are very powerful antioxidants. Go for broccoli; red, yellow, and green peppers; dark green leafy

How to Quell Your Sugar Cravings

While you're changing to a diet that is lower in sugar, you can help balance your brain biochemistry and quell your sweet cravings simultaneously by taking the amino acid L-glutamine, which appears to help prevent the mental fatigue that can result from sugar withdrawal. (Take 1g per day with lunch, or see Resources for other products.) Some research also suggests that L-glutamine helps alcoholics avoid alcohol—the ultimate sugar buzz.[21]

Artificially sweetened products may also help with sugar cravings. The sweeteners I like the best are acesulfame potassium and stevia. Acesulfame is in the same general chemical category as saccharin, but so far, at least, there are no data to suggest any adverse effects. Since acesulfame is stable when heated or in liquid form, it can be used in cooking or to sweeten coffee or tea. Stevia is a natural sweetener made from an extract of the leaves of the South American plant *Stevia rebaudiana*. It is usually sold in US health food shops as either a liquid or powdered leaves, and it tastes bitter if you use too much. Stevia is also stable in liquid or when heated. (Stevia is not available in the UK – see Resources for US suppliers.) Though I feel that some other artificial sweeteners are quite safe, they have not yet stood the test of time. It's probably best to use them sparingly.

A variety of other very satisfying low-carbohydrate products are also available that can help you switch to a healthier diet without feeling deprived. Some women find that using artificial sweeteners results in an increase in food binges. I haven't found this to be true for me. Though some authorities suggest that we should eliminate all artificial sweeteners, I'm not ready to do that and may never be. In any case, I know they're far healthier than the biscuits and other desserts I used to consume regularly.

vegetables such as kale and spinach; and tomatoes. Pigment-rich blueberries have been found to have the highest concentration of antioxidants compared to forty other fruits and vegetables.

Studies suggest that the carotenoid content of tissue may be the most significant factor in determining life span in primates, including humans.[22] Though beta-carotene (the vitamin A precursor found in carrots, other yellow-orange vegetables, and dark leafy greens) has received the most attention and is the carotenoid most commonly found in multivitamins, other carotenes that have little or no vitamin A–type activity exert much greater antioxidant protection. Alpha-carotene (usually found in the same foods as beta-carotene) is approximately 38 per cent stronger as an antioxidant and ten times more effective in suppressing liver, skin, and lung cancer in animals.[23] Even more powerful is lycopene, the red pigment found in tomatoes. Some US studies have shown a 50 per cent reduction for all cancers among elderly people reporting a high tomato intake.[24] Food processing doesn't destroy lycopene, so tomato juice and canned tomato products also offer protection.

Every day the list of benefits from the natural antioxidants found in pigment-rich foods grows. They help balance hormones, protect the skin from sun damage, keep the skin and eyes radiant, maintain the lining of the blood vessels, and help prevent varicose veins. They also boost the immune system and help the body resist cancer and other degenerative diseases.

In addition to being good sources of cholesterol-lowering fibre, fruits and vegetables are also good sources of lignans, which are meta-bolised into phytohormones that help balance hormones and metabolise excess oestrogen. Linseed is by far the richest source of lignans and is also very rich in essential omega-3 fats (see pages 184–6).

High-glycaemic-index fruits and vegetables such as potatoes, sweetcorn, and bananas have a lot of nutrients in them, though their antioxidant content isn't as rich as that of the foods I've mentioned previously. You don't have to eliminate them completely. Just remember that the more processed they are, the higher their glycaemic index. A baked potato is an entirely different food from a potato crisp or chip, and it is far healthier. And fresh corn on the cob in season is a better choice than canned sweetcorn, which is often processed with added sugar in the form of corn syrup. Though fresh vegetables are always the best choice, research has shown that even canned and frozen varieties still contain many nutrients.

What Should I Drink?

The answer is water, pure and simple. Too many women avoid water in the mistaken belief that they will put on weight if they drink too much. Then they end up dehydrated, and it shows in their skin. In fact, you need lots of water to help your body eliminate the breakdown products of fat if you are trying to lose weight.

If you don't like the plain flat kind, go for designer waters with lime or another flavour. Iced tea is another healthy choice. I keep a jug of decaffeinated green tea in the refrigerator at all times. It's loaded with antioxidants, and it contains phytohormones that have been shown to build bone. You can also drink diluted fruit juice occasionally (watch the carbohydrates – it's easy to drink too many). It's nice mixed half and half with sparkling water and is a good alternative to a cocktail. An occasional caffeine-free diet drink won't hurt unless you are sensitive to aspartame.

Eat Healthy Fats Each Day

Over the past two decades we've gone overboard with the low-fat approach to diet. As the population has substituted carbohydrates for a moderate amount of healthy fat, we've simply become fatter and fatter.

Back in the 1980s and early 1990s, when the low-fat craze reached its peak, I watched patient after patient come in complaining of sallow skin, brittle fingernails, weight gain, difficulty fighting infections, inability to concentrate, and fatigue. None of these women was getting enough healthy fat in their diets, having been brainwashed into thinking that all fat was the enemy. Now we know differently.

Essential fatty acids (EFAs) are indispensable for human development and health. Our bodies cannot synthesise EFAs, so we need to consume them in our foods. There are two essential types of EFAs: omega-6 fats and omega-3 fats. Omega-6 fats occur in relative abundance in the foods we eat. However, the current Western diet is woefully deficient in omega-3 fats. This is partially a result of our food choices, with trans fats and refined carbohydrates often displacing omega-3 fats. In addition, because of agricultural practices, the fats in eggs and meat do not contain nearly the percentage of omega-3 fats that they used to. Farm animals raised on wild grasses instead of grain have a healthier, leaner body composition. Animals, like humans, get fat on diets composed mostly of grain, especially if they aren't allowed to roam.

Omega-3 deficiency often begins in utero, when our only source of these fats is our mothers, who are likely to be deficient in them already. Ideally, the omega-3 fats, particularly a fat known as DHA, are found abundantly in human breast milk, but DHA is absent in most baby formulas used in the West. Research is rapidly accumulating that implicates DHA deficiency in the epidemic of attention deficit disorder in both children and adults. This essential fat is also one of the reasons why children who were breast-fed as infants have been found to have higher IQs than formula-fed babies.[25] Gratifying improvements in learning ability and mood stabilisation have resulted when both children and adults have had their diets supplemented with omega-3 fats.

In addition to their role in nervous system and brain function, omega-3 fats also favour the production of series 1 and 3 eicosanoids, thus limiting the production of the pro-inflammatory series 2 eicosanoids. It's not surprising, then, that supplementing the diet with omega-3 fats in either foods or pills has been shown to alleviate conditions associated with eicosanoid imbalance, including arthritis, PMS, eczema, breast tenderness, acne, diabetes, brittle fingernails, thinning and brittle hair, psoriasis, dry skin, and the sex hormone imbalance so common during perimenopause.

Good sources of omega-3 fats include pumpkin seeds, sunflower seeds, linseed or linseed oil, organ meats (eg liver and kidney), cold-water fish or fish oil supplements, and docosahexaenoic acid (DHA) supplements. Nuts are also a good source, and they make a very satisfying low-carbohydrate snack – I take them to films instead of high-carbohydrate popcorn. Just make sure you enjoy them in moderation – no more than a handful once or twice per day.

TRANS FATS: THE BAD ACTORS OF THE FAT WORLD
The most dangerous fats by far are the trans fats – the partially hydrogenated fats and oils that aren't found anywhere in nature. They are present in margarine, which is made by blowing hydrogen into liquid

vegetable oil at very high temperatures and pressures. Trans fats contribute directly to the overproduction of pro-inflammatory eicosanoids and have therefore been found to contribute to the development of cancer and heart disease.

Unfortunately, trans fats are added to just about every type of packaged baked good because they don't get rancid nearly as quickly as unprocessed fats. This prolongs the shelf life of the product. Since such products are also invariably high in refined carbohydrates, it's best to simply eliminate them from your life. (If you have them once in a while, pray over them first.)

SATURATED FAT: AN OVERRATED THREAT

I don't feel that saturated fat is the culprit we've made it out to be as far as heart disease is concerned. If you're following a diet that keeps your insulin and blood sugar levels normal, then saturated fat isn't likely to become a problem. After all, the epidemic of heart disease didn't start in the West until margarine – which is a trans fat, not a saturated fat – was added to the diet back in the 1940s. Before that, lard and butter were widely used, and heart disease was rare. Studies of the Atkins diet, which can be high in saturated fat, have shown that it doesn't appear to contribute to cholesterol and heart problems. Some women, however, are sensitive to the arachidonic acid found in dairy foods, eggs, and beef. It contributes to a larger amount of series 2 eicosanoids in these individuals, and they suffer from menstrual cramps and arthritis when they eat these foods. The symptoms go away when they eliminate these foods. Other women have no problem. As with all things, I'd suggest that you enjoy saturated fat in moderation.

You don't have to count fat grams if you are keeping your carbo-hydrate level relatively low. In the absence of excess insulin, it appears that fat in your diet is not stored as fat. But the minute that fat is combined with sugar or starch – as in a doughnut, for example – the pounds pile on!

COOKING AND SALAD OILS

Most salad and cooking oils contain omega-6 fats, and since an excess of omega-6 fats can lead to the overproduction of pro-inflammatory eicosanoids, I suggest that you limit their use. Substitute linseed oil or olive oil whenever possible. (Olive oil is a monounsaturated omega-9 fat with metabolic effects that are neutral when it comes to eicosanoid

Educate Yourself

All of the following books contain meal plans and recipes that have helped thousands of women lose or maintain their weight. All of them will balance hormones as well as insulin and eicosanoid levels. I recommend that you go to a library or your local bookshop and look through a few of them. Then choose the one that speaks to you.

Protein Power, Michael R. Eades and Mary Dan Eades (Thorsons, 2000).

The Protein Power Lifeplan, Michael R. Eades and Mary Dan Eades (Warner Books, Inc., 2000).

Recipes for Change: Gourmet Wholefood Cooking for Health and Vitality at Menopause, Lissa DeAngelis and Molly Siple (Plume Books, 1998).

Sugar Busters: Cut Sugar to Trim Fat, H. Leighton Steward, Morrison Bethea, Sam Andrews, and Luis A. Balart (Vermilion, 1998).

Syndrome X: Overcoming the Silent Killer That Can Give You a Heart Attack, Gerald Reaven (Simon & Schuster, 2000).

The Glucose Revolution: The Authoritative Guide to the Glycemic Index, Jennie Brand-Miller, Thomas Wolever, Stephen Colagiuri, and Kaye Foster-Powell (Hodder & Stoughton, 2000).

Eating Well for Optimum Health: The Essential Guide to Food, Diet, and Nutrition, Andrew Weil (Little, Brown & Company, 2000).

Dr Atkins' New Diet Revolution, Robert C. Atkins (Vermilion, 1999).

balance.) You can also use a little clarified butter – also known as ghee – for cooking, since it won't burn. My favourite salad dressing is made by mixing a little balsamic vinegar with some high-quality olive oil. For variety, try light sesame or nut oils.

Stoke Up Your Metabolic Fat and Carbohydrate Burners

We all have two metabolic 'burner systems' in our bodies – one for fat and one for carbohydrates. We need to make sure that the pilot lights on both of these are lit, so to speak.

Let's start with the internal fat burners within our cells – the mitochondria. When you eat fat with low-glycaemic-index carbohydrates or with no carbohydrates at the same meal, your body will not secrete much insulin. As a result, the fat you eat will not be stored in the body as fat – unless your body is overproducing insulin because of the effects of stress or an excess of food.[26] However, if you consume fat along with high-glycaemic-index carbohydrates, your insulin levels soar and the consumed fat is stored as fat. This is why it's always wise to eat high-glycaemic-index carbohydrates without fat, limit portion size, and eat when relaxed and happy. When you eat fat without insulin present, your body will break down either the fat you eat or the fat on your hips into molecules known as fatty acids. These fatty acids get taken into the mitochondria, where they are broken down further into chemicals known as ketones.

Fatty acids cannot get into the mitochondrial furnace, however, without the help of a substance known as L-carnitine. L-carnitine also helps prevent toxic fatty acid metabolites from building up in the heart, substances that can set the scene for angina and arrhythmia. L-carnitine is manufactured in the body and is also found in some red meats and some leafy vegetables. For reasons that are not entirely clear, some individuals don't seem to make enough L-carnitine to burn their fat effectively. With my family history, I've started to take this nutrient daily, both to help me burn fat and to protect my heart. (See also chapter 14, 'Living with Heart, Passion, and Joy'.) The usual dose of L-carnitine is 500–2,000mg per day.

The mineral chromium has been shown to make insulin receptors more sensitive, helping you to burn carbohydrates more efficiently. It also helps to regulate the number of insulin receptors on the cell membrane. Many Westerners has low levels of chromium because of soil depletion and a diet too high in refined foods. But it's easy to supplement in your diet. Take either chromium polynicotinate or picolinate. The dose to take for a weight problem is 200–700mcg per day.

A number of other nutrients, such as green tea, coenzyme Q_{10}, and alpha-lipoic acid, have also been shown to be helpful for fat burning. Unfortunately, much of the research showing their effectiveness has been done on men, and it's difficult to assess their value for peri-menopausal women. It certainly cannot hurt to try them, since they help in other important ways. Their antioxidant activity, for example, is well documented.[27]

Protect Yourself with Antioxidants

Every day, more and more research is showing the benefits of vitamins and minerals, especially those known as antioxidants. Antioxidants combat cellular damage from free radicals, which is one of the key underlying mechanisms leading to chronic conditions such as heart disease, cataracts, macular degeneration, and many cancers.

Free radicals are highly reactive unstable molecules that have lost one electron and are aggressively seeking a replacement – a process that, in your body, results in damage to everything from your DNA to the collagen layer of your skin. You can't escape from free radicals completely, because they are a by-product of normal metabolism. They are formed in our bodies when, for instance, molecules of fat react with oxygen in a process similar to the one that turns fat rancid or makes iron rust. But free radicals are also formed by exposure to ozone, tobacco smoke, car exhaust, chemicals given out from new carpets, and other pollutants. Exposure to radiation, insecticides, and excessive amounts of sunlight can also lead to the formation of free radicals. Free-radical damage results in cellular inflammation and the release of too many of the 'bad' eicosanoids that appear to be involved in virtually every disease process known.

The body was designed to fight off free-radical damage in the same way that your immune system is designed to fight viruses and bacteria. One mechanism that your body uses to fight free-radical damage is to repair the damage once it's done. Another mechanism is to 'scavenge' the free radicals before they cause harm: to supply the extra electron they need before they can take it from vulnerable tissue. This is what antioxidants do.

WHERE TO GET ANTIOXIDANTS

Antioxidants are found abundantly in fresh fruits and vegetables, especially the brightly coloured ones. The amount of antioxidant in a given fruit, vegetable, grain, or protein source depends upon the soil in which it is grown or on which its food source is grown. Organically grown fruits and vegetables that are picked and eaten when ripe have the highest amounts of antioxidants and minerals in them.

Food is the best source for our antioxidants. They seem to work synergistically – that is, they're more powerful in balance with one another and with other nutrients as they occur naturally. However, if you don't manage to consume five servings of fruits and vegetables a day, supplements can still provide significant protection.

Perimenopause Supplement Programme

Although some doctors still insist that we don't need supplements if we eat a sound diet, more and more evidence is suggesting that this simply isn't true. Over the years I've seen hundreds of patients who have been helped by a good supplement programme such as the one below.

Following this programme means that you'll have to give up the idea of getting everything you need in one tablet a day. It's simply not possible to pack all those nutrients into one or even a few tablets – you'll probably end up taking ten or more capsules or tablets per day. Think of them as food, not medicine.

Antioxidants

Vitamin A (as beta-carotene)	15mg/day
Vitamin D	350–800IU/day
Vitamin E as mixed tocopherols	400–800IU/day
Vitamin C	1,000–5,000mg/day
Glutathione	2–10mg/day
Alpha-lipoic acid	10–100mg/day
Coenzyme Q_{10}	10–100mg/day
DHA	100–400mg/day

B Complex Vitamins

Thiamine (B_1)	8–100mg/day
Riboflavin (B_2)	9–50mg/day
Pyridoxine (B_6)	10–100mg/day
Niacin	20–100mg/day
Biotin	40–500mcg/day

Folic acid	400–800mcg/day
Vitamin B$_{12}$	20–250mcg/day
Pantothenic acid (B$_5$)	15–400mg/day
Inositol	10–500mg/day
Choline	10–100mg/day

Minerals

Calcium   500–1,200mg/day (amount depends on calcium content of diet)

Magnesium	400–1,000mg/day
Boron	4–12mg/day
Chromium	100–400mcg/day
Copper	1–2mg/day
Iron	15–30mg/day
Manganese	1–15mg/day
Zinc	6–50mg/day
Selenium	50–200mcg/day
Potassium	200–500mg/day
Molybdenum	10–20mcg/day
Vanadium	50–100mcg/day

Trace minerals – usually from marine mineral complex

Optimising Midlife Digestion

Digestive problems, especially in the form of bloating and flatulence, are very common in women. Sometimes they begin at midlife and sometimes they develop only later, when you are in your sixties or seventies. I recently talked to one of my mentors from childhood, a woman who at the age of ninety still teaches yoga at a nursing home. One of her biggest problems is constipation and heartburn, but she is otherwise doing well.

Being a Gut Reactor:
Digestion and Your Third Emotional Centre

One of the first things you need to do in order to heal your digestive problems at midlife is to shore up your third emotional centre. The third emotional centre is located in the solar plexus area, and the health of this area affects all our organs of digestion, including the stomach, liver, gall bladder, pancreas, small intestine, and upper large intestine. Women with substantial weight problems usually have unresolved issues in the third emotional centre.

The health of the third emotional centre depends on a balance between responsibility to ourselves and responsibility to others, and also on our sense of self-esteem. It is adversely affected whenever we feel overly responsible for the welfare of others or when we avoid taking responsibility altogether. Gloria, a patient I've followed for years, illustrates the conflicts in the third emotional centre very well. Gloria is the oldest of four children. Her mother always told her that she was responsible for her siblings because she was the oldest and should 'know better'. Whenever any of her siblings was injured or got into trouble, she was blamed. As a result of having this responsibility placed on her at a relatively early age, Gloria developed a very acute 'gut feeling' about when things were about to go wrong. This ability has served her well in her job as an executive assistant at a large hospital. Nevertheless, she still suffers from digestive upsets whenever there are conflicts at work – conflicts for which she always feels responsible. She once told me that she always seems to be caught in the middle between her boss and a colleague, and this conflict quite literally goes into the middle of her body. It is not surprising that Gloria has problems with her weight and her blood sugar, and that she tends to overeat whenever she feels bad about herself for not doing enough at work. In fact, she does far more than most, but she still feels as though she hasn't done enough.

At midlife our job is to learn how to take care of ourselves instead of everybody else. If we don't learn how to do this, we soon learn that no one will do this for us. But as we begin to go about learning this important skill, we often find ourselves feeling guilty. Who will do everything around the house or the office if we don't? This feeling of guilt hits us right in our solar plexus, which is also the body centre associated with self-esteem and personal power.

Self-esteem comes from feeling good about ourselves in the world. It is effectively created by developing skills in the outer world of work – one of the reasons why so many midlife women heal their lives and their digestion when they go back to college and get the degree they didn't finish after school. Our third emotional centre is also related to how good we feel about our relationships, our bodies, our homes, and our lives in general. Sometimes a lifetime of weight

What to Do About Bloating

During perimenopause there is a shift toward fat-accumulating hormones (cortisol and insulin) and away from fat-mobilising hormones (oestrogen and growth hormone). If your body is under stress of any kind, this shift will worsen. In addition, your abdominal fat cells have more cortisol receptors on them at midlife, so fat is preferentially directed towards them. This often results in fluid retention and bloating.[28] Try the following to reduce bloating:

- *Decrease consumption of high- to moderate-glycaemic-index carbohydrates.* Yet another product of the 'bad' series 2 eicosanoids is excess stomach acid. A diet lower in carbohydrates and higher in fat and protein very often results in complete and fast relief of heartburn and indigestion.

- *Eat three to five small meals per day.* Consuming large quantities of food elevates insulin levels and makes bloating worse – even when the foods are healthy.

- *Include some protein, healthy fat, and low-glycaemic-index carbohydrates in every meal or snack.* However, fruit is best eaten alone. Consuming it with fat causes bloating and indigestion in many women.

- *Eliminate all breads and baked goods for at least a week.* See if this makes a difference. Many women are sensitive to gluten.

- *Drink plenty of water.* It helps the body rid itself of toxins.

- *Leave at least three hours between your last meal and bedtime.* Going to bed on a full stomach can cause acid reflux.

- *Stop or cut right down on alcohol.* Alcohol is a gastric irritant.

> • *Use enteric-coated peppermint.* This supplement can be
> very soothing for digestion problems. Take 2–3 capsules
> between meals. If rectal burning occurs, reduce the
> dose.

and self-esteem problems are solved at midlife as we finally learn the self-acceptance that is part of self-esteem.

MELBA: STRESS AND ANTACIDS

Melba was forty-two and perimenopausal when she first came to see me. She had worked for ten years in a stressful job. After several months of working in this job, Melba began to feel abdominal pain, bloating, and indigestion. After a routine check at her doctor's surgery, she was told to 'reduce stress' and eat a high-carbohydrate, low-fat diet. Her problem became worse, but a colleague introduced her to the world of antacids. Soon she would not travel without a few packets of Tums in her handbag. At first she noticed immediate relief upon taking antacids, but then after a while she began to take them earlier and earlier in the day, until she was taking antacids from nine until five, when she left her job. Over time, however, she noticed that she began to feel weak and tired, and she lost her appetite. In addition, her bowel movements became irregular. When she first came to see me for a routine annual gynaecological check-up, I suspected that some of her problems were related to both her diet and her excessive use of antacids. Within a week of eliminating refined carbohydrates and grain products, and also learning some stress-reduction skills, Melba was able to cut down on her antacid use. Some days she didn't need them at all.

Avoiding Antacid Addiction

Many women are addicted to antacids and acid medications such as ranitidine (Zantac). Antacids have been known for many decades to be useful for indigestion, and even in the treatment of ulcers. There are several types of antacids; most contain either aluminium hydroxide or magnesium hydroxide. Neither of them is without side effects. Aluminium hydroxide neutralises stomach acid but tends to produce constipation. Prolonged and regular use may reduce the body's phosphate levels, with resultant fatigue and loss of appetite. In addition to this, it is still a matter of debate whether aluminium consumption contributes to Alzheimer's disease, so it's best to avoid it whenever possible. Magnesium hydroxide, on the other hand, produces loose stools or diarrhoea in some individuals. Although some antacids combine both aluminium and magnesium, there may still be side effects.

Other antacids, such as Tums, have calcium carbonate as their main ingredient. Though these can help with indigestion, over time they cause acid rebound, a condition in which the excess calcium actually stimulates increased acid secretion. In addition, chronic excessive calcium carbonate intake is associated with a pattern of abnormal blood chemistry known as milk alkali syndrome, producing elevations of blood calcium, phosphate, bicarbonate, and other abnormalities. Over time, kidney stones and even progressive kidney disease may result.[29] The irony is that while many people believe that indigestion and heartburn are due to excessive stomach acid, which is why they are led to take antacids in the first place, chronic indigestion results, in part, not from excessive stomach acid, but from *deficient* stomach acid. And if stomach acid is chronically deficient, it can lead to nutritional deficiencies of vitamins such as B_{12}, which can set the stage for both chronic anaemia and dementia.

If you have an imbalance of protein and carbohydrate in your diet, with refined carbohydrates predominating, this diet may be promoting a decrease in the production of gastric acid and overproduction of series 2 eicosanoids, which may be (1) suppressing your immune system, (2) increasing inflammation in the stomach lining, and (3) increasing stomach discomfort and other pain. Since it is well documented that high blood sugar results in a decrease in gastric acid secretion, it's not surprising that refined carbohydrates are a set-up for indigestion. Hundreds of individuals who switch to a diet of decreased carbohydrate and increased protein for weight loss have noted a complete disappearance of gastritis, reflux, and indigestion. I have personally experienced this since changing my diet. I used to have to take Tums after dinner sometimes, and I never connected it with the bread I was eating until my problem disappeared along with the bread and rice (and biscuits, I might add). This diet has been shown to improve the quality of the protective mucus in the stomach lining and also to normalise muscular control, preventing reflux and spasm.

If you find yourself taking antacids regularly, here's what I'd suggest.

- *Get off the antacid merry-go-round.* If you need to take one, use one without aluminium.

- *Take your antioxidants.* Low levels of vitamin C, vitamin E, and other antioxidant factors in gastric juice have been shown to encourage the growth of *Helicobacter pylori,* a bacterium whose overgrowth is associated with ulcers. Higher antioxidant intake may prevent these bacteria from growing and also improve the healing of the stomach and intestinal lining.

- *Try deglycyrrhised licorice (DGL).* DGL may also help reduce *H. pylori* and stimulate the body's natural internal defences. Unlike antacids, DGL does not reduce acid in the stomach. DGL improves both the quality and quantity of protective substances that line the intestinal tract, increases the life span of intestinal cells, and improves the blood supply to the intestinal lining.[30] DGL is available in natural food shops.

- *Take the right calcium supplement.* Though the calcium in Tums is better than no calcium at all, you're much better off taking a calcium supplement that also contains magnesium and vitamin D, which help the body efficiently utilise calcium.

- *Try SeaCure or Sea Plasma.* SeaCure is a polypeptide supplement made from predigested whitefish; it appears to nourish the bowel wall directly during the absorption process. It can be very easily absorbed by anyone who can take food by mouth, no matter how ill they are. SeaCure has helped many of my patients recover from a broad range of digestive problems, including chronic indigestion, irritable bowel syndrome, and ulcerative colitis, as well as the side effects of chemotherapy. It also provides the many well-documented benefits of eating fish. The recommended dose is three capsules in the morning and three capsules in the evening.

Sea plasma is a phyto-plankton which provides a highly

nutritious and digestible food. It is also a concentrated source of natural beta-carotene.

The Final Frontier:
Accepting Our Bodies

Ultimately, our digestive, food, and weight problems will not be healed completely until we have accepted our bodies unconditionally. Part of creating health at midlife is to regain the body acceptance and self-esteem that most of us lost when we entered adolescence. This is not inconsistent with wanting to make changes – and in fact may facilitate them. May the following story from one of my newsletter subscribers inspire all of us about what is possible when we cultivate enough compassion and self-acceptance and resolve to heal our third chakra at last.

TRACEY: RECONNECTING WITH BODY ACCEPTANCE AT MENOPAUSE

I disconnected from my body when I became pregnant at eighteen, an unmarried first-year in college who dropped out for my 'shotgun wedding'. I hated being pregnant – it was a daily reminder of my guilt and shame at having had sex before marriage, out there for the whole world to see and know. I never caressed my big belly, rubbed my aching feet or back, felt the wonder and magic that was going on inside me. I looked at myself totally nude only once and felt nothing but shame and disgust.

From that point onwards, Tracey was anywhere from 3 to 6 stone overweight and at war with her body. In retrospect, she reasoned that the extra weight was a way to keep herself safe from sexual relationships, since the negative self-image it created kept intimacy at arm's length. Over the years, with maturity and years of self-discovery and therapy, Tracey slowly realised that she no longer needed such protection. Now, at the age of forty-seven and in the midst of perimenopause, her insights have clarified. She wrote:

I remembered something I said to my therapist many years ago. We were talking about what I liked about my body, and I honestly couldn't say there was anything I liked. I said, 'Well, look at me – I look pregnant!' And it's true. In varying degrees of heaviness since my pregnancy, my body has always looked pregnant, patiently waiting for me to love it, which I never did when I was actually pregnant. Now I can mourn the loss of enjoying the real experience and move on. I love my essence. I'm very happy with who I am inside. I've come to understand that my physical body is the way my essence can have presence in this world. Therefore I can celebrate it now – I can reconnect my essence with my body. I can celebrate that my hands and senses allow me to express creativity and my body allows me to express my love.

No matter what your size, shape, percentage of body fat, or BMI, you and I, like Tracey, can start right this minute to express gratitude to our bodies for being home to our souls and allowing us to express our uniqueness on the earth at this time.

EIGHT

Creating Pelvic Health and Power

*P*erimenopause is the most common time for women to develop problems with their pelvic organs, ranging from heavy bleeding to fibroids and urinary incontinence. It is also the most common time for women to undergo hysterectomies or other surgical procedures to treat these conditions.

Though numerous approaches help alleviate midlife pelvic symptoms, women can heal fully only when they acknowledge the message behind the symptoms. The emotional and energetic reason that so many women have midlife pelvic problems is associated with the rising need to undergo individuation at midlife and to transform the relationship struggles that tend to make themselves known in the organs of the second emotional centre: the genitals, lower bowel, lower back, and bladder. As the transforming kundalini energy rises through us, it often stops in our pelvic organs to create symptoms that will nudge us to address the money, sex, and power issues that are related to this area of our bodies. Whether or not we need surgery or other treatments, perimenopause is a crucial time to develop pelvic power by claiming and shoring up our boundaries, and by assuming more dominion over our creative energy.

What Is Yours, What Is Mine, What Is Ours?
Reclaiming Our Boundaries

The health of the second emotional centre is tied in to our creative drives: how well do we balance going after what we want in the world with spending time and energy on our relationships? As I've pointed out, young women are both biologically and culturally predisposed to funnel a great deal of creative energy into maintaining relationships. Men, on the other hand, are biologically and socially programmed to focus on the outer world. However, as the energy in our bodies shifts during perimenopause, many women begin to turn their focus towards more worldly accomplishments. Men of the same age often turn inwards and become more interested in relationships and nurturing.

Given both our cultural heritage and our shifting creative drives, it is not surprising that boundary conflicts often emerge as we begin, sometimes for the first time, to go after what we really want. This always requires us to claim or reclaim the healthy personal boundaries that allow us to access our power and autonomy.

BETTY: UNMET CREATIVE NEEDS

Betty was forty-two when she first came to see me for recurrent urinary tract infections. She seemed surprised when I asked her what was going on in her life and what gave her life meaning, but she clearly welcomed the chance to talk.

Betty had graduated from university over twenty years before and had made her living as a freelance writer before her marriage. She clearly had a keen mind and lots of ambition. When she was thirty-two Betty met a wonderful man named Ralph who was supportive of her writing. Ralph's dream was to run his own business, a family restaurant.

In the first year of their marriage, Betty became more flexible with her usual productive writing schedule. After all, Ralph needed help interviewing personnel for his restaurant. And could she help set up the accounting books? – it would take just a week or so, he said. But what started out as a week expanded into a month, and so on, until it became a nearly full-time job.

Despite Ralph's stated support for her writing, Betty's projects invariably took a back seat to the needs of his restaurant. As she started missing deadlines, commissions began to dry up. More and more of her waking hours were spent on his business – which he was now calling 'their' restaurant. Somehow, inexorably, 'his' had turned into 'theirs'. And 'hers' (Betty's writing career) had nearly disappeared.

As midlife adults, it is imperative that we assume responsibility not only for our current circumstances, but also for the often outmoded beliefs that created them – beliefs that usually result from childhood programming. When I asked Betty about her family history, she told me that her father had been very demanding and invasive when she was growing up. He had a finger on every detail of their lives, and he kept after her about how she spent every minute: 'You should be working on your homework now', 'When are you going to do the washing-up?' 'Why aren't these clothes being put away as soon as you get home?'

Betty's body had registered this invasion of her second emotional centre at an early age. She was only eight when she started to have bladder infections. They continued intermittently until she left for university, after which they cleared up for nearly twenty years. Five years into her marriage, they began again.

As she told her story, Betty realised that her bladder and its symptoms were part of her inner wisdom letting her know that her life was out of balance. She had been overrun by her father as a child, and she had re-created a similar pattern with her husband. In addition to checking out her urinary system thoroughly, I suggested that it was time for Betty to begin shoring up her leaky boundaries.

How Healthy Are Your Boundaries?

Every single one of us has experienced some violations of our personal identity – attempts to control how we think, dress, spend our money or our time, use our creativity, pursue a career. As children, we do not have the ability to form our own boundaries, and we need our parents to help us make healthy choices. But as we get older, we need more and more distance between our own choices and those of our parents. Individuation actually begins when we are two or three years old, which is why toddlers delight in saying no. In many cases, however, this process is incomplete, leaving us with less-than-ideal boundaries – which we may not even be aware of until the wake-up call of perimenopause.

Whatever our history, we must learn to live with healthy respect for our own boundaries – and for those of others. When we do, we'll have an easier time creating health in our second emotional centres.

Become Aware of Ongoing Boundary Problems

What events seem to make your symptoms worse? What makes them better? When was the last time you felt really healthy? Betty noticed, for example, that her UTIs disappeared completely when she was at university and during the first few years of her writing career – times when she did not feel required to compromise her creativity to meet the needs of a loved one.

A boundary violation may be so unconscious or subtle that you do not notice it. For example, one of my patients couldn't buy shoes without checking with her husband first. When I questioned her about this, she said, 'Well, he's paying for them, isn't he?' I pointed out that the shoes were for *her* feet, not his. Consider the following questions:

Can you buy an article of clothing without asking your partner's opinion or permission? Do you feel guilty if you do so?

Have you ever made a major purchase (such as a camera or appliance) without first running it by your mate? Does your mate make such decisions without consulting you?

Does your mate have the right to veto your decisions? Do you have an equal right to veto his or hers?

If you bring a purchase home and your mate doesn't like it, do you feel you must return it?

At election time, do you and your mate decide together for whom you are both going to vote? How do you resolve any differences of opinion?

Do you find yourself eventually giving in to your mate's preferences for how to spend time and money?

Do you defer your career development needs for the sake of your partner's business or well-being?

If your mate makes more money than you, does that automatically mean that his or her career is taken more seriously and gets more support than yours?

Are you constantly on the receiving end of criticism or unsolicited advice from your mate or family about how you should live your life?

Sometimes awareness alone can help create healthier boundaries. However, if you think your boundary problems are affecting your physical health, it is almost always helpful to discuss your situation with a trusted friend or counsellor. He or she can help you get clear on what healthy boundaries look and feel like in a relationship, and, most important, whether you are likely to be able to create them in your current relationship.

Hormonal Imbalance: Fuel to the Fire

The emotional imbalances that demand our attention at perimenopause are fuelled by – and in turn contribute to – hormonal imbalance at a cellular level. This hormonal imbalance is characterised by a relative excess of oestrogen, not enough progesterone, and, often, too much insulin, all of which can also result in the overproduction of androgenic hormones. Stress of all kinds, emotional, physical, or nutritional, also leads to an imbalance in the evanescent cellular hormones known as eicosanoids, such as prostaglandins and cytokines, which govern every aspect of cellular metabolism. These same midlife metabolic imbalances also contribute to physical conditions such as fibroids, cramps, endometriosis, adenomyosis, and heavy bleeding. Some women have all of these simultaneously.

Whether your problem is an asymptomatic fibroid or heavy bleeding, the dietary and nutritional supplement approach to these conditions is identical, because both oestrogen dominance and eicosanoid imbalance are related to the same dietary factors. Follow the guidelines in chapter 7 with regard to refined carbohydrates, protein, types of dietary fat, and essential vitamins and minerals. In the sections that follow, I will discuss additional medical approaches to each pelvic condition.

Menstrual Cramps and Pelvic Pain

Starting in the teenage years, about 50 per cent of all females suffer from menstrual cramps (dysmenorrhoea). During perimenopause, the tendency towards cramping may worsen because of hormonal imbalance and the conditions associated with it, such as fibroids and adenomyosis. My own menstrual cramps started when I was about fourteen and occurred on the first two days of each cycle until I had my first child. They went away for a couple of years (which is very common because of the changes that pregnancy makes in the uterus) but came back in my mid-thirties. My cramps responded to acupuncture and dietary change, and by the age of forty I had recovered from them completely.

Too Many 'Bad Eicosanoids'

Cramps result when the uterine muscle and the endometrial lining produce too much of the eicosanoids called prostaglandin E2 and F2-alpha. When these prostaglandins are released into your bloodstream (usually within an hour or two after the onset of your period, but sometimes even before) you begin to experience the effects of this hormone: spasm in the uterine muscle, sweating, hot flushes, feeling cold alternating with feeling hot, loose stools, and possibly feeling faint. A gel made of prostaglandin E2 is used to induce labour, and it can produce exactly the same symptoms you get when your period starts. However, in the case of cramps, the eicosanoid imbalance starts in your own body and is affected by the food you eat and the amount of stress you're under, among other factors.

The Wisdom of Cramps

Are your cramps trying to get you to slow down, rest, and tune in to yourself? Slowing down and resting can help balance eicosanoids. How do you view your menstrual cycle? Is it merely a biological inconvenience for you – or do you see it as part of your wisdom?

The menstrual period is a natural time for rest and renewal. It's nature's way of slowing you down so that you can replenish your body for the next lunar cycle. In many ancient cultures, and even in some contemporary societies such as parts of India, women were expected to take it easy during their periods. But in this society all of us have been taught to try to be efficient, upbeat, and at 100 per cent energy all the time. No wonder our wiser bodily processes try to get our attention! Women are lunar. Our bodies and our energies quite naturally follow the phases of the moon. Though this has been considered a sign of female weakness, once you begin to listen to your body, you will find that your cyclic energy shifts are a source of inspiration. If we have not been doing this regularly in our twenties and thirties, our pain can become particularly acute during perimenopause, when the wake-up call to health becomes louder. As one of my perimenopausal patients said, 'If I just slow down, take a long bath, and take care of myself, I rarely suffer during my cycle. But when I try to ignore my needs, my body – and my cramps – really does try to get my attention.'

As you learn to slow down during your premenstrual and menstrual times, not only will your cramps diminish, you'll often find that your intuition is at an all-time high. Insights may come to you more easily. And you'll begin to look forward to this special time.

Keep the following in mind. Whenever the majority of a population – in this case, the majority of women – suffers around a perfectly normal function like menstruation, you can be sure that there is a cultural blind spot in operation. Waking up and seeing the blind spot – and how it might be related to your cramps – is part of embracing your woman's wisdom.

Treating Pelvic Pain and Cramping

• *Follow a hormone-balancing diet (see chapter 7).*

• *Eliminate all dairy foods (cheese, ice cream, cream, milk, yogurt) for two months.* Though I do not have any statistics on this, I've seen many women get rid of their menstrual pain altogether (even in cases of severe endometriosis) by eliminating dairy foods, which are high in arachidonic acid, from their diets. Some are able to prevent cramps by avoiding dairy products just for the two weeks before their periods. During perimenopause, when periods so often become irregular, you may need to stop dairy products altogether for a few months to experience the benefits.

• *Eliminate red meat.* Red meat, like dairy foods, is high in a fatty acid eicosanoid precursor known as arachidonic acid, which results in symptoms such as cramps and arthritis in susceptible individuals. Eliminating it from your diet can cut down on the inflammatory eicosanoids associated with cramping and endometriosis pain.

• *Take additional supplements.* Follow the supplement programme outlined in chapter 7, with special attention to the following:

Magnesium: 100mg taken as frequently as every two hours during times of actual pain has been shown to help relax smooth muscle tissue and therefore decrease cramping. Do not exceed 1,000mg per day.

Omega-3 fatty acids: Omega-3 fats are precursors for series 1 and 2 eicosanoids. Consume at least one of the following:

- Fatty fish (100g) three or four times per week

- DHA, 100–400mg per day

- 4tbsp ground fresh whole organic linseed per day

- 1tbsp fresh linseed oil daily

Vitamin C: 1,000–5,000mg per day. Increase when cramping occurs.

- **Acupuncture and Chinese herbs.** Acupuncture has been scientifically shown to alleviate menstrual cramps and pelvic pain.[1] I have seen its benefits hundreds of times in my practice, and I personally found it extremely helpful for severe cramping in my late thirties. I also took individually prescribed Chinese herbs for about a year. If you cannot locate a trained practitioner of traditional Chinese medicine near you, it is safe to try Bupleurum (Xiao Yao Wan, also known as Hsiao Yao Wan). Indeed, many of my patients have done very well with it. (See Resources section.) Take four or five of the tiny tablets four times per day during the two weeks before your period is due, and continue through the first day of bleeding. It may take two to three months to see full results. Yunnan Bai Yao is a traditional Chinese medicine that can stop heavy bleeding within one to two weeks – sometimes sooner. Take one to two capsules, four times daily.

- **Castor oil packs.** Lying down with a castor oil pack on your lower abdomen for sixty minutes two to four times per week is often very helpful for both treatment and prevention of cramps and pelvic pain. Edgar Cayce, the renowned medical intuitive of the early to mid-1900s, recommended this immune-system-enhancing treatment for all kinds of conditions. (See Resources section.) *Note:* Do not use these if they increase your pain or if you are bleeding heavily.

• *Nonsteroidal anti-inflammatories (NSAIDs).* Nonsteroidal anti-inflammatory drugs such as ibuprofen (Motrin, Brufen), naproxen sodium (Naprosyn, Synflex), and ketoprofen (Orudis) work by partially blocking your body's production of prostaglandin F2-alpha. (So does aspirin, but through a slightly different mechanism.) For best relief, NSAIDs must be taken *before* you get uncomfortable. If you take them only after the pain has begun, the prostaglandin will already be in your bloodstream. The drug stops production of prostaglandin F2-alpha, but it cannot stop the effect on your cells once the prostaglandin has been released.

• *Contraceptive pills.* All pelvic conditions tend to quieten down when the natural hormonal cycles are put to sleep by the steady-state synthetic hormones in contraceptive pills. Take the lowest-dose pill available. Avoid contraceptive pills altogether if you are a smoker.

Heavy Bleeding

Many women develop heavy and irregular bleeding in the years before menopause because oestrogen dominance causes the lining of the uterus to overgrow. Emotional stress of all kinds can make this worse. Instead of the normal monthly build-up and shedding of the uterine lining, too much endometrial tissue builds up and then breaks down in a disordered way that results in spotting or irregular heavy bleeding.

What do I mean by heavy bleeding? Many women experience a heavier flow on the first or second day of their periods, which slows them down a bit, but I consider this within the realm of normal. (You may still wish to try some of the gentler treatments listed.) However, if your bleeding prevents you from leaving the house or participating fully in your life for more than two days per month, if you routinely soak through a couple of tampons and a pad all in place at the same time and then through your clothes or your nightgown, or if you've been diagnosed with iron deficiency anaemia, you need to take action.

The Wisdom of Bleeding: Are You Leaking Life Energy?

I always ask my patients with heavy bleeding if they are leaking their life's blood into any dead-end job or relationship that doesn't fully meet their needs. Are you giving more than you are receiving in return? Is someone or something draining your energy by being a kind of Dracula? Take some time alone, sit right down on the earth, and pray for guidance and a boost of energy for yourself.

Physical Causes of Heavy Periods

In addition to hormonal imbalance, physical conditions may impede the normal uterine contractions that help stop menstrual blood flow each month.

Fibroid tumours are the most common physical reason for excessive bleeding. Whether or not a fibroid causes bleeding depends upon its location in the uterine wall. Bleeding is most often caused by submucosal fibroids, which are located right under the endometrium, the mucous membrane that lines the uterus.

Adenomyosis is another condition that can cause heavy bleeding. Adenomyosis results when the endometrial glands that line the uterus grow into the uterine muscle (the myometrium). When this happens, little lakes of blood form in the uterine wall that do not drain during menstruation. Over time, the uterus enlarges and becomes boggy, spongy, and engorged with blood, disrupting the normal uterine contraction patterns.

Since both fibroids and adenomyosis are associated with excess oestrogen, minimal progesterone, too much prostaglandin F2-alpha, and often, too much insulin, hormonal and physical factors are often present at the same time.

Treatment Choices for Heavy Bleeding

Before you start any treatment programme for heavy bleeding, I recommend that you have a physical examination and a cervical smear if you haven't already had one within the year. Though the vast majority of cases of heavy bleeding are benign and can be treated with the advice I'm about to give you, you want to be sure that you don't have some other condition that is contributing to your problem.

• *Diet and vitamins.* Follow the hormone-balancing diet outlined in chapter 7, with special attention to supplemental antioxidants and

B vitamins. These help strengthen your blood vessel walls and help your liver break down and clear excess oestrogen from your body.

B complex: Take the mid to high range of the B vitamins on pages 218–19. These help neutralise excess oestrogen.

Vitamin E (mixed tocopherols): 400IU, twice per day.

Vitamin C complex with bioflavonoids: 1,000–5,000mg per day.

Vitamin A (as beta-carotene): 15mg per day.

Supplemental iron: In many women with heavy bleeding, the primary symptom is fatigue from iron deficiency anaemia. Get your blood count checked. If it's low, take iron. The recommended daily allowance is 15mg per day. You may need to take three to four times this amount until iron levels are restored. (Iron supplementation itself has been shown to decrease menstrual flow in some women.)

The best, most absorbable iron supplement I've found is ANR Iron 27+. It is time-released, doesn't cause stomach upset or constipation, and is easily and readily absorbed. It has helped many women in my practice keep their blood counts normal – something they were previously unable to do with other iron supplements. It has even saved some women from needing surgery. This is not available in the UK, but see Resources for a US supplier.

• *Acupuncture and Traditional Chinese Medicine.* See discussion on pages 187–90.

• *Castor oil packs.* See the discussion on pages 234–5.

• *Natural progesterone.* A prescription-only cream that contains 1.5–3 per cent natural progesterone can be used to decrease heavy bleeding. Rub 1/4-1/2tsp into your palms or on the soft areas of your skin two times per day starting two to three weeks before your period is due. Stop when your period begins, then start again one to two weeks later. If this approach is going to work, you should see results after about three months. For some women, 1.5–3 per cent natural progesterone isn't strong enough to counteract their own oestrogen. In this case, ask your doctor for a stronger prescription, such as Crinone gel, which comes in 4 per cent and 8 per cent strengths.

• *NSAIDs.* Take a nonsteroidal anti-inflammatory drug, such as ibuprofen (Motrin, Brufen), naproxen sodium (Naprosyn, Synflex), or ketoprofen (Orudis), daily starting one to two days before your period, and continue it regularly through your heaviest days. Use the lowest dose that gives you results. The NSAIDs have definitely been shown to decrease menstrual blood loss because of their ability to interrupt excess prostaglandin F2-alpha.

• *Synthetic progesterone.* When natural progesterone doesn't work, it is sometimes necessary to use a strong synthetic progestogen such as norethisterone (Primolut N). (This is the only circumstance in which I recommend the synthetic.) This is especially true if you have a fibroid that bleeds and you haven't been able to stem your problem with gentler approaches. Primolut N for heavy periods is prescribed at a dose of 5mg two or three times daily for the week before your period is due. Then you give your body a rest for three weeks and start again. Usually a three-month cycle of the progestogen will result in a significant decrease in excessive bleeding. Primolut has fewer side effects than many progestogens and anyway these are usually acceptable compared to losing your uterus.

• *Contraceptive pills.* Many women who are having heavy, irregular periods due to fibroids, lack of ovulation, excess oestrogen relative to progesterone, or a combination of these conditions often do well on contraceptive pills. Although they do not result in a true cure, they are a good option when the alternative is surgery.

• *D&C (dilatation and curettage).* This standard surgical treatment for heavy bleeding involves scraping the uterine lining and removing excess tissue. It frequently decreases the problem, for reasons that aren't entirely clear. It is often used also to diagnose the specific condition causing the bleeding.

• *Endometrial ablation.* In this surgical procedure, the lining of the uterus is obliterated with a laser or with cautery. Because the procedure destroys the endometrial lining, it often results in complete cessation of periods or very light periods. It should never be used by anyone who wants to maintain her ability to have children.

Endometrial ablation works very well for many types of intractable bleeding and may be done as a day case, though it involves a general anaesthetic and you may be required to stay in until the next day because of this. The procedure should be done by someone highly skilled, with extensive previous experience. Ask your doctor to refer you appropriately.

I've referred a number of women for this procedure. For some it provides great relief. One of my newsletter subscribers wrote to me: 'Three months ago I underwent an endometrial ablation and tubal ligation. At the age of forty-four this sterilises me two ways, for which I'm grateful, and has remedied the constant bleeding and clots for weeks on end. I now have no more periods! Yeah!'

MARTHA: INTRACTABLE HEAVY BLEEDING

Martha wrote me the following about her midlife bleeding problem:

> I am forty-two years old. I weigh about 13^1/2 stone on God-given big bones, exercise regularly, am generally healthy. My problem has been described as flooding. I have seen several doctors about this. They prescribed a double dose of contraceptive pills that I took for four months with no result. I have had a biopsy done, with negative results. My cervical smears are normal.
>
> My periods last twelve days and are very heavy with lots of clots. There is constant bleeding in between. I consulted a herbalist, who thought that because of my 3 excess stone, my fat cells could very well be overproducing oestrogen. That is why the pill and the progesterone cream that I have used have not helped the constant bleeding.
>
> I have read Susun S. Weed's book *Menopausal Years: The Wise Woman Way*. In it she suggests using homeopathic remedies such as lachesis. I am also drinking raspberry leaf tea and using shepherd's purse. I am taking iron, as that has been low. Also *Lactobacillus acidophilus*, calcium, magnesium, and a good multiple vitamin.
>
> The bleeding still has not stopped. I am becoming pretty tired of all of this, and as you can well imagine, my desire for sex is

low with me having to constantly wear a pad. The bleeding has
been going on for four months. Do you have any suggestions
that may help?

I suggested to Martha that she seek help from an acupuncturist
right away and also continue taking iron. I also recommended a
Chinese patent medicine called Yunnan Bai Yao that is superb for
helping flooding problems. (See Resources.) It generally works within
a week or two. I also suggested that she lose 10–20lb, which could
significantly reduce her excess bodily oestrogen production.

It is possible that Martha has an undiagnosed submucosal fibroid.
The diagnosis is made with ultrasound or with a procedure known as
hysterosalpingogram, in which dye is injected into the uterine cavity
under X-ray visualisation. If this is the case, she may need a surgical
approach such as endometrial ablation or fibroid removal done via the
vagina. I've also seen her type of problem respond well to a D&C
done in the operating room.

The main point here is that there are many, many approaches to
controlling heavy bleeding during perimenopause. In every case, it's
helpful to have a diagnosis and treatment plan with alternatives to
hysterectomy. Here is the bottom line: every perimenopausal woman
who is experiencing heavy bleeding needs to know that there are
many safe and effective treatment options. Hysterectomy, which
amounts to killing the messenger, should be a last resort.

Fibroids

Benign fibroid tumours of the uterus are present in 30–50 per cent of
women. They occur in women of all races and backgrounds, but they
are more common in women of African-American or Caribbean
descent. Fibroids arise from the smooth muscle and connective tissue
of the uterine muscle itself. Though they can occur in women as
young as their late teens or early twenties, they are most often
diagnosed when a woman is in her thirties or forties.[2]

The majority of fibroids do not cause any real problems. In other
words, they are just there. Sometimes, depending upon their location,
you will be able to feel them. They feel like a smooth lump in your
lower abdomen, just above your pubic bone. Because the female

FIGURE 13: TYPES OF FIBROIDS

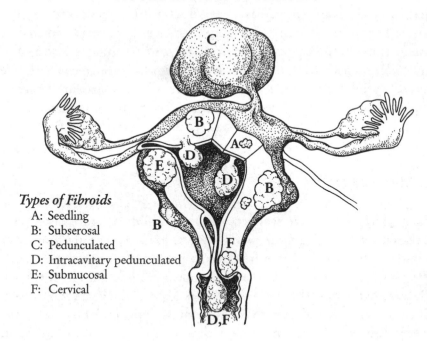

Types of Fibroids
A: Seedling
B: Subserosal
C: Pedunculated
D: Intracavitary pedunculated
E: Submucosal
F: Cervical

pelvis can accommodate growths the size of a newborn baby, it is obvious that small and even large fibroids don't necessarily lead to any problems. In other words, you may not even be aware that you have one unless you have a pelvic examination or pelvic ultrasound. Your periods may not be any different, and chances are you won't experience any pain or other symptoms. Fibroids may grow dramatically during perimenopause because of oestrogen dominance (their growth is stimulated by oestrogen), but they often shrink just as dramatically after menopause – nature's treatment.

The Wisdom of Your Fibroids

Though there are well-established dietary and hormonal reasons why so many women have fibroids, the baseline energetic patterns that result in fibroids are related to blockage and stagnation of the energy of the second emotional centre. Women are at risk of fibroids (or other pelvic problems) when we direct our creative energy into dead-end relationships that we have outgrown. When my own fibroid appeared at the age of forty-two, for instance, I knew that it was related, in part, to my staying in a one-on-one direct patient care

practice for several years longer than I really wanted to. I was afraid
that I wouldn't be respected as a 'real' doctor if I wasn't doing surgery
regularly and maintaining a full surgical practice. Though I longed to
channel my creativity into more writing and teaching, I also feared
my colleagues would resent me if I worked only part time. This is the
classic second emotional centre double bind. Our simultaneous
ambition and need for love and approval create a logjam in the
creative centre of our bodies that, under the right circumstances,
becomes a fibroid.

ELLEN: BIRTHING HER CREATIVITY

Ellen, thirty-eight, was married with two children and worked as a
research associate at a local university. She loved everything about her
job, from the subject matter itself to the people she worked with daily.
She was proud of the fact that her colleagues sought her out when
they needed help with their own projects. But as the years progressed,
Ellen found herself drawn to working more independently. Unfortunately, because she had become 'indispensable', it was very difficult
for her to set those other projects aside to birth her own individual
creation. Her fibroid tumour was diagnosed at about this time.

Over the next several years, her fibroid continued to grow as she
found herself torn between the needs of her own particular research
and the needs of her colleagues, children, and husband. During a
surgery visit in which she consulted me about possible surgery for the
fibroid, I asked her to consider where she was 'leaking' her energy.
She said that a large part of her identity and sense of self-esteem came
from being there for others. She told me that if she was to go off and
work by herself, she was afraid that she wouldn't feel as useful – and
that others would think she was selfish. As we talked about this, she
realised that she had to make some long-overdue changes in her
schedule and in her priorities. Then she told me that she wanted to
give herself another six months before having any surgery.

The next time I saw her, her fibroid hadn't grown any further and
was even a bit smaller. But more important, Ellen had told her
colleagues what she was and was not willing to do for them – and had
simultaneously made some big steps towards pursuing her own
projects. In other words, she had started to birth her own creativity.

If you have or have had a fibroid, ask yourself the following questions. What are the creations within me that I want to put out in the world before I'm no longer here? If anything at all were possible, what would my life look like? If I had six months to live, what relationships would I release from my life immediately? Which ones would I give more of my time and attention to? What relationships truly feed and nourish me? Which ones drain my energy? Write your answers in a journal. Discuss them with supportive friends. Deep within you, you have all the answers you need. You just need to be open to hearing them.

Treatment of Fibroids

The first thing to consider is that a fibroid may not need to be treated. A watch-and-wait attitude is not unreasonable in many cases; you can live with fibroids for years with no adverse health consequences if they are not bothering you. What may well bother you, however, is simply knowing that you have them. Given our cultural inheritance about our pelvic organs, the perception that something *will* go wrong is often a bigger risk to a woman's well-being than the fibroid itself.

It would do most women a world of good to take their fibroids less seriously. At the time your fibroid is diagnosed, you usually will not know what has caused your second-chakra imbalances. Understanding comes retrospectively. Instead, commit yourself to learning from the process, whatever course of treatment you decide upon.

An essential element of this learning experience is to release self-blame. It is never helpful to hold the idea that you have a particular illness or symptom because you are 'doing something wrong'. If you knew ahead of time what the condition was trying to bring to your attention, you wouldn't have had to manifest it. And in fact, all physical conditions have genetic, dietary, environmental, and emotional components simultaneously.

On the other hand, there are times when you may wish to seek treatment for a fibroid. Though most fibroids will shrink after menopause is complete, you may not want to live with a growth that makes you look pregnant until that time comes. If you find, as I did, that you are dressing to disguise your fibroid, and your menopause is six or more years away, then you may want to take action. And, of course, if your symptoms include pain, heavy bleeding, cramping, or backache, you'll definitely want relief. Thankfully, the treatment options are extensive.

DIETARY CHANGE AND SUPPLEMENTS

Any dietary or alternative approach that works to balance excess oestrogen or enhance the flow of energy *(chi)* through the pelvis often works for fibroids as well as for heavy bleeding or menstrual cramps. These include acupuncture and Chinese herbs, phyto-oestrogens from sources such as soya or linseed, dietary change, and oestrogen-balancing supplements (see chapter 6). Exercise such as yoga is also helpful.

Such approaches are always worth a try, as this letter from a newsletter subscriber attests:

> I have been suffering for years with multiple uterine fibroid tumors, approximately 25–30 in number in the wall of my uterus. For two weeks out of every month I had excruciating, unbearable pain. I was unable to sleep, would lie down curled up in a ball, and literally sweat in agony. In 1991 and 1992 I had laser surgery through the laparoscope twice, and the surgeon was only able to remove three or four of the larger fibroids. Then I read your book and have been religiously following your advice to cut out dairy products and take B complex vitamins as well as 800mg of magnesium. As a result, if I could, I would give you my firstborn child in gratitude! My pain is gone! Though I was planning reconstructive surgery, I changed my mind when I realised that your suggestions were working. I feel like a completely new woman – reborn, revitalised, and empowered.

HORMONAL TREATMENTS

• *Bioidentical progesterone.* Progesterone skin cream helps to counter oestrogen dominance. It is available in a 1.5–3 per cent strength (trade names ProJuven and ProGest (see chapter 5 'Hormone Replacement Therapy')). The usual dose is 1/4–1/2tsp rubbed into your palms or on the soft areas of your skin once or twice per day, three weeks on and one week off. If you are having regular periods, time the application so that your week off corresponds to the week of your period. If your periods are irregular, I suggest coordinating use of the progesterone cream with the phases of the moon, to which every human life is attuned. Plan to be off the progesterone during the new moon – the time when women were most apt to have their periods before the advent of artificial lighting. Some women do best using the cream every day, with no week off.

Some women may need a higher dose. Stronger natural progesterone is available as a 4 to 8 per cent vaginal gel (trade name Crinone)
from your doctor.

Most women do well on transdermal progesterone, which is
absorbed into the bloodstream directly.

• *Contraceptive pills.* Contraceptive pills are a combination of
synthetic oestrogen and progestogen that can smooth out the
oestrogen dominance that so often causes fibroids to grow or become
symptomatic. Because they consist of synthetic hormones, I'd suggest
that they be used only after more natural approaches such as dietary
change or acupuncture and herbs have failed, or in situations in which
a woman is unwilling or unable to try a more natural approach.

• *GnRH agonists.* GnRH agonists such as nafarelin (Synarel) or
leuprovelin (Prostap) act at the level of the pituitary gland and put the
body into a state of artificial menopause. This lowers oestrogen levels
and shrinks fibroids. Side effects include all the symptoms of late
perimenopause, such as bone loss, hot flushes, and vaginal dryness,
but these can sometimes be effectively countered with low-dose
hormone therapy that doesn't cause fibroids to grow.

GnRH agonists can be quite effective as alternatives to surgery for
some women. I do not recommend them if you have a family history
of Alzheimer's disease, because the rapid withdrawal of oestrogen
from the brain may not be advisable in susceptible women.

SURGICAL TREATMENTS

• *Myomectomy.* Fibroids can often be removed surgically. The size
and location of a fibroid will determine the surgical route. Fibroids
that are located just under the uterine lining deep within the uterus,
for example, can sometimes be removed vaginally. Others can be
removed via laparoscopy (sometimes known as belly-button
surgery). Large ones, such as the one I had, usually require abdominal
surgery.

If you decide to have your fibroid removed surgically, the procedure should be done by a gynaecologist who is philosophically
aligned with your desire to keep your uterus. When he finished my
surgery, my gynaecologist told me, 'Well, I'm happy to report that
you now have completely healthy and normal pelvic organs. I didn't

have to remove a thing except the fibroid!' That's exactly what I wanted to hear.

Having your fibroids removed can be a very empowering experience. As one of my newsletter subscribers wrote to me:

> After having fibroids surgically removed, I also removed most negative issues from my life. It is wonderful! No headaches, no cramps, no backaches. I am still working on more dietary changes, but the ones I have already made have made me more positive, stronger, and carefree. I am also a praying person. So with this, and lifestyle changes, I am well on my way to healing and growing up at the age of forty!

• *Fibroid embolisation.* Uterine artery embolisation (UAE) is a relatively new treatment for fibroid tumours that involves injecting a substance (usually polyvinyl alcohol particles) into the uterine artery. This causes clotting of the blood supply to the fibroid, which then shrinks over time. The procedure is done in hospital, under the care of the gynaecology department. To reach the uterine arteries, a catheter is threaded into the femoral vein of the thigh. Most centres report good outcomes, with a worldwide success rate of about 85 per cent. All types of fibroid symptoms, including heavy or irregular bleeding, uterine enlargement, and symptoms related to the size of the fibroid, such as urinary frequency, have responded.

The average patient who undergoes this procedure can expect a 40–60 per cent decrease in uterine size after about six months, but even those women who have no reduction in uterine size report improvement in symptoms such as heavy bleeding. Although no long-term follow-up data are yet available, UAE has a low risk of complications compared with myomectomy or hysterectomy. However, some serious complications, such as renal failure or an allergic reaction to the clotting agent, have been reported.[3] If this procedure appeals to you, ask your doctor to refer you to a hospital where UAE is frequently done.

• *Hysterectomy.* Hysterectomy should be the last resort for fibroid treatment, reserved for those women who, in addition to their fibroids, also have intractable bleeding or pain problems that simply have not responded to other measures. When this is the case, hysterectomy can be a real blessing, dramatically enhancing the quality of a woman's life.

CAROL: THE NEED TO LET GO

Carol was forty-six when she first came to see me for a second surgical opinion. Carol had multiple fibroids in her uterus that were causing her to bleed heavily each month, resulting in chronic anaemia and fatigue. For the past four years she had tried desperately to keep her uterus, clinging to the hope that she'd be able to have a child of her own one day. Carol's condition had deteriorated to the point that keeping her uterus had become her career. In fact, she had even lost her job because of constant absenteeism for doctor's appointments and episodes of heavy bleeding that required her to leave work. Though Carol had tried contraceptive pills, synthetic hormones, and multiple D&Cs to control the bleeding, nothing had helped. Her condition was too dangerous to suggest alternative treatments such as diet or acupuncture. I suggested that her health and overall well-being would best be served by a hysterectomy. (If I were to see her now, I would suggest uterine artery embolisation.)

Carol's uterine condition was preventing her from actually living her life. She was stuck in a holding pattern consisting of pouring her life's blood (literally) into unrealised hopes and dreams that had little or no chance of manifesting. Like all of us at midlife, Carol needed to let go of an unrealised dream from her past (having a biological child), allow herself to grieve fully, and then finally move on. Though this is never easy, sometimes it is the most healing choice.

An Empowered Approach to Surgery or Invasive Procedures

When you feel that you have been involved with the choice to have surgery or UAE and really know your options, then you've stepped out of the victim role and into the partnership model. This shift alone improves your chance for a good outcome. You can continue that partnership mode by reading *Prepare for Surgery, Heal Faster* by my colleague Peggy Huddleston. Peggy has written the definitive manual for how to have a healthy and empowering surgical experience. I personally used her approach when I had my own fibroid surgery. (See Resources.)

Hysterectomy for the Wrong Reasons

Make sure that you get a second opinion if someone gives you one of the following reasons for having a hysterectomy for a fibroid.

1. *'You should have surgery before your fibroid gets any bigger. If you don't, your fibroid may grow and make the surgery much more difficult in the future.'*

Unless a small tumour is causing intractable bleeding or fertility problems, it does not need to be removed. Not all fibroids are destined to grow, and even if they do, studies have shown that surgery to remove a uterus with large fibroids poses no increased risk to the patient. If necessary, the fibroid can be removed (see the section on myomectomy on page 245) leaving the uterus, and the blood supply to the ovaries, intact.

2. *'Your fibroid may become cancerous'* or *'We cannot be sure it is* not *cancerous unless it is removed.'*

It is extremely rare for a fibroid to be cancerous (the incidence is less than one in a thousand). If a fibroid tumour does become cancerous, it is called a uterine sarcoma, and currently the prognosis for this condition is very poor, which means that diagnosing it via surgery will not greatly increase your chances of survival. In fact, the chances of dying from complications of hysterectomy, though small, are statistically a little greater than the chances of having a uterine sarcoma.

3. *'Your ovaries can't be seen on ultrasound.'*

If you have had an ultrasound examination (or even an MRI) to confirm the diagnosis of a fibroid, one of your ovaries may not be visible because it's hidden behind the fibroid. Since doctors may be held liable for failing to diagnose an ovarian problem if it's present, they may suggest surgery to be absolutely certain that your ovary is OK.

However, if you have no reason to believe that your ovaries are diseased, you can ask simply to be followed by your doctor. Remember, inability to see an ovary on ultrasound doesn't mean that something is wrong with it – it just means that there are limits to technology! In this situation, some women will want to have laparoscopic surgery so that the pelvis can be examined from the inside with a light. (The uterus and ovaries can also be biopsied during this procedure.) Others will feel comfortable trusting that they are OK. Make whichever choice brings you the most peace of mind.

Should You Have a Hysterectomy?

Fibroids and heavy and irregular bleeding are the most common reasons why women have hysterectomies at midlife. Though hysterectomy is sometimes necessary, far too many women have them when they could have resolved their symptoms more easily and naturally using other means. In addition, there is great value in keeping our pelvic organs intact when possible.

In an ideal world, every girl and woman would be taught the value of her pelvic organs from an early age; their benefits would be as well studied as those of the male organs, research on safe and effective natural alternatives to bleeding and pain would be common, and hysterectomy with or without removal of the ovaries would be a very rare operation performed only when all other alternatives fail. This mind-set is currently in place when it comes to male sexual organs. As a result, orchiectomy, the removal of the testes, is performed only as a last resort, though it is a very effective treatment for prostate cancer. And removal of the penis is just about unheard of, even in cases of penile cancer.

Unfortunately, the uterus and the ovaries have been the target of bad press for so long that many women have internalised a fear of their pelvic organs. Recently I overheard a woman I'll call Jane talking to her friends at a party about her impending hysterectomy. Her fibroid was the size of a small orange, she told them, and she wasn't having symptoms. But, she explained, 'I'm fifty, and at my age it's just a matter of time before something happens in that area. I might as well get it out now.' Many doctors reinforce these fears. A patient who came to me for a second opinion to avoid hysterectomy for a fibroid had been told by her gynaecologist that her uterus (which had produced a healthy baby girl only seven months earlier) was 'not her friend'.

The Greek word *hystera* (womb) was used in ancient times to describe all manner of women's suffering, both psychological (hysteria) and physical, believed to be caused by the uterus. In the 1800s after the advent of anaesthesia, hysterectomy became an enormously popular cure for women's ailments and was performed for just about anything that a woman's husband, father, or doctor thought was wrong with her: overeating, painful menstruation, psychological disorders, and most particularly masturbation, promiscuity, or any erotic tendency.

Surgical removal of the uterus remains one of the most commonly performed operations in the UK – both doctors and their patients

FIGURE 14: PELVIC ORGANS WITH SUPPORTING MUSCLES

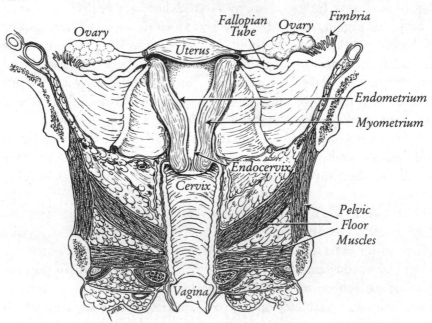

Strong pelvic floor muscles are an essential part of pelvic power.
© 2001 by Northrup and Schulz

have been taught that these organs are dangerous at worst or expend-
able at best. One in three women in the US has had a hysterectomy by
the age of sixty. This is a staggeringly high number. And about 43 per
cent of women have their ovaries removed at the same time as their
uterus, to prevent the possible development of ovarian cancer, despite
the fact that the vast majority will never get ovarian cancer, but could
definitely benefit from the hormones produced by the ovaries
throughout their lives.

Good Reasons to Keep Your Uterus, Cervix, and Ovaries

• Your uterus, cervix, and ovaries all work together to provide your
body with hormonal support throughout your entire life. They also
share much of the same blood supply. When the uterus is removed,
the function of the ovaries is affected even if the ovaries are left in. Up
to 50 per cent of women who have had hysterectomies lose the function of their ovaries earlier than they normally would – and they go
through menopause earlier, thus increasing their risk of heart disease
and osteoporosis.[4]

• Ovaries are the female equivalent of the male testes. As such, they
are an important producer of androgens, the hormones that are
involved in normal sex drive. Some studies have shown that up to 25
per cent of women have decreased sex drive following removal of the
ovaries. Removal of the ovaries literally castrates the female – and it is
called that in the medical literature.[5]
    Many doctors routinely remove the ovaries at the time of hyster-
ectomy in order to prevent ovarian cancer. If a woman has a strong
genetic risk of ovarian cancer, this may be a sound decision. But
the vast majority of women will never get ovarian cancer, and the
routine removal of normal ovaries as prevention is a very high price to
pay.

• Natural menopause, with ovaries and uterus intact, is a normal
physiological event that takes place over a period of six to thirteen
years. As your ovaries gradually shift function, the adrenal glands
naturally take over some hormone production, as does the body fat.
When a woman has her uterus, or uterus and ovaries, removed, her
body goes through an instant menopause, which can be a shock to the
hormonal system.

• The uterus itself undergoes rhythmic contractions during orgasm, which contribute to the depth of sexual pleasure that many women experience during lovemaking. Some women who have had a hysterectomy complain that orgasm is not as satisfying any more.

• The cervix (the lower portion of the uterus that protrudes into the vagina) is part of the normal pelvic floor and helps to support the bladder. The nerves that go to the bladder are intimately connected to the cervix. When hysterectomy with removal of the cervix is performed, these nerves can be damaged, resulting in an increased risk of urinary incontinence.[6]

• Only 10 per cent of hysterectomies are done because of cancer. That means that up to 90 per cent of the time, a woman's pelvic organs are removed for benign disease – disease that can often be treated effectively by non-surgical approaches.

Unearthing Your Hysterectomy Legacy

Over the years I've found that all the education and information in the world won't change a woman's life as long as she's operating from old, unconscious, and unexamined beliefs. Each of us carries a unique personal legacy passed down to us from family members. This is especially true when it comes to women's pelvic organs, a subject that has been shrouded in secrecy and misinformation for generations. Here are some questions to help you uncover your hysterectomy legacy.

Which of your family members, if any, have had hysterectomies? Why? Do you know what was going on in their lives at the time? Do you know what their diagnoses were and what symptoms they were having? Would it be possible to find out? Do you feel that you can't ask because this information is 'too personal'? Does a belief in 'better living through surgery' run in your family?

One of my patients believed that she would need a hysterectomy some time during her forties because 'all my sisters had them then'. As a result, she became overly focused on her pelvic organs at midlife, noting every irregular or heavy period and every twinge. Ultimately, her mind–body connection – plus her unhealthy lifestyle – created enough symptoms so that she actually wanted a hysterectomy 'for relief'.

If, after going through these questions honestly, you still believe that hysterectomy is the best solution for you, then it well may be.

If You've Already Had a Hysterectomy

If you've had a hysterectomy and didn't know that you had any other choice, I know that it's upsetting to hear that the surgery may not have been in your best interest. One of my newsletter readers said:

> After reading your article on the benefits of keeping your ovaries and uterus, I wept. I was only forty-five when I had my hysterectomy for a fibroid that wasn't really bothering me at all. They took my ovaries, too. But that was twenty years ago. I didn't know that I had any other choice. And I also realised that I had never fully grieved for the loss of my pelvic organs. I have now completed that process, and I can let it go and move on.

The first step to healing after hysterectomy is to appreciate any benefits you've experienced from having the surgery. In a landmark study in Maine in the US, it was found that hysterectomy for non-cancerous conditions of the uterus, such as bleeding and pain, was positively associated with improving the woman's quality of life in the vast majority of cases.[7] I want to stress that in this particular study, all of the women were given a choice: to have the surgery or to not have it and be followed. I referred many women to this study and even performed some of the hysterectomies that were included in the data. Many of the women who chose surgery were convinced that they'd be better off with a hysterectomy. Some had lived with pelvic discomfort or heavy bleeding for years that was cured by the surgery. Others actually had an improvement in their sex lives following the surgery. The moral is this: hysterectomy can be a healing surgery under the right circumstances.

Yes, your uterus and ovaries are important, but always remember that you are more than the sum of your organs. Your spiritual body, the field of electromagnetic energy that surrounds and nourishes your physical body, is always whole and intact. You cannot destroy this essential part of yourself, no matter what happens to your physical body.

Appreciate the fact that your body has the ability to rebalance your hormones and maintain its health if you follow a healthy diet, exercise regularly, and use natural hormone replacement strategies that match as nearly as possible what your body normally produces.

If you had a hysterectomy that you now regret, realise that you probably made the best decision you could have under the circumstances that were present at the time. Give yourself credit for that. Our medical care system and its beliefs simply reflect those of the culture we're all a part of. And we can't help but be affected by these beliefs, at least to some degree. Maybe you would have avoided your hysterectomy if you had known more – but you didn't have that knowledge. Let any emotions you have around this issue come to the surface, even if they aren't pleasant ones. (One of my patients had a recurrent fantasy that she wanted to injure or even kill the surgeon who did her surgery. When she allowed herself to feel these unlady-like revenge fantasies fully and express them out loud, she was able to release herself from the past and get on with her life, eventually for-giving herself and the surgeon.)

You can heal from anything – even events as life-changing as losing some body parts to surgery. And when you heal, your story can help someone else on her journey towards health. One of the most helpful things you can do to improve your health right now is to look back on the events leading up to your hysterectomy and see if you had any issues with boundaries or creative drive at the time. Making this link can be very empowering and will also give you greater appreciation for the wisdom of your body.

Strengthen Your Urinary Health and Pelvic Floor Muscles

At midlife, the loss of hormonal support in the vagina and lower urinary tract is often accompanied by the loss of muscle tone in the pelvic floor. As a result, many women experience urinary problems, ranging from loss of urine when coughing or sneezing to recurrent urinary tract infections.

While you're learning how to create healthy boundaries in your personal relationships, you can also develop the muscles in your pelvic floor by doing Kegel exercises or using vaginal weights regularly. This not only strengthens the pelvic floor, but also increases blood flow to the vagina, bladder, and urethra, making the tissue more resilient. This will improve both your sex life and your bladder control.

Keeping Dry: Keeping or Regaining Bladder Control

Urinary incontinence, the involuntary leakage of urine, is a major health problem. It is estimated to affect approximately thirteen million people in the US. Though 10–30 per cent of women aged fifteen to sixty-four experience urinary incontinence at least some of the time, the condition tends to increase in frequency with age. It often makes itself known during perimenopause, when a great deal can be done to make sure it doesn't progress. By the time women reach the age of sixty-five and over, the overall rate of incontinence increases to about 15–35 per cent.[8]

Though the problem does affect men, it affects women five times as often. Many women feel too embarrassed to bring it up with their doctors and therefore don't know about many of the new and effective treatments that are available. To compound the problem, many doctors aren't up on the latest treatments, either. In an editorial in the *Journal of the American Medical Association,* Dr Neil M. Resnick wrote, 'Most physicians have received little education about incontinence, fail to screen for it, and view the likelihood of success as low.'[9]

This doesn't mean that you should suffer in silence. Urinary incontinence is easily diagnosed and often treatable with excellent results. Read through the treatment options outlined below and see which ones speak to you. Then discuss them with your doctor. If possible, seek out someone who specialises in the evaluation of female urological problems and ask to be referred to them. Determining exactly what type of incontinence you have will allow you and your doctor to create an individualised plan of action.

Stress urinary incontinence (SUI) is the most common type of incontinence. It is diagnosed when a woman loses urine while performing any activity (such as laughing, standing up quickly, or exercising) that increases her intra-abdominal pressure and thus overrides the ability of her urethral sphincter to stay closed. This may result from problems with the sphincter muscle itself or from the fact that the angle of the urethral tube has changed, becoming too mobile to function properly – a condition known as urethral hypermobility. A number of factors that are increasingly common in perimenopause lead to this situation:

- Weakened pelvic floor muscles. Unless you exercise regularly and include your pelvic floor muscles, then these muscles, like your biceps, may be weaker than they should be.

- Thinning of the tissue of the outer urethral area, from oestrogen deficiency.

- Nerve damage resulting from childbirth, major pelvic surgeries, a history of radiation, smoking, or excess intra-abdominal fat that pushes the urethra out of the proper position every time you urinate. Innervation of the urethral sphincter also tends to decrease with age, but age alone does not inevitably lead to loss of function. (Research has shown that nerve density in this area varies widely in perimenopausal women.)[10]

- Underlying neurological disorders such as multiple sclerosis can result in other types of incontinence.

Whatever the exact cause of your problem, there are a lot of solutions besides spending the rest of your life wearing incontinence pads!

Non-surgical Incontinence Solutions

• *Keep a record.* Keeping a record will help both you and your doctor to learn which substances and situations may be contributing to your incontinence. Record how often you experience the problem, any activity that precedes it, how much urine actually leaks, whether or not you experience a warning beforehand, if it wakes you up at night, and whether it follows the ingestion of certain foods, drinks, or medications. Sometimes you can alleviate your problem just by becoming aware of when it happens and making adjustments.

Many women also have an increased urinary output on the first day of their period, when they get rid of all that premenstrual fluid. On these days, stress incontinence will always seem worse because your bladder fills more quickly.

• *Reduce or eliminate caffeinated drinks.* Many women have stress incontinence only when urine output is increased from drinking coffee or tea. Even decaffeinated coffee is a diuretic – and so is cold weather (I never drink a cup of coffee in the morning if I'm going skiing, otherwise I'll have to stop at a bar after every other run). Coffee is also a known bladder irritant. I've been able to help some women resolve their incontinence problem completely just by providing them with this information.

• *Medication.* Since there is a great deal of overlap between pure urinary stress incontinence and urge incontinence, many women are also offered medication to relax the bladder muscle. (See section on urge incontinence, page 261.)

• *Strengthen your pelvic floor.* Many women are able to resolve or greatly improve their incontinence by strengthening the muscles of the pelvic floor and urethra, so that they can withstand increases in intra-abdominal pressure without giving in. Strong muscles in the pelvic floor also increase blood flow and innervation of the pelvic organs. That is exactly what Dr Kegel had in mind in 1948 when he told his patients to practise vaginal contractions in preparation for childbirth. Ideally, every pregnant woman should be doing Kegels regularly both before and after birth so that these muscles will be strong enough to withstand the rigours of childbirth. When Kegel exercises are done properly and consistently, they work very well, and often improve your sex life as well. Some studies report that up to 75 per cent of women are able to overcome stress incontinence with Kegels alone.[11]

Unfortunately, the vast majority of women who are told to do Kegel exercises are not instructed in how to do them properly – which is why so many women think they don't work and why the reported results are so variable. Here's how: squeeze the vaginal muscles (the same muscles you use to stop the stream of urine) and hold for a slow count of ten (ten seconds). Relax for a count of five, then repeat. Do five sets three times per day. And keep at it. Results are noticeable in three to four weeks.

Kegels will not work if you contract your abdominal, thigh, or buttock muscles at the same time that you are squeezing the vaginal area. In fact, this only increases intra-abdominal pressure and aggravates the problem. Check yourself by putting one or two fingers in your vagina as you squeeze. These are the only muscles that should be contracting. Put your other hand on your lower abdomen as a reminder to keep your belly soft and relaxed.

There's an even easier way to do Kegels that doesn't require counting to ten or focusing on which muscles to contract. In this method, which is based on ancient Chinese techniques, you insert a weighted cone into your vagina and simply hold it in place for at least five minutes twice a day, gradually working up to fifteen minutes twice a day. You start with the heaviest cone that you can easily hold in for one minute, gradually move on to the heavier cones, and finally shift to a maintenance programme. (Cones range in weight from 15 to 100g.) Holding the cone in the vagina automatically uses just the right muscles. I have been recommending these cones for years and my patients have had excellent results with them, provided there are no complicating factors such as infection, neurological damage, or use of diuretic medications or caffeine. About 70 per cent of women can expect improvement or cure within four to six weeks of consistent use.[12] (See Resources.)

• *High-tech pelvic floor rehabilitation (biofeedback and EMRT).* Biofeedback-assisted behavioural treatment provides immediate audio and visual feedback to reinforce your control of your pelvic muscles. It has shown excellent results, ranging from 50 per cent to 89 per cent improvement after six to eight weeks. It has been shown to be far more effective for incontinence than medication, and it is generally available from physical therapists specially trained in the technique.[13] The disadvantage is that it requires the use of rectal or vaginal probes. Another technique known as extracorporeal magnetic resonance therapy (EMRT) has recently been approved by the US FDA. This device, known as Neocontrol, uses a magnet built into a special chair. Magnetic energy is targeted on the pelvic floor muscles and increased slowly to create a magnetic field. The resonating magnetic flux will, in turn, induce electrical depolarisation of nerves and muscles, resulting in contraction and exercise of exactly the right muscles. Studies have shown a 77 per cent improvement in patients tested so far.[14]

• *Oestrogen cream.* The outer third of the urethra is oestrogen-sensitive, just as is the vaginal tissue. In post- or perimenopausal women with stress urinary incontinence, oestrogen cream placed on the top surface of the outer third of the vagina has been shown to enhance nerve function and blood supply to the urethra, which in turn increases muscle size and strength. About 50 per cent of women who have incontinence associated with oestrogen depletion will be cured or greatly improved simply by re-oestrogenising their urethral area. This success rate increases for women who also strengthen their pelvic floor simultaneously.

While systemic HRT also works to relieve urinary symptoms, I recommend oestriol vaginal cream for this purpose. It is extremely effective when applied locally, and it doesn't result in any appreciable absorption into the bloodstream. That makes it ideal for any woman who is worried about the risks of oestrogen, including those with a history of or risk factors for breast cancer. Oestriol vaginal cream is available by prescription from any chemist that carries natural hormones. The usual strength is 0.5mg/g. (See Resources.)

• *Alternative devices.* Over the past few years a variety of urethral prosthetic devices have been developed. These devices are very useful for stress incontinence caused by urethral hypermobility and are especially good for those women who have incontinence only during specific activities such as golf or aerobics. These devices may be available in the UK soon, so keep asking your chemist. In the meantime, I suggest you order from the US.

The Impress Softpatch (from UroMed, US – see Resources) is a single-use soft foam patch that is coated with an adhesive. It is placed over the urethral opening to create a seal that stops mild to moderate leakage.[15]

Fem-Assist (from Insight Medical) and CapSure Shield (from Bard Urological) are silicone devices that fit over the urethral opening like a suction cup with the help of an ointment that helps seal them in place. These are only available in the US at present, but you can order them. The mild vacuum that results from the suction effect gently supports the surrounding tissue and squeezes the urethra shut. Once in place, these devices are concealed within the labia, so they can be worn with leotards or bathing suits. When you wish to urinate, you simply pull the device by the edge to remove it. It can then be washed with soap and warm water and reapplied. A single device can be used for a week before disposal.[16]

Some urinary incontinence devices work by stabilising the bladder base and re-establishing a normal angle between the bladder and urethra. Products available include the Incontinence Ring Bard's Contiform is a non-silicone, non-allergic vaginal device designed to elevate and support the bladder neck. (You may have noticed that it's more difficult to urinate with a tampon in. This is because the tampon elevates the bladder neck.) This device is meant to mimic the effect of a minimally invasive surgery known as urethropexy, which permanently tacks the bladder neck into place. The device comes in three sizes. When you first use it, buy the New User Pack which contains all three sizes. Thereafter you can simply buy replacements of the size which suits you. You can wear it all day or just when doing activities which may cause problems. It can be used for up to 30 days before you need to replace it, and should be removed and cleaned each night. You should be able to obtain Bard's Contiform from your chemist.

Many users of these devices report a heightened sense of self-confidence and freedom. The devices can be used on an as-needed basis and are virtually risk-free. They can also be used temporarily while you're strengthening your pelvic floor muscles.

Further information and advice can be obtained from the Continence Foundation (see Resources).

Surgical Techniques to Relieve Bladder Symptoms

• *Standard surgical procedures.* There are a variety of tried-and-tested surgical techniques for treating stress urinary incontinence that give long-term success rates of 80–95 per cent in the hands of an experienced surgeon. In all of these procedures, sutures are placed in the tissue near the urethra to elevate the bladder neck so that it functions properly. The disadvantage of these approaches is that they require an abdominal incision and a fairly long recovery period.[17]

• *Minimally invasive procedures.* A whole host of new surgical techniques have recently been developed to help permanently reposition the bladder neck so that urethral function is restored. They are done laparoscopically on an outpatient basis. Short-term results with the new techniques are also favourable, with a cure rate of about 82 per cent. Long-term results are not yet available.[18]

• *Injectables.* A variety of agents, including body fat or bovine collagen (Contigen Bard Collagen Implant – see Bard in Resources), can be injected around the urethra under local or general anaesthesia. These injections increase the volume of urethral tissue, allowing it to close properly and prevent the passage of urine during times of increased intra-abdominal pressure such as coughing, laughing, or change of position. They are effective immediately and can be done as an outpatient procedure. A skin test is necessary four weeks prior to the procedure to be certain that there will be no allergic reaction to the material. Alternatively ask for a new product Pelvicol (Bard), which is a cellular porcine (pork) dermal collagen tissue, which can be used in the same way and has no allergic risk. It usually takes two or three injections over time to get the desired result, and they may eventually have to be repeated. The improvement or cure rate ranges from 82 to 96 per cent, depending upon the type of incontinence being treated.[19]

Irritable Bladder: Urge Incontinence

Some incontinence is caused by involuntary contractions of the bladder muscle (the detrusor muscle). These involuntary contractions cause strong, sudden urges to urinate and the feeling that you might be about to wet yourself – which sometimes happens. Women with an overactive bladder often find themselves missing out on normal activities because they have to go to the lavatory so often and worry whether or not one will be available.

Urge incontinence is commonly treated with drugs such as tolterodine (Detrusitol) that inhibit detrusor contractions. Side effects include headache, dry mouth, dry eyes, constipation, and indigestion. Though this type of medication can be very helpful, there are other options.

Sometimes bladder irritation is caused by the localised lack of oestrogen in the bladder and urethral area associated with perimenopause and menopause. The problem resolves with local or systemic oestrogen therapy.

Irritable bladder syndrome can also be associated with stressful psychological situations such as taking an exam, being assessed at work, or worrying about some aspect of your life that isn't working. Many perimenopausal women find that they repeatedly have to get up at night to urinate when their sleep is interrupted by chronic worry or anxiety. In my experience, there is an exquisite connection between the 'worry-and-obsess' area of the brain and the bladder. Happily, we each have the ability to interact consciously with this area and get it to cooperate with us.

Biofeedback-assisted behavioural training, for example, has been shown to reduce involuntary incontinence episodes by about 80 per cent (drug therapy results in a 68 per cent reduction).[20] In one controlled study, women were asked to keep a voiding diary in which they recorded the time of day of the urgency and what they were doing at that time, so that their voiding patterns and the circumstances surrounding them would become clear. They were then taught how to identify their pelvic muscles and contract and relax them voluntarily while keeping abdominal muscles relaxed (the same as with Kegels) – a procedure that took only one session. Women were then taught to respond to the sensation of urgency by pausing, sitting down if possible, relaxing their entire bodies, and then contracting their pelvic muscles repeatedly to diminish urgency, inhibit detrusor muscle sensation, and prevent urine loss. When the urgency subsided, they were taught to proceed to the toilet at a normal pace. Women were encouraged to practise pelvic muscle contraction at home in various positions and also during activities when urge incontinence is most apt to occur. Finally, they were taught to practise interrupting or slowing their urine stream during voiding once per day.

Recurrent Urinary Tract Infections

Urinary urgency and frequency are often the result of recurrent urinary tract infections.

• Get a medical check-up to ensure that you don't have some anatomical problem that is contributing to your infections. Make sure that the outer third of your urethra is well oestrogenised. Your doctor should be able to evaluate this during a pelvic examination, because the urethra runs right under the top part of the vagina and is easily felt and observed. If there is any evidence of thinning of the outer urethra, get a prescription for oestrogen cream (see pages 258–9).

• Drink copious amounts of water or unsweetened (or artificially sweetened) cranberry juice the minute you feel any bladder symptoms. The extra liquid helps encourage frequent urination, which tends to flush out any bacteria lurking in the system, and cranberry juice renders bacteria less able to establish an infection in the lining of the urethra or bladder.

• Try cranberry capsules available at natural food shops. Take as directed. Cranberries contain a substance that prevents bacteria from sticking to the bladder wall, thus decreasing the risk for recurrent infection.

• Take a probiotic regularly to help recolonise your gut with 'friendly' bacteria. Because the anus and urethra are so close anatomically, encouraging the growth of favourable bacteria in one area of the body also helps the other. My favourite probiotic is PB 8, which doesn't have to be refrigerated.

• If these approaches don't work, consider a course of acupuncture and Chinese herbs. This treatment works very well for recurrent UTIs.

There you have it. I hope this information has given you hope and some peace of mind about the problem. Don't resign yourself to using incontinence pads the rest of your life when so many other solutions are available. You are not alone – incontinence is more common than diabetes. It is also often easier to treat! But you have to take the first step. Ask for help.

NINE

Sex and Menopause: Myths and Reality

Remember the first time you fell in love? You thought you had discovered the moon and the stars. The lyrics of the songs on the radio seemed as though they had been written especially for you. And chances are you felt so high and full of life that you didn't even feel much like eating. When a woman falls in love, she begins to experience an almost overwhelming influx of energy, filling her with exhilaration, benevolence, vigour, creativity ... and an eager, often insatiable sexual desire.

This can't-eat-can't-sleep feeling is not limited to young women experiencing their first love. It can be experienced at any age, any time we are able to connect at a deep emotional and spiritual level with another person. When that kind of connection is made, we bask joyfully in the knowledge that we are two people seeing, and being seen, as our truest selves.

This wonderful feeling of connection is something we have been led to believe can be experienced only by those in love. Our culture, through its books, films, and media images, promotes love and sex as the major, if not exclusive, route to happiness. But this is only part of the truth. When we are fully open to the energy that created the universe in the first place – which is another way of saying, when we are in love with our own lives – then we can re-create the chemistry of being in love simply by tuning in to the vitality of the world around us and in us. It's everywhere – in the beauty of nature, the pursuit of a cause we believe in, the exercise of our creative powers.

Falling in love with life itself, whatever form it takes, is an experience so powerful that I've known it to cause even women who were well past menopause to start getting their periods again.

In other words, if we think of sexual energy in the largest possible context – as life force, or as Source energy – then the relationship between the two becomes clear: the health and vitality of our sexuality is inexorably linked to the health and vitality of our lives.

The Anatomy of Desire

By the time we reach midlife, the challenge for each of us is to be able to access that in-love feeling in other ways besides looking to another person for fulfilment and gratification. The call goes out for each of us to expand our personal repertoire for accessing Source energy in our lives. Many men have opted to negotiate this developmental step by forging new sexual relationships with much younger partners. We women have only recently been granted anything close to equal opportunity in this regard. In the film *Moonstruck,* the character played by actress Olympia Dukakis wants to know why men, and her husband in particular, cheat on their wives. She gets the answer when her daughter's somewhat eccentric fiancé tells her, 'Because they are afraid of death.' Many men at midlife rejuvenate their fading life force through the bodies and fertility of younger women. In so doing, these men bypass a critical developmental stage: learning how to tap into Source energy directly.

Many women who are in the midst of negotiating this step for themselves find that their sex drive decreases for a while. In one study, 86 per cent of women reported some form of sexual problem during the years immediately before and after menopause, usually in the form of loss of sexual desire, often associated with vaginal dryness, dyspareunia (pain during penetration and intercourse), painful spasms in the vaginal muscles (vaginismus), loss of clitoral sensation, and touch sensation impairment.[1]

A menopause-related deficiency of hormones most often gets the blame, but the truth is, ferreting out the cause of sexual problems can be challenging. Sexual function is a complex, integrated phenomenon that reflects the health and balance not only of the ovaries and hormones, but also of the cardiovascular system, the brain, the spinal cord, and the peripheral nerves. In addition, every factor that affects sexual function has underlying psychological, sociocultural, interpersonal, and biological influences of its own.

Interestingly, of the 14 per cent of women who reported no sexual problems in the study mentioned above, one-third admitted that they had had sexual problems previously but that the problems had resolved themselves when the women found new sex partners. So much for hormone replacement being the sole viable solution to midlife libido problems! Resolving problems in an existing relationship can have an effect on sex life that's comparable to that of a new sex partner – when a woman reaches a *true* partnership with the man (or woman) she loves, she experiences a boost in her life energy, which translates to an equivalent boost in sexual energy.

In turn, an active and joyful sex life can have amazingly restorative effects on life force. Nothing illustrates the parallel circuitry between sexual energy and life energy better than the power of sexuality to heal when it is able to express itself freely. In her 1999 book *Reclaiming Goddess Sexuality: The Power of the Feminine Way,* Linda Savage writes about her experience of recovering from Crohn's disease, a chronic disease involving inflammation of the gastrointestinal tract that can result in weight loss, bloody stools, bloody diarrhoea, and an increased risk of bowel cancer. Her weight had dropped to 6 stone when she met a man with whom she began a very remarkable relationship. Within a few weeks all traces of her Crohn's were gone. She attributes her recovery entirely to the healing power of sexual energy, which is simply one of the many forms the life force takes.

This doesn't mean I'd recommend running straight out and having sex in order to heal yourself of a disease. The only way sexual energy can act as a healing force is if you experience it in the context of an unconditionally loving relationship in which your body, your soul, and your psyche are all cherished by another – or by yourself. *Remember, you do not necessarily have to have a partner to experience the rejuvenating energy of your own sexuality.*

With all this in mind, it is also important to remember that as a woman traverses the perimenopausal transition and all the changes it invites, her libido may seem to go underground for a time, while she reprioritises her life and the manner in which she uses her energy on a day-to-day basis. This is a perfectly normal diversion of life energy – an investment that can yield great dividends – but it is only

Midlife Changes in Sexual Function

All of the following changes in sexual function have been associated with perimenopause. Reading through the list, you can quickly appreciate that change itself – and not the nature of the change – is the one common theme.

- Increased sexual desire

- Change in sexual orientation

- Decreased sexual activity

- Vaginal dryness and loss of vaginal elasticity

- Pain or burning with intercourse

- Decreased clitoral sensitivity

- Increased clitoral sensitivity

- Decreased responsiveness

- Increased responsiveness

- Fewer orgasms, decreased depth of orgasm

- Increase in orgasms, sexual awakening

temporary. There is no reason for a diminished sex drive to become a permanent feature in the life of a menopausal woman.

Sexuality at Menopause: Our Cultural Inheritance

Like it or not, our sexuality has been, and continues to be, influenced by a male-dominated culture with an inherent double standard. In a recent best-selling book on how to slow the ageing process, for example, the quality of a man's sex life and its purported effect on his health was determined solely and meticulously by the annual number of orgasms – with a figure over three hundred being considered the most healthy. When it came to women, the author never bothered to tabulate or quantify how many orgasms a year could promote longevity. We got points only for being 'satisfied with quantity and happy with quality' of orgasms. Why is there such a plethora of data about men and so little about women?

The double standard is also apparent in the fact that men can buy Viagra at any of hundreds of Internet sites without seeing a doctor, while women still can't get contraceptive pills anywhere without a prescription.

Along those same lines of phallocentric reasoning, I recently read about an ongoing study testing Premarin vaginal cream as a kind of 'female Viagra' for women whose husbands are already on Viagra. The premise is that women's sex drive decreases at midlife because of vaginal thinning and dryness. Inserting Premarin cream in the vagina, the researchers posit, will result in a re-oestrogenisation of the vagina, making the experience of sex more comfortable for the woman (who, we assume, is already having intercourse regularly with a Viagra-enhanced penis). When I discussed this study with Dr Mona Lisa Schulz, her response was: 'Applying vaginal oestrogen cream to the vagina and expecting this to be the female Viagra is a joke. All you're doing is reducing the vagina and female sexuality to a runway that requires de-icing for the plane to be able to take off more comfortably.' For most women, sexual desire is related to far more than the oestrogenic state of the vagina (though oestrogen cream certainly helps some women). Female sexual response is related to a woman's total being: emotional, psychological, and spiritual, in addition to physical and hormonal. And we are profoundly affected by touch, taste, and smell as well as emotions. All are part of our sexuality.

I am reminded that our word *vagina* is derived from the Latin word meaning 'sheath for a sword'. It would appear that we have not come very far in this respect since the ancient Romans. We still see female sexuality predominantly in terms of how well our bodies meet and satisfy the needs and desires of males, rather than ourselves. That attitude, and the beliefs associated with it, finds its way into every aspect of our lives, including the medical research upon which women's health treatments are based.

In a recent study entitled 'Vaginal Changes and Sexuality in Women with a History of Cervical Cancer', the authors note that women who had been treated for cervical cancer experienced changes in their vaginal anatomy and function that had negative effects on their sexual function, including decreased lubrication, decreased elasticity, and decreased genital swelling during arousal. The authors said that the women experiencing these changes reported them to be 'distressing', and then went on to make the following observation:

> Although numerous studies have documented the distress associated with the loss of a breast, changes in the vagina have been neglected in this respect. A [literature] search performed in mid-1998 with the combined terms 'cancer', 'breast', and 'distress' yielded 197 references. In contrast, a search in which the term 'vagina' was substituted for 'breast' yielded only two references. One might assume that vaginal changes would affect sexual function at least as much as the loss of a breast. An obvious reason for the predominant interest in the breast is that, in developed countries, breast cancer is more common than cancer of the female genital organs. Nevertheless, the paucity of literature on the effect of vaginal changes is noteworthy, and it may not be irrelevant to speculate about nonscientific reasons. For men, female breasts have aesthetic as well as sexual value, which may influence research policies in academic medicine, where male investigators predominate.[2]

Overcoming Cultural Barriers:
The First Step Towards Waking a Sleeping Libido

Although progress is being made, change in our culture's attitude about women and sexuality is slow in coming, and many women have never felt as though they had permission to explore their own sexual energy on their own terms. In *Reclaiming Goddess Sexuality*, Linda Savage writes:

> [Women] want the beauty of the context of sexual encounters to be more important than the act. They want to be touched in slow, sensual ways. They want to be ravished with intense passion that demonstrates how much their partners need them, rather than just needing an orgasm to relax. All in all, women want to be adored as precious feminine beings.[3]

The fact that this need is incompletely met for women in our culture is what drives the multi-million-pound romance novel industry. Many women are absolutely addicted to these stories, because they invariably show women being adored for who they are, not just for their bodies.

LORI'S STORY: WHAT I DID FOR LOVE

Over the years, Lori had become gradually aware that her sex life with her husband, Roy, was not meeting her needs. 'There was never any cuddling, caressing, nothing to get me in the mood. And he wanted it at least once a day – the harder his day had gone at work, the more he needed it. For him it was a tension reliever. For me it had become mechanical and pretty much unsatisfying.' With the help of a marriage counsellor, Roy became aware of Lori's needs, and together they learned techniques that opened up a whole new world for them both. 'The sex became great,' Lori wrote. But Roy's needs for regular 'pressure release' after work didn't go away, and to engage in that sort of sex seemed to Lori like a step backwards. 'To be honest, it made me angry,' she reported. 'I felt like screaming, "Haven't you been listening?"' Their counsellor, in subsequent sessions, led Lori to believe that to be in a fair partnership, she must be willing to meet Roy's needs, too.

Generally speaking, Lori's counsellor was correct. All couples must learn how to compromise in order to satisfy the needs of each person, and sex is no different from any other area of need. But there were parts of Lori and Roy's story that deeply concerned me when I first spoke to Lori, who came to see me about hormone replacement therapy at the age of forty-five, when she started skipping periods.

I wanted to be sure Lori didn't believe that it was her 'job' to relieve Roy's tension and stress by allowing her body to be used in this way every day. I validated her anger at this and told her that it was her barometer, letting her know that the problem it signalled was real and needed to be addressed. Second, I suggested that when an individual needs that much sex to medicate his (or her) stress, something is wrong in his (or her) life. I asked if their therapist had suggested that Roy examine his life, his job, and his stress levels. Lori said that she had raised this in therapy but had been told that this was an individual, not a couples, issue. Since Roy had refused individual therapy, there was nothing further she could say on this subject during their sessions.

This is a perfect example of what can happen when couples therapy goes awry. Fully 96 per cent of all couples therapy involving hetero-sexual relationships is initiated by the woman, who usually holds it over her husband's head as a last-ditch effort to save the marriage. He goes in, usually reluctantly, often feeling, 'It's her problem, but I'll go along,' and unable or unwilling to understand that his own issues are part of the couples dynamic.

Candidly, many therapists have told me that if the man's issues were addressed directly, he'd be sufficiently uncomfortable that he'd probably terminate therapy altogether. So the therapist tries to keep him engaged with so-called couples issues. Too often, the woman's individual concerns also get subverted to the needs of the 'couple'. This kind of therapy can go on for years, relieving the relationship tension just enough so that the couple stays together, while the funda-mental power dynamic of the relationship never changes because key individual behaviours never change. When this happens, there's no chance for the transformational power of true partnership.

To create a true partnership, Roy needed to see that he was using Lori sexually as an opiate, to medicate himself for stress. There was no way Lori could have a sense of true communion or of being cher-ished by him as long as stress relief was the main energy driving his lovemaking. Though it would be perfectly reasonable for them to compromise with a 'quickie' now and again, for Roy to make a daily pattern of using sex to self-medicate for stress sounded like sexual addiction and dysfunction to me. It was certainly undermining Lori's ability to feel good about their sexual relationship. Roy needed to take responsibility for his own stress reduction needs, and he needed a wider repertoire of behaviours to accomplish this. This might include exercise, meditation, or even masturbation. Though wives have been expected to serve their 'wifely duty' in this way for centuries and have acquiesced for fear that he might go elsewhere to 'get his needs met', there is no place for these assumptions today if a couple is to reach the joyful communion that's possible at midlife.

At the time of her next annual examination, Lori told me that over the past year Roy had begun to realise he needed to change his job if he didn't want to follow in the footsteps of his father, who had died at the age of sixty, only one year after retiring from a job he had hated. He had also found several ways of achieving stress reduction, including going to twice-weekly yoga classes and joining a basketball league at work. Thanks to these changes, Roy's blood pressure and cholesterol dropped to normal, and he began to feel better about himself, knowing that he had been able to assert this kind of control over his life and free himself of the pattern that had probably helped bring about his father's premature death. Once Lori saw that he had become more emotionally self-sufficient, she found him more sexually attractive – to the point that she was actually initiating sex.

What Viagra Tells Us About Our Sexuality

Viagra and the enormous publicity surrounding it speak volumes about the values of our culture. There is no question that this drug can be a boon to quality of life for many couples in which the male partner suffers from erectile dysfunction. But enhanced sexual performance through medical manipulation of the male's genitals only cannot heal a relationship that is not working.

Our culture is quick to forget the holistic nature of sexual function and how profoundly it is enhanced when a couple is truly connected via their hearts and minds. The sex researchers Masters and Johnson have described how the excitement and plateau phase of the sexual response can be prolonged if the connection between the man and woman is not only genital but also related to heart and mind. At midlife many couples find that they have the time and the desire to be fully present to each other in this way, and as a result they experience the best sex of their lives. I've heard their stories repeatedly in my surgery. But for some, making love is just another task on the to-do list. Sex therapist Dr Patricia Love wrote:

Sensuality, the ability to be comfortable in one's body, suspend time, and communicate through the skin is what is missing in many marriages . . . . All too often husbands and wives go to bed feeling distracted and numb, reflexively groping for each other's genitals. The unspoken goal is to go from neutral to orgasm in 15 minutes like a car zooming from zero to sixty.[4]

This results in what sex therapists call 'spectatoring', which is a mental disconnection during lovemaking, thinking more about work or household chores than about the partner beside them. For the man, this may translate to erectile difficulties; for the woman, difficulty reaching orgasm. The man who looks first to Viagra to 'save' him may be discounting the importance of making a connection with his lover. A woman involved with a man who feels he needs Viagra for psychogenic impotence would be wise to ask herself about the quality of their connection. Those things that remain unspoken between them, the issues and feelings that are too uncomfortable to talk about, may be blocking full erection and orgasm, and may also be putting their health at risk in other areas.

VICTOR AND VIAGRA: GINNY'S LAMENT

Ginny and Victor had been married for thirty years and had a pretty happy relationship. Victor had always prided himself on his virility, and he and Ginny had enjoyed a vigorous sex life for years, making love about three times per week. When he reached fifty-five, however, Victor noticed that his erections were not as hard as they used to be, and it sometimes took him longer to achieve them. Occasionally he even found that he was unable to sustain an erection long enough to bring Ginny to orgasm. He and Ginny had gradually slowed down in their lovemaking to about once every two weeks. This didn't bother Ginny, particularly because she was very busy starting a new catering business – something she'd always dreamed of. Her business was taking off, and now that their youngest child had left home for college, her life was no longer focused solely on the needs of her husband and children. But Victor, who was planning to retire in a year or two, was not nearly as happy with his life. It seemed that just as he was starting to slow down, Ginny was taking off in the outside world.

   Victor sought a consultation with his doctor, who prescribed Viagra. Victor was elated with the results. Ginny wasn't. The Viagra introduced a 'mechanical' element to their sex life that had never been present before. She didn't like having to be sexually available just because Victor had taken his pill, and she began to spend more and more time away from home, partly because she was having so much fun at work, partly because she didn't want to have sex 'on demand'. When asked how she felt about Viagra, Ginny replied, 'I think we were better off without it. I love Victor and it really didn't bother me when it took him a little longer to get hard. I usually knew how to help. Now I feel as though a vital emotional component of our love-making has been replaced by a pill.'

Their situation is not unusual. Victor's change in sexual function is, in part, related to his sense of decreasing power in the outer world, even though it is his own choice to retire from work. Though Viagra is probably a relatively safe solution for him for a time, he would be best served by finding a new life's purpose into which to pour his energy. Otherwise he won't be able to keep up with his wife, in the bedroom or otherwise, without resorting to a drug for support. That doesn't mean there aren't valid indications for Viagra. Rather, it is to point out that sexual function is related to much more than the size and duration of an erection.

Menopause Is a Time to Redefine and Update Our Relationships

Five years ago I would have written all of this while thinking it did not apply to me. Similarly, many of you may be thinking, 'That's interesting, but my relationship with my significant other is good', and you may be right, overall. For many of us, the relationships we have maintained over the years have served us well and have been mutually beneficial, even passionate. But it is very often necessary to renegotiate some of the terms of the old relationship as you enter the transformative years of midlife. No matter how good that relationship may have been, what worked for you in your 'previous' life will, in all likelihood, need some updating in order to serve the person you are becoming.

One area in which the necessity for change may become apparent is in the waning of a woman's libido. Just as wild animals refuse to breed in captivity unless everything is in balance in their environment, a woman and her significant other may notice problems in their sexual intimacy if their relationship is in need of rebalancing. Menopause is also a time when what a woman wants from a relationship begins to change.

As we have seen, it is usually the woman who sacrifices career and personal growth for the sake of maintaining and nurturing the family, even if she works full time outside the home. Not only the unwritten rules of society but the hormones flowing through her veins encourage her to give high priority to family, nurturing, nesting, and protection of loved ones. At menopause the hormonal changes are only part of a woman's ongoing transformation, which begins at an energetic level and triggers changes not only in her biology but also in her perception, intuition, neural pathways, emotions, creative drive, and overall focus. While she spends the first half of her life giving birth to others (literally and figuratively), everything about her menopausal transition suggests that the second half of life is when she is meant to give birth to herself.

If, through the lens of your transforming self, you discover that you are not in love with your life, your libido may suffer as a result. In fact, a fading sex drive may be one of the first places a red flag will pop up, as a signal of a fading love of life – a waning life force. Only if both you and your significant other are willing to question what is no longer viable in your relationship and work together on the necessary remodelling can you open the door to rejuvenation of your life energy and the rekindling of your passion, sexual and otherwise. Healing will require a bilateral effort – both you and your partner must be willing to ask, and hear the answers to, some difficult questions in order to restore and renew your relationship.

Terminal Busyness Leads to Exhaustion and Waning Libido

Someone sent me the following anonymous posting from the Internet. This one paragraph summarises the plight of many midlife women – and the difference between their lives and those of their husbands.

Mum and Dad were watching TV when Mum said, 'I'm tired, and it's getting late. I think I'll go to bed.' She went to the kitchen to make sandwiches for the next day's lunches, rinsed out the popcorn bowls, took meat out of the freezer for supper the following evening, checked the cereal box levels, filled the sugar container, put spoons and bowls on the table, and started the coffeepot for brewing the next morning. She then put some wet clothes into the dryer, put a load of clothes into the wash, ironed a shirt, and secured a loose button. She picked up the newspapers strewn on the floor, picked up the game pieces left on the table, and put the telephone book back into the drawer. She watered the plants, emptied a waste-paper basket, and hung up a towel to dry. She yawned and stretched and headed for the bedroom. She stopped by the desk and wrote a note to the teacher, counted out some cash for the field trip, and pulled a textbook out from hiding under the chair. She signed a birthday card for a friend, addressed and stamped the envelope, and wrote a quick shopping list. She put both near her handbag. Mum then cleansed her face, put on moisturiser, brushed and flossed her teeth, and trimmed her nails. Her husband called, 'I thought you were going to bed.'

'I'm on my way,' she said. She put some water into the dog's bowl and put the cat outside, then made sure the doors were locked. She looked in on each of the kids and turned out a bedside lamp, hung up a shirt, threw some dirty socks in the laundry basket, and had a brief conversation with the one still up doing homework. In her own room, she set the alarm, laid out clothing for the next day, and straightened up the shoe rack. She added three things to her list of things to do for tomorrow.

About that time, her husband turned off the TV and announced to no one in particular, 'I'm going to bed,' and he did.

MARY: OVERCARE AND BURNOUT SEND LIBIDO UNDERGROUND

Mary was a registered nurse. As the eldest of five children from an Irish Catholic family, she had always been expected to take care of her parents and younger siblings. When her mother died suddenly, Mary's alcoholic father, a man in the early stages of dementia, came to live with Mary and her husband, Jeff, a police officer. Despite having four other siblings, Mary had never questioned her role as the designated family caregiver. But the increased need for 'alone time' so many women experience at menopause led Mary to feel not only a total loss of sexual desire, but also complete emotional burnout. She had recently been diagnosed with hypothyroidism and was suffering from weight gain, depression, lethargy, fatigue, dry skin, and the desire to sleep all the time. Though her family doctor had prescribed thyroid hormone replacement, Mary saw little improvement in her depression. And despite normal oestrogen, progesterone, and testosterone levels, her sexual desire remained non-existent.

When a woman is experiencing caregiver's burnout, her body is often, quite literally, running on empty. She may have insufficient levels of many nutrients, such as the B vitamins and magnesium, which contribute to her fatigue. And her adrenal glands may be producing either too much cortisol or, after years and years of unabated stress without replenishment, too little cortisol. Either way, the end result is physical exhaustion. Sleep, not sex, is what women like Mary find themselves fantasising about.

I prescribed a programme for Mary that focused on her rejuvenation from the inside out. I told her that she needed to get help at home at least two days per week. She also needed to improve her eating habits, cutting right down on refined carbohydrates like cakes, sweets, and biscuits and increasing her intake of protein, essential fatty acids, and fresh fruits and vegetables. I also suggested a high-potency multivitamin and told her she needed to go to bed by 10 o'clock every night. Mary had known all along that her life needed to change, but, she told me, she was relieved to finally have a medical authority supporting her in the changes she would have to make if she was going to resume optimal functioning – which would include the rekindling of her libido. If she didn't stem the chronic draining of her life force by getting adequate rest, exercise, and nutrition, then her libido, like every other aspect of her health, would pay the price. It's too bad that so many women who have taken on the caretaker role need a doctor's 'prescription' to give them permission to live more healthfully.

Hormone Levels Are Only One Part of Libido

One of my colleagues underwent a hysterectomy (uterus removed, ovaries left intact) at the age of forty-eight, a procedure that is associated with measurable declines in oestrogen and testosterone because the surgery compromises the blood supply to the ovaries. This is the reason given for the fact that many women experience some sexual problems following hysterectomy. But my colleague, who had started a new relationship just prior to her surgery, couldn't wait to get out of the hospital and back into bed with her new love. She told me, 'When you have someone waiting for you whom you're madly in love with, you can bet you're not likely to have much problem with desire or lubrication, or anything else.' On the other hand, if you are in a relationship that has been problematic for years, a relationship in which you have had little or no interest in sex but put up with it anyway, you can bet that your body will do anything it can to keep you from having to get back into that position again. It is well documented, for instance, that unassertive women in dysfunctional sexual partnerships experience limited genital arousal and few if any orgasms. Sexually assertive women, on the other hand, report higher levels of sexual desire, orgasmic frequency, and greater satisfaction with both their sexual and marital relationships.[5]

Psychiatrist and neuroscientist Mona Lisa Schulz points out that sexual impulses and desire are controlled, in part, by the frontal lobes of the brain, and anything that changes frontal lobe activity can affect libido – in either direction. In the frontal lobe dysfunction known as depression, libido is often decreased. But in the frontal lobe dysfunction known as dementia, sexual impulses can run rampant, sometimes resulting in socially embarrassing behaviour. An example of this is a nun I once treated who had developed an uncontrollable urge to masturbate all the time. Although she was not distressed by this, her community was. She eventually ended up under the care of a neurologist, for dementia.

Changes in libido can, of course, be triggered by declining hormone levels, especially in women who have undergone medical or surgical menopause.[6] In my professional experience, however, fading life force is equally likely, if not more so, to be at the root of declining sexual desire. Two influences are universally underestimated in terms of their potential impact on libido: the state of a woman's relationship with her sexual partner, and her overall emotional and spiritual love for life. And, interestingly, both of these factors may well have the potential to change hormone levels in and of themselves.[7]

A woman with a strong current of life force, who is in love with her life, can continue to have a strong libido regardless of what her hormones are doing. This fact is supported by research that shows that the hormonal changes of menopause, per se, are not the cause of decreased libido. In fact, the relationship between hormones and libido may be a chicken-and-egg question, as it seems equally plausible for a faltering life force to be the result, rather than the cause, of a dying sex life.

Therefore I want to encourage every woman to consider the health and vitality of her connection with life – her connection to Source energy – along with the more conventionally accepted hormonal issues as she evaluates her sex life and the possibility that it may need help at this stage of her life.

Secondary Libidinal Support: Oestrogen and Progesterone

With all that said, it is possible for a woman to experience a fading libido during and after menopause even if she is involved in a true partnership, one that supports her life force rather than drains it. If a woman is in love with her life, if her life force – a repository for sexual energy – is free-flowing and vigorous, then a weakening libido may be due to secondary, hormonal factors.

As we learn more about the roles of oestrogen and progesterone in the maintenance of bodywide functions such as circulation, nerve transmission, and cell division, it becomes clear how declining levels of these hormones can contribute to changes in sexual response.

• The entire nervous system is surrounded with oestrogen-sensitive cells.[8] It stands to reason, then, that a decrease in oestradiol levels can have a dampening effect on nerve transmission during sex. Research has shown that oestrogen deprivation can lead to actual peripheral neuropathy – a form of nerve dysfunction that makes a woman less sensitive to touch and vibration. Oestradiol replacement can restore this sensitivity to levels that approach those seen in women who are still menstruating.

• Declining levels of oestradiol and progesterone can have an effect on a woman's potential for sexual arousal, sensitivity, sensation, and orgasm, because at optimal levels these hormones increase the flow of blood to the sexually sensitive areas. In other words, a woman's physical response to sexual stimulation may be slower and less likely to build to orgasm because of decreased speed and volume of blood supply to the sexually sensitive areas, which may in any case be less sensitive than before because of the nerve dysfunction sometimes caused by oestrogen deprivation.

• Oestrogen levels that are too low can lead to cell atrophy in the genital region, which can cause thinning of the vaginal and urethral tissue, with the result that intercourse becomes painful. Women with oestrogen depletion may also experience urinary problems such as recurrent urinary tract infections or even stress urinary incontinence.

• Vaginal fluid production during sexual arousal and intercourse is also an oestrogen-dependent process. If oestrogen is low, there may be a reduction of vaginal fluid, resulting in vaginal dryness and painful intercourse. Because a woman's level of sexual arousal tends to be judged by the amount and ease of vaginal lubrication achieved, lack of vaginal fluid can lead to the perception that she has low sexual arousal. While sexual arousal may be negatively influenced by the anticipation of pain, libido is not the real issue in these circumstances.

• Progesterone has additional effects on libido that have not been as well studied as those of oestrogen but are no less important. Its effect seems largely to be one of maintenance, valuable in keeping a woman's existing libido from declining. Moreover, as a precursor of oestrogen and testosterone, progesterone is important for maintaining high enough levels of these other hormones for optimal sexual pleasure. A normal balance of progesterone also acts as a mood stabiliser and supports normal thyroid function, thereby enhancing the libido both emotionally and metabolically.

The bottom line is this: a deficiency of oestrogen and/or progesterone can decrease a woman's libido by orchestrating physical changes that, quite simply, make the sex act less pleasurable. Dryness and thinning of the vaginal wall can result in physical discomfort during intercourse, as can vaginal muscle spasms. Changes in nerve function can numb ordinarily sensitive body parts, and changes in blood circulation can decrease the physical response when stimulation occurs, making it ever more difficult to reach orgasm.

Research has shown that libido-dampening effects are most likely to occur when a woman's blood levels of oestradiol (our body's most biologically potent natural oestrogen) drop below 50pmol/l. Salivary oestradiol levels can also be used, with 1pg/ml being the lower end of the threshold for normal sexual function.[9] Blood flow to the vulva and vagina is dramatically increased when supplementation brings oestradiol back to these levels, and often this is enough to restore sexual response. With the help of a woman's health care provider, achieving this level is simple. Depending on the individual woman, a transdermal oestradiol patch (usually the 0.1mg strength) or 0.5 to 1mg oral oestradiol taken twice daily is adequate, gentle, and consistent in restoring oestradiol levels to that comfortable threshold. And in the early stages of perimenopause, when many women have declines in progesterone levels but oestrogen levels that are still within the normal range, 1/4tsp of natural progesterone cream massaged into the hands or soft skin twice a day can have a restorative effect on a subtle downturn in libido.

JEANNETTE: WHERE DID MY SEX DRIVE GO?

'Dave and I have been through some rough times,' Jeannette said, 'but I really feel our relationship has grown along with us – we're better than ever. The trouble is, I just don't have any desire to make love. I love Dave, I really do, but I could go the rest of my life without having sex and I wouldn't care.'

Now forty-five years old, Jeannette had noticed some early signs of perimenopause. She hadn't had any hot flushes or vaginal dryness, but her periods, which used to come 'like clockwork,' were more erratic, and she thought she might have had some night sweats ('either that or I just had on too many covers').

Salivary hormone testing revealed that Jeannette's oestrogen levels were still well within the rather broad limits of the normal range, but her progesterone level was on the low side, and her testosterone level was significantly below normal for a woman her age. After some discussion, we decided to boost her progesterone levels with a 1.5–3 per cent natural progesterone cream, 1/4tsp massaged into her hands and wrists twice a day. For her testosterone supplementation, Jeannette opted for an oral testosterone pill. 'It made all the difference,' she reported. 'I find that I'm in the mood more often, and even if I'm not in the mood, I can get aroused a lot faster than before.'

Testosterone: The Hormone of Desire?

Although much has been written in the popular press about testosterone's role in sex drive, a deficiency of testosterone is probably the least common cause for a woman's waning libido, coming in at a distant fourth place behind relationship issues and progesterone and/or oestrogen decline. Part of the reason testosterone has received so much attention, however – apart from the fact that testosterone is universally thought of as a male hormone – is its very specific effect. While oestrogen and progesterone play a supportive role in a woman's healthy libido, supplemental testosterone can directly and quickly stimulate the sex drive in both men and women if the reason for the diminished libido has to do with lowered testosterone levels.

Contrary to popular belief, however, testosterone levels do not fall appreciably after menopause. In fact, in most (but not all) women, the postmenopausal ovary secretes *more* testosterone than the premenopausal ovary. Still, testosterone levels do undergo a gradual decline in some women, beginning in their late twenties and continuing through midlife, and it is possible for levels to dip low enough to quash libido.

Sometimes the decline in testosterone – and hence in libido – is sudden, rather than gradual. This can occur following removal of, or loss of function of, the ovaries. The same can happen if the adrenal glands are exhausted (see chapter 4). That's because the ovaries and the adrenals (as well as the liver and the body fat) all produce the steroid hormones collectively known as androgens, one of which is testosterone. If you've had a loss or sudden decrease in ovarian function secondary to chemotherapy, radiation, or surgery, then you may find that your libido dramatically decreases because your body has not had time to shift androgen production to the other body sites that make it. Women with this problem often complain of 'not feeling like myself any more . . . it's as if my life energy has somehow gone'. And they lose their libido – their sex energy – as well. The reason this doesn't happen to *all* women who lose ovarian function is that some women's bodies *are* able to make the move to other androgen production sites without much interruption in the hormonal output. But for those whose bodies don't adjust as easily, prescription supplemental hormones may be required to restore their androgen levels.

In women with testosterone levels that have declined significantly, for whatever reason, supplemental testosterone often does have the desired effect on libido. Studies have shown that 65 per cent of menopausal women with depleted testosterone who received testosterone supplementation experienced an increase in libido, increased sexual response, increased frequency of sexual activity, increased sexual fantasies, and increased sensitivity of erogenous zones.[10]

However, in my experience, results are completely satisfying only if a woman's intimate relationship is healthy and mutual. This is particularly true at midlife, when a woman is less likely to sweep resentments under the rug. When her significant relationship is in trouble, testosterone supplementation is much less likely to be effective in stimulating her sex drive.

If, however, you think your decline in libido may be related to lowered levels of testosterone or one of the other androgens, you may want to have your testosterone and/or DHEA levels checked. This can be done through saliva testing. Ask your doctor to arrange salivary samples for you, or submit a salivary sample on your own. (Salivary testing is available through Higher Nature Ltd; see Resources.)

If your levels turn out to be low, your physician can prescribe natural testosterone, available through a formulary pharmacy (Boots the Chemist). Natural testosterone can be used either as a capsule or as a vaginal cream. The usual starting dose is 1 to 2mg every other day, gradually increasing if necessary. Another option is to take the supplement DHEA at a dose of 5 to 10mg once or twice per day. In some women this hormone, which is a precursor for testosterone, will raise testosterone levels sufficiently to improve a waning sex drive. (For more information, read *The Hormone of Desire: The Truth About Sexuality, Menopause, and Testosterone*, by Susan Rako.) DHEA is also prescription only in the UK, but can be bought in small quantities from the US (see DHEA in Resources).

Aids to Lubrication

Some women at midlife find that, although the spirit is willing, the body is not. Their libido is unchecked, but for reasons they don't understand, they no longer get sufficiently lubricated. There are a variety of treatments that can help with this problem.

NATALIE: SUSTAINING ONGOING RELATIONSHIPS

Natalie first came to see me when she was fifty-two. Her husband, Brad, accompanied her on her visit. Natalie's health was good, but she had been having problems with intercourse. She couldn't seem to get lubricated before intercourse, which made lovemaking difficult. And she had also had a couple of episodes of urinary burning and frequency that felt like urinary tract infections (UTIs).

As I watched Brad and Natalie interact, it was clear that although Brad was uncomfortable talking about the situation, he was genuinely concerned about his wife. He didn't want to hurt her, but he couldn't understand what had gone wrong with their lovemaking. And both expressed fear that their sexual problem could spread, causing them to become distant from each other in general. I performed a pelvic examination on Natalie and found that her vaginal wall was significantly thinned, which would make it less resilient and more sensitive to irritation and discomfort from the stretching and friction inevitable during intercourse. Her vaginal thinning also explained the UTI symptoms, given that vaginal thinning is associated with thinning and irritation of the outer third of the urethral passage as well. Natalie's examination also showed an obvious lack of natural lubrication, which would make intercourse more traumatic for her and less pleasurable for both partners. Suspecting that Natalie was in perimenopause, I took a vaginal sample and sent it to the lab for what is known as a 'maturation index', a test to see how many cells are well oestrogenised and how many aren't. I also had her oestrogen, progesterone, and testosterone levels tested. Her testosterone was well within normal range, but her oestrogen and progesterone were low. Her maturation index confirmed that she had what is called atrophic vaginitis, a term that simply refers to a lack of oestrogen in the cells of the vaginal lining, making it thin and inflamed.

I explained to Natalie her treatment options and ultimately prescribed oestriol cream for the vagina, plus progesterone cream to be applied anywhere on her skin. By retesting her levels and adjusting her dosage according to how she felt, over a three-month period we established optimal baseline oestrogen and progesterone levels for that particular stage of Natalie's life. In a follow-up visit within a month, Natalie reported that their sex life was 'back to normal'. This is exactly what I had expected would happen. Treating bona fide perimenopausal vaginal dryness and thinning is safe, easy, and very effective.

GRACE: BEGINNING A NEW RELATIONSHIP

Grace was fifty-five when she came to see me for a check-up. Her husband, with whom she'd enjoyed a monogamous relationship for twenty years, had died five years before. Her marriage had been a happy and fulfilling one, and she did not actively look for a new partner after his death. She enjoyed a busy life teaching tennis, gardening, and travelling. But then she was reintroduced to a man who had been one of her boyfriends at school and whom she hadn't seen for many years. He, too, was widowed – his wife had died several years before. Since they lived a fair distance apart, they began writing letters and phoning each other. Her visit to me was prompted by his invitation to spend a few weeks at his house. He had told her he wanted her to consider marrying him. Though she wasn't exactly planning on having sex with him during her visit, she wanted to be prepared. Like many women, Grace was worried that her vagina had 'shrivelled up' from so many years of disuse. I assured her that her vagina was designed to be functional for her entire life, even though it might need some initial help after years of abstinence. (This is not always the case. Women who masturbate in ways that involve vaginal penetration often maintain excellent vaginal function even when not in a relationship that involves sexual intercourse. And of course, many women achieve orgasm without vaginal penetration.)

Grace had been postmenopausal for five years and had decided not to take hormone replacement therapy because she had no family history of heart disease or osteoporosis, her bone density was excellent, and she wanted to avoid any increased risk of breast cancer. Because she still had no compelling reason to start hormone replacement therapy, I saw no need in her case to prescribe it.

On pelvic examination, however, Grace's vagina looked a bit reddened, and the lining, called the vaginal mucosa, appeared somewhat thin. Sometimes this condition is associated with painful intercourse, and sometimes it is not – it depends on the individual. It was entirely possible that Grace would be able to have intercourse with no problem at all, but on the other hand, given the newness of her situation, I felt it was best if she had a couple of options. Grace agreed that she didn't want to take chances. Though she had not experienced any sensation of vaginal dryness or discomfort for the past ten years, she wanted to be sure that she'd be able to have comfortable intercourse.

I offered two options: a prescription for vaginal oestriol cream, or a very effective and safe non-hormonal lubricant. Grace chose the vaginal oestriol cream so that by the time she got to his house three weeks later, her vaginal tissue would be very well oestrogenised and thicker than it now appeared. She also wanted to come back to see me just before leaving so that I could assess her progress. The hormone oestriol is a natural oestrogen that does not stimulate the growth of breast or uterine tissue as strongly as the other oestrogens, oestrone and oestradiol. It can be given orally as a pill or locally to relieve vaginal dryness. Given locally in the vagina only, it is safe to use even if you've had breast cancer, uterine cancer, or ovarian cancer, or are concerned about getting these oestrogen-related problems. Oestriol has a very beneficial local effect on the oestrogen-sensitive tissues of the vagina. (Other conventional oestrogens, such as Premarin cream or Vagifem vaginal tablets, also work well for vaginal thinning and dryness, but the oestrogen in these can act as a growth factor in breast and uterine tissue, which may be of concern if you've had cancer in one of these organs. However, at low doses they don't appear to cause any appreciable problem. Like oestriol, these creams can also be very helpful in treating urinary incontinence that stems from localised lack of oestrogen.)

I prescribed daily use of the cream for one week, to build up what is called the cornified layer of epithelium in the vagina, then one to three applications per week afterwards, to maintain the suppleness, resilience, and moistness of her vaginal tissues. I also told her that if she began having regular intercourse, the blood supply to her vagina would increase. This, combined with the repeated stimulation and stretching of her vagina, would result in a much decreased need for the cream – possibly to the point of being able to eliminate it completely, with just a touch of a non-prescription lubricant as needed.

Non-prescription Help with Lubrication

With or without the use of prescription oestriol, there are several choices of lubrication available that work well for relieving vaginal dryness. Good old K-Y jelly is available at every chemist, though this water-soluble lubricant may not be enough for some, and for others it can form an annoying residue. Other lubricants that work very well are Sylk, made from kiwi fruit, and Women's Group Formulas Vaginal Lubricant, which contains a number of soothing herbal extracts such as marigold. (See Resources.) A number of herbal remedies taken systemically can also help restore vaginal lubrication: black cohosh, wild yam, dong quai, or chaste berry are good examples. Vitamin E suppositories are effective, too. And many women find that their vaginal resiliency and moisture are restored when they start eating whole soya foods regularly – the higher the daily dose of isoflavones, the more effective. (Note, however, that oil-based lubricants may weaken latex condoms and diaphragms, making them less effective.)

Another approach to vaginal health is to do Kegel exercises regularly to stimulate and strengthen the muscles of the vaginal floor. They're easy to do, and they can be done any time, anywhere; nobody can tell what you're doing. Studies have shown that in addition to increasing blood supply (which will increase vaginal wall thickness as well as lubrication), these exercises can improve libido by increasing clitoral tumescence and sensitivity and increasing the strength of orgasm. As a happy side effect, Kegel exercises also can help prevent, or reverse, urinary incontinence (leakage). (See chapter 8.)

Telling the Truth

At midlife, more and more women become comfortable with telling the truth about their sexuality – to themselves and to others. Here are some areas you might want to re-evaluate.

- *Come to terms with your own sexuality.* All humans are sexual by nature – it's part of being human. Women undergo vaginal lubrication at regular intervals during sleep, and men get erections. But how you choose to express your sexuality when you're awake will depend upon many factors, including your upbringing, your hormone levels, your general overall health, and your level of satisfaction with your sexual partner, if you currently have one.

- *Stop keeping score.* What is a normal sex life? Only you can answer that question for yourself. To help you find your personal truth about this issue, let me remind you that we live in a society that often confuses quantity with quality. Even the medical profession equates the quality of one's sex life with the frequency of intercourse. This is a gross disservice to couples everywhere, many of whom will inevitably feel they don't measure up. For perspective, you may find it comforting to know that a recent study from the University of Chicago in the US pointed out that it's pretty common for couples to have intercourse three times per month and be completely satisfied with that. Ask yourself the following question, and answer it honestly: if your life were ideal, how much time would you like to devote each week to being sexual – either with yourself or with a partner?

- *Respect your inherent sex drive.* Sex therapist Dr Patricia Love notes that people can be divided into three different categories when it comes to innate sex drive: high, moderate, and low.[11] Individuals with relatively high testosterone levels (high Ts) tend to have a higher sex drive than those with lower levels (low Ts), while those with low T levels often find that after the initial honeymoon period of a relationship wanes, it takes a lot of energy for them to initiate or become interested in being sexual. Because it's not uncommon for a high-T individual to be attracted to a low-T person, there's a good chance that a couple's sexual appetites may differ from time to time. But this doesn't make either of them 'wrong' or 'abnormal'.

And although our culture teaches us there is something wrong with us if we can't keep our sex life at its original fever pitch, the truth is that the initial emotional and physiological high of a new sexual relationship eventually needs to be replaced by a more consciously created and sophisticated form of passion and intimacy.

• *Practise safe sex.* Many of today's perimenopausal women came of age during the sexual revolution of the 1960s, when, for many, having multiple sexual partners was common. And many were married or in monogamous relationships by the time the AIDS epidemic emerged in the early 1980s. If you've been divorced or widowed since then, you may have little awareness of the risk you face from unprotected sex. In the US 11 per cent of new HIV infections are among people over fifty, and from 1991 to 1996 HIV in that population rose more than twice as fast as among young adults.[12]

It is all too easy to assume that anyone you would partner is probably not infected. You may be a good judge of character, but a sexual partner is only as safe as every partner he or she has ever had. Remember also that there are many other STDs out there, including incurable conditions such as genital herpes, genital warts, and hepatitis B. Perimenopausal and postmenopausal women are at greater risk of contracting all STDs than are younger women. The decrease in vaginal lubrication and the thinning of the vaginal walls make it easier for microscopic tears to occur during intercourse, creating an entry point for bacteria and viruses.

Safe sex means keeping your partner's body fluids out of your vagina, anus, and mouth. Body fluids include semen, vaginal secretions, blood, and the discharge from STD lesions, such as herpetic sores. Though most people reduce the concept of safe sex to the use of a condom, it is really much larger than that. It includes being honest with yourself about the risk you face from unprotected sex with a partner whose STD status is unknown to you. It also includes waiting to have sex with someone until you know each other well enough to discuss your sexual history, and such issues as using a condom and/or getting a blood test. Though this kind of conversation is rarely easy, it is a good test of the intimacy that is possible between you and your partner.

• *Use contraception if required.* I've seen all too many change-of-life pregnancies in women who were absolutely sure they could not get pregnant and who thought nappies and car seats were out of their lives for good. Even if you are skipping periods regularly, you can still be ovulating. The general rule is that you should use contraception for a full year after your last menstrual period. Obviously, you won't know exactly when that is until you have reached the one-year mark.

Nine Steps to Rekindling Libido

Psychiatrist Helen Singer Kaplan, a pioneer in the field of human sexuality, originated the term 'hot monogamy', using it to refer to the potential for enduring sexual passion in a committed, monogamous relationship. Dr Patricia Love has identified nine factors that can help sustain that state of desire. As she explains in her book, *Hot Monogamy,* they all interconnect with each other, so that progress in one area will have beneficial effects in the others.[13]

1. *Communication.* Even if you and your partner haven't talked much about your sexual relationship until now, being able to talk easily about sexual changes will become increasingly important. Simply letting your partner know what is going on with you is a good first step, and it can pave the way to discussing adjustments you'd like to make.

2. *Mood.* At midlife, women can take responsibility for getting in the mood, even if desire doesn't arise as spontaneously as it used to. A fifty-six-year-old colleague told me that for her, 'getting older means *deciding* to have a sex life, instead of being *driven* to it'. (For help in this regard, see 'Sensuality', below.)

3. *Intimacy.* Take time to make the personal connection. There is nothing more conducive to a good sex life than the ability to share one's thoughts and feelings with one's partner on a regular basis. One of the really nice things about midlife is that we often have more time to spend with our partners than ever before. That time can translate into a second honeymoon. One of my male colleagues and his wife went on a prolonged European holiday recently – their first signifi- cant time away since their four children were born. When I asked him

about the trip, he told me, 'We got acquainted all over again. I remembered why I had married her in the first place.' Another one of my patients described how rejuvenating it was to be able to make love without children in the house. She laughed and said, 'We can be loud!'

4. Technique. It takes skill and practice to learn what arouses your partner and what arouses you. Learning to pleasure yourself to the point of orgasm is an invaluable skill when it comes to making love with a partner, because you've already discovered, and can teach, what works for you and what doesn't. If you don't know how to do this, read *For Yourself,* by Lonnie Barbach. (See Resources.)

5. Sexual variety. Both you and your partner need to explore your willingness to add creativity and novelty to your lovemaking.

6. Romance. You and your partner need to learn how to show love for each other in concrete ways. Flowers, cards, special nights out, and so forth are all part of what it takes to keep romance alive.

7. Body image. Patricia Love describes body image as 'your inner image of your outer self'. Many of us don't feel good about our bodies because we've learned to compare ourselves with the airbrushed, perfect models we see in the media. This is especially true when our bodies start changing at midlife. When we feel bad about our bodies, it is very difficult to be fully present for lovemaking. If body image is a problem for you, use my mirror exercise. Stand in front of a mirror twice a day for thirty days, look deeply into your own eyes, and say out loud, 'I accept myself unconditionally right now.' This may sound silly, but it works – and it can instantly point out to you the areas in your life that need love and compassion.

8. Sensuality. To enhance your libido, you must be willing to relax and involve all your senses in your lovemaking.

Sight. According to feng shui, the Chinese art of placement, the bedroom should be a place of rest and relaxation, not a place to pay bills or watch television. The bedroom should also be a sensual place. To help make it so, choose bedroom wall and sheet colours with your partner that will enhance the romance of your surroundings.

Many couples enjoy watching sensual films together. Because taste varies so widely in this area, I hesitate to make any suggestions. Many of my patients also like erotic literature, which tends to leave more to the imagination than graphic films. Here are two of my favourites, both of which have great erotic sections: *The Valley of Horses*, by Jean Auel, and *Outlander*, by Diana Gabaldon.

Note: Be selective when it comes to erotic material and make sure that the books, photos, or books you look at are not degrading to women in any way. Nothing is a bigger turnoff. Lovemaking should be an activity that enhances the well-being and self-esteem of both partners. If you are currently with a partner whose sexual demands feel degrading to you in any way, get outside help.

Smell. Women are more attuned to the sense of smell than men are, and we often prefer different odours than men do. You and your partner will need to be honest with each other about odours one of you might find offensive, such as sweat, bad breath, and the like. Aromatherapy can be wonderful – but you must agree on a scent.

Touch. Practise giving each other foot and shoulder rubs. Learn to *receive.* You'd be amazed at how many women have difficulty lying still and receiving pleasure in this way. Practise telling your partner what feels good and what doesn't.

Taste. Many options are available in this area if it appeals to you, such as flavoured oils.

Sound. Use sensual music to set the mood. Turn on the answering machine to intercept the phone, make sure that the children aren't around or that the door is locked, and so on. Nothing is more distracting for most women during lovemaking than the fear that one of the children might walk in at any minute.

9. *Passion.* Dr Love notes that it is not possible to be passionately in love with a person you don't know. She describes passion as the 'ability to combine intense feelings of arousal with love for your partner'. However far we may have strayed from this state, it is certainly a destination to which we can all aspire – an example of what is possible at midlife as our kundalini energy rises to our hearts and we achieve a fusion of sexuality and spirituality not just in our genitals, but in our hearts and souls as well.

Remember, the brain is the biggest sex organ in the body. Talk to your partner, take risks, be vulnerable, laugh together. Dare to enter the brave new world of hot monogamy together. If you don't currently have a partner, cultivate a sensual relationship with yourself.

TEN

Nurturing Your Brain: Sleep, Depression, and Memory

The changes that go on in women's brains at midlife prepare us for living with more wisdom than ever before. This new wisdom gets wired in our brains as we move from the alternating current of our menstruating years to the more direct current available after menopause. As this natural adjustment takes place, we may find ourselves experiencing disturbing symptoms, ranging from insomnia and depression to forgetfulness. Rather than succumbing to the common cultural view that we are about to begin the long, slow glide into senility and depression, we need to realise that the brain changes we are experiencing are usually normal – temporary bumps in the road that can be alleviated when we have the courage to see them as messages from our inner wisdom. No study has ever shown that menopause per se increases one's risk for any mental disorder, whether depression, forgetfulness, or anxiety, unless we are already predisposed to them. Perimenopause *amplifies* our brain and thought patterns, highlighting the areas that need support and change.

Fighting or trying to control mental symptoms with denial, drugs, or even overdependence on mental techniques such as meditation is ultimately doomed to fail. Instead we need to heed the messages behind our symptoms, support ourselves fully with sound information, and, when necessary, be willing to take life-changing action.

Given our culture's love affair with control, this approach takes a great deal of courage and faith. Some women have to go through painful breakdowns before they are ready to relinquish this struggle for control.

PRUDENCE: THE ANXIOUS SIREN

Prudence, a corporate lawyer married to a college professor, first came to see me when she became pregnant with her first child, at the age of thirty-four. Prudence and her husband appeared to be the perfect couple, with the kind of dual-career lifestyle to which many of us aspire. Prudence's pregnancy, labour, and birth were normal, but postpartum she fell into a dark depression that lasted for about six months. During this time she sought help from a psychiatrist and went on antidepressants for about a year. She subsequently remained stable except for rather severe PMS symptoms such as anxiety, mood swings, and cravings for sweets that lasted from mid-cycle through to the first day of her period. Prudence was able to control these symptoms with progesterone cream, diet, and exercise. I never pressed her further to see what was going on in her life that might be precipitating her PMS symptoms. Her programme was working, she was satisfied, and I intuitively felt that Prudence was not interested in looking more deeply into her life or her psyche. That all changed at perimenopause.

When Prudence began skipping periods in her mid-forties, she couldn't seem to deal with her PMS symptoms any more. She didn't know exactly when to use the progesterone cream, and her former self-discipline when it came to diet and exercise disappeared. In addition to this, she often found herself unable to get to sleep at night. But Prudence had another worry that completely surprised me: every time she skipped a period, she worried that she might be pregnant. Since her husband had had a vasectomy after their child was born, I knew that something had definitely changed in her life.

When I asked Prudence if there was anything unusually stressful going on, she admitted to me that she was having an affair with a colleague. She said, 'I don't know what has come over me. I never thought I'd ever do anything like this. But I feel possessed. When I'm with David, I feel young and wild – as though a part of me has awakened that I didn't even know existed. I'm interested in sexy black underwear for the first time in my life. I sit at my desk, and when I should be going over legal briefs, I fantasise about my next business trip with him. I feel higher than a kite when we're together or even just thinking about him. But when I have to be home and we can't see each other for a while, I crash. I feel anxious and depressed and I can't sleep.'

At first Prudence simply wanted my opinion about contraception and also whether or not she should go back on antidepressants or start using sleeping pills. She also wanted to know what effect medication might have on her newly recharged sex drive. Though I agreed that drug therapy of some sort might be an option to help her symptoms, I also wanted to help Prudence make the link between her perimenopausal mental symptoms and her life.

Why was she having the affair now? At first she told me that her marriage was fine and that her husband was a good man. But after a few minutes she broke down in tears and told me that he had not been promoted in his job and had become more difficult to live with over the past year or so. As is so often the case, Prudence's husband was also going through a midlife crisis of sorts, but he preferred not to talk about it. This was especially difficult for Prudence because her own work life was better than ever. In fact, given her husband's discouragement and apparent depression, she increasingly preferred being at work to being at home.

I asked Prudence what the affair had done for her. She thought it over for a moment and replied, 'It makes me feel alive, powerful, and sexy in a way I haven't felt before.' Prudence's uncharacteristic affair allowed her to move into a part of her brain – the temporal lobe – that had probably been relatively shut down since her late teens or early twenties but which, as we've already seen, becomes increasingly activated during perimenopause. Neuroscientist Dr Mona Lisa Schulz points out that this area of the brain is associated with ecstasy, sensuality, and creativity and that its messages are often overridden by our frontal lobes – the centres in our brains associated with rules, regulations, and conventional morality.

At midlife our bodies and brains cry out for balance. Those who have been overly intellectualised and controlled need to break free and become more fluid and spontaneous, while those who have lived in the moment, pursuing pleasure and creative self-expression with abandon, now need to rein themselves in with more structure and self-discipline if they are to stay healthy.

Though I don't prescribe midlife affairs, I do recognise how therapeutic a passionate out-of-control experience of some kind can be for women like Prudence. Unfortunately, an affair rarely provides a healthy structure for relinquishing the need for control and learning how to trust and work consciously with ecstasy and creativity. Ultimately it becomes another means of controlling joy by allowing yourself to feel it only through sex, and only within contrived, secretive parameters.

I suggested to Prudence that she spend a few months thinking about the following questions, either alone or with the help of a therapist or other professional. Did she love her husband? Did she intend to stay married to him and grow old with him? What were the circumstances that led to the affair? What feelings had it brought up for her? Did she believe that it was possible to feel the ecstasy of the affair in other parts of her life? Was her affair important enough to her to risk losing the life she had built with her husband? Was she willing to see the link between her symptoms and her life?

Prudence told me she'd think about what I had said. She then went to see a psychiatrist for her depression, anxiety, and insomnia. Over the next two years she went through a series of medications, none of which worked for very long and all of which gave her side effects. After having been given prescriptions for Prozac, Celexa, Effexor, Xanax, Valium, Elavil, and Desyrel, Prudence was finally offered Nardil, a monoamine oxidase inhibitor (MAOI), which required her to be on a special diet. After all these attempts at trying to find peace through pills, many of her symptoms were still present.

Prudence did not return to my surgery for a check-up until two and a half years later. Her affair had come to an end, she told me, and she was still married. When I asked her how her husband was doing, she told me that he had found another teaching job but seemed to be just marking time until retirement. When I performed the physical examination, I found a small but distinct lump in her left breast that concerned me. I referred Prudence to a local breast care centre for diagnosis and possible treatment. Before she left, Prudence began to sob. Through her tears, she said, 'I feel as though my body is totally out of control. The more I try to control my symptoms, the worse things get. I have no idea what to do next.' I told Prudence that she had finally reached 'breakdown to breakthrough' – a place that, while uncomfortable, is usually the first step towards living more fully.

Prudence is finally working with a therapist to confront the aspects of her life that require changing. Her breast lump turned out to be carcinoma in situ, and she is being monitored regularly by a breast surgeon. Her diagnosis leaves her with uncertainty about the future: medical science still can't identify which cases of carcinoma in situ will become invasive cancers later on and which won't. Prudence's body had presented her with a dilemma that simply couldn't be solved with more control or more information. She finally surrendered and knew that she had to take her life and her health one day at a time.

Midlife teaches us a liberating truth: many aspects of our lives, including our mates, our families, our children, and our jobs, are simply not under our control. True mental health always involves striking a balance between certainty and ambiguity. At midlife the kinds of certainty and control that often served us well earlier in our lives must now make way for another way of being in the world. We must learn to trust our inner wisdom, a reality that we cannot see, taste, touch, or measure – let alone control.

Enhancing Midlife Sleep

Midlife women often go through changes in their sleep patterns, not unlike those we experienced at adolescence. Some of us find ourselves needing more sleep than ever, some suffer from insomnia, and some find that sleep simply isn't as refreshing as it used to be.

Unfortunately, insomnia makes the entire midlife transition harder. Insufficient sleep increases our levels of corticosteroids and catecholamines, stress hormones that can, over time, throw off our hormonal balance and depress our immune system. Studies show that 20–40 per cent of women have sleep disorders and are far more likely than men to have insomnia after the age of thirty-five.[1] Perimenopausal women often need more sleep than do men of the same age.[2]

Sleep restores both physical and mental energy. Experimental animals have been shown to die from sleep deprivation. Insufficient sleep leaves us obviously drowsy, fatigued, and irritable. We also suffer from decreased concentration, lowered efficiency, decreased work motivation, and a higher rate of errors in judgement. When we are sleep-deprived, we are more accident prone, since our brains will fall into 'micro-sleeps' that may not be apparent to those around us.

Insomnia Is Often a Message from Our Inner Guidance
At menopause, insomnia and fatigue are frequently the result of unprocessed and unresolved emotions such as anger, sadness, or anxiety, which often accompany the enormous changes of midlife.

The brain chemicals that are important for sleep undergo changes in many women at menopause, and they are also profoundly affected by our feelings.

For example, it is not uncommon to be so exhausted emotionally after a fight with a spouse that despite going to bed early and sleeping for ten hours, you still feel tired. One of my patients realised that her insomnia was associated with chronic worry about her daughter's seeming inability to find a career and a living situation that suited her. Her sleep problem resolved when she decided to stop enabling this twenty-three-year-old by allowing her to live at home without making any contribution to the household. She insisted that her daughter find a job – any job – and learn how to support herself in the world.

One of my perimenopausal patients could not understand why she was having trouble sleeping. She said she was not having hot flushes or sweats, did not drink coffee, and wasn't really stressed. I asked her if she slept better when she was not in the same bed as her husband. She said, 'Yes. I've noticed that I do.' I told her that this was a sign from her inner wisdom. She replied, 'But what am I supposed to do? You can't not sleep with your husband.' I told her that although I couldn't tell her what to do about her sleeping arrangements, she still needed to be aware of the connection. She might consider sleeping separately for a while. She would learn a lot by how her husband responded to this suggestion.

How Much Sleep Is Enough?

Our inherent biological rhythms are also taxed by the demands that modern life makes on our sympathetic nervous system, which is responsible for keeping us alert. We forget that the electric light bulb has only been around for a very short time, evolutionarily speaking, and most of us weren't meant to stay up until midnight every night. Taking naps, sleeping late on dreary mornings, or going to bed at sunset are regarded with disdain in our culture. Instead, we worship hyperactive individuals who work sixteen hours a day, and we even boast about how little sleep we get!

At medical school, particularly after lunch as I was sitting in lectures, I would fantasise that there was a bed up on the podium, where I could sleep while the lecturer droned on. Some of this fatigue was from low blood sugar; I was eating too many carbohydrates. But even with a better diet, I couldn't have stayed alert on only five to six hours of sleep a night. Whenever I get too little sleep I feel extremely groggy in the morning and have difficulty getting motivated to do my work. It's important to be flexible and compassionate about our needs when life makes extra demands. Like it or not, what we really need during those times of unusual demands is to get into bed and let our parasympathetic nervous systems restore us. The much-maligned midday nap can be profoundly rejuvenating. Some corporations have even found that the productivity of their employees goes up when they are allowed to nap. Sleep is an indispensable bodily function, as important as breathing and eating. Although doctors and scientists don't really know exactly why sleep is so important physiologically, most agree that it is critical for bodily rest, for consolidation of learning and memory, and also as a way to help us sort out in our minds and bodies the things we have learned and experienced during the day. You've probably noticed how a good night's sleep helps you integrate new information or even new physical skills, like exercise or dance moves that you may have struggled with the day before. When we allow ourselves to 'sleep on' something, we're actually allowing ourselves to make connections in our sleep that we couldn't have made before.

Research has shown that our most restful sleep takes place when we are following our internal biological rhythm. For me that means getting up with the sun and going to bed relatively early, between nine and ten at night. I always find that I am at the peak of my productivity and happiness when I am following this pattern. However, this takes discipline. I am always tempted to use those evening hours to have some time for myself. Think back on a time in your life when you felt clearest and most rested. What time did you go to bed and what time did you wake up? In other words, synchronise your daily clock with your biological one.

Many of my menopausal patients have been dismayed when they find that the amount of sleep that sustained them a year or two earlier seems inadequate now. I personally have found that I need more sleep now than I did a few years ago. But I also know that this is my body's way of getting the restoration it needs, given all the changes that are happening in my life. During both adolescence and perimenopause, it is a biological truth that we need more sleep than at other times in our lives. It is important for a woman to recognise this, honour it, and get the rest she needs, any way she can.

Tips for Better Sleep

The following are some suggestions for better sleep during perimenopause. What works for one person may or may not work for
another, so you should expect to go through some trial and error.
Experiment with such sleep aids as meditation, deep relaxation
exercises, listening to soothing music, or sipping a mug of warm
chamomile tea. Whatever your routine, be sure to keep it free of
'performance anxiety' – don't think about how few hours of rest
you'll get if you don't fall asleep right away, don't look at the clock,
and above all don't give in to your mental to-do list and get busy. You
might end up establishing a night-owl habit that will be that much
harder to break in the long run.

• *Cool your hot flushes.* Hot flushes and night sweats are by far the
most common reasons for sleep deprivation during menopause.
Unless you're able to take a nap during the day, your first priority
should be to cool your hot flushes so that you can get the rest you
need at night.

As I've explained, hot flushes and night sweats are triggered by
neurotransmitter changes in the brain that result, in part, from erratic
oestrogen levels or by wide deviations in the balance between
oestrogen and progesterone levels (even when total oestrogen is
normal). In addition to maintaining hormonal balance, progesterone
also has a calming effect on the central nervous system, particularly on
the brain.[3] It follows, then, that unbalanced oestrogen can be a cerebral
irritant, affecting the body in much the same way as adrenaline.

Sleep disturbances are one of the most common reasons for me
to prescribe natural progesterone cream, oestrogen replacement,
acupuncture, or herbal remedies (alone or in combination) to help a
woman stabilise her hormone levels. But keep in mind that erratic
hormones are not the only factor in sleep disturbances. Hot flushes
are also exacerbated by underlying unresolved stress and anxiety and
the unfinished business that fuels these symptoms.

• *Eat for better sleep.* The number-one rule of thumb is: do not go to
bed on a full stomach. Lying horizontal when your stomach is full
can cause gastric reflux, which occurs when pressure from the
stomach's contents overwhelms the lower oesophageal sphincter and
food (or stomach acid) comes back up the oesophagus. The result is

heartburn, sour stomach, a bad taste in the mouth, and, possibly, asthma-like respiratory distress. The ideal is to wait three hours after eating before going to bed (or reclining on the sofa).

On the other hand, a carefully chosen snack before going to bed can be good for you. A snack that is relatively high in protein and low in carbohydrates, or high in complex (unrefined) carbohydrates, is usually well tolerated. This would include fresh fruit, cheese, brown rice, a baked potato, lean meat, tofu, or cottage cheese. Notice what this list does not include: biscuits, leftover pie, cakes, ice cream, or crisps. Refined and processed foods simply do not promote rest, relaxation, and the sort of deposits that need to be made in your health bank while you're rejuvenating yourself for the next day.

Taking antioxidant supplements once or twice a day can also support refreshing sleep.

• *Avoid caffeine.* Even one cup of coffee in the morning can disrupt sleep that night. Caffeine is cleared from the system much more slowly in women than in men. In addition to its effects on the central nervous system, caffeine, especially in coffee, is a bladder irritant: it will wake you up at night to urinate.

• *Avoid alcohol.* Alcohol is a sedative, but it also disrupts the brain-stem sleep mechanism, resulting in rebound insomnia – meaning that you are more apt to awaken in the middle of the night because your body will need more sedative to get back to sleep.

• *Get regular exercise.* Among a host of other benefits, regular exercise improves one's ability to get a good night's sleep. However, vigorous exercise within three to six hours of bedtime is counter-productive. The increased activity boosts the metabolism and stimu-lates the central nervous system, making restful sleep more difficult to achieve. Relaxation exercises, on the other hand, such as hatha yoga and meditation, can be very helpful. Experiment with your own body's response to before-bed activities. As a general rule, the hour or two before bedtime is best spent winding down.

• *Sleep in the dark.* Electric lights, headlights of passing cars, even moonlight streaming through your window can disrupt a good night's sleep. If lack of pure darkness is disturbing your sleep, pull your curtains across and make sure that you can't read the face of your alarm clock. Seeing what time it is can cause anxiety if you have a tendency towards insomnia. You might want to try wearing an eye mask, as I do, if I'm in a place where I can't make the room dark. For added comfort, I scent mine with calming lavender oil.

• *Cover your bedroom mirrors at night, or remove them.* If you have mirrors in the bedroom that you can see when lying down, they can be a deterrent to sleep. The reflections in them can make you feel jumpy and unsafe. According to the principles of feng shui, the ancient Asian art of working with the environment, mirrors enliven a room and increase the energy flow in it. Obviously, this is exactly the opposite of what you want in a place designed for sleep and relaxation. One solution is to put curtains over your mirrors that can be drawn back during the day.

• *Develop, and adhere to, a going-to-sleep ritual.* Sleep aids such as melatonin or valerian (see page 303) can be great for getting you through one or two restless nights, but you need to establish and adhere to a going-to-sleep ritual based on good overall sleep habits. This is known in the trade as 'good sleep hygiene'.

First, count backwards from your preferred wake-up time to establish a bedtime that gives you sufficient sleep. Keep to this bedtime every day, even at weekends, so that your body clock can stabilise.

Get out of your everyday clothes and into something more comfortable (even your pyjamas) up to a half-hour before sleep, to give your body the signal that it's time to start winding down. Do your bathroom rituals at least half an hour before bedtime, too, including brushing your teeth, washing your face, and taking bedtime medications, so you can go straight to bed without reawakening yourself with these tasks.

• *Be your own editor.* Don't read, watch, or listen to anything that might be disturbing before bedtime, because this can activate your sympathetic nervous system, thereby taking the rest-and-rejuvenation functions of the parasympathetic nervous system offline. (When I went to see the film *Titanic* with my kids, I couldn't sleep that night because of visions of freezing, drowning victims.) Also, please get the television out of the bedroom. On an energetic level, even having a television set up in your bedroom means that you are only a switch away from all the worries of the world.

• *Avoid emotionally stressful discussions or potentially difficult phone calls near bedtime.* For some, however, an urgent unresolved issue with a loved one will result in a sleepless night. The point here is to know yourself and consciously decide which approach works best for you.

• *Get the hamster wheel out of your head.* One of the most common sleep detractors is the hamster-wheel-in-the-head syndrome: stewing over worries, things not said, things not done, or things on the list for tomorrow. When I get into one of these states, I get out of bed, take kava kava or valerian (see page 303), step into a warm bath, and read a good book. Then, when I am sleepy, I consciously send God's love into my sleep and into my dreams. After about a half hour I go back to bed, and I don't look at the clock.

• *Put your worries to bed.* Another way to get rid of the hamster wheel is to write down everything that is bothering you just before you turn out the light. Then turn your worries over to the higher power of your choice, asking this power to guide you towards solutions to your problems while you sleep. Then imagine that when you wake up the next morning you'll have a healthier perspective and be inspired to the right action to change your situation for the better.

• *Improve your sleeping surface.* Many people try to get a good night's sleep using mattresses that have lost their support years before.

Prescription Sleep Medications: Caution

Use prescription sleep medication sparingly if at all. Some UK doctors still prescribe sleep medications of the benzodiazepine class of drugs, such as diazepam (Valium), lorazepam (Ativan), and temazepam (Temazepam), but many do not, being aware of the risk of addiction. These work by binding to GABA receptors in the brain to produce a calming effect. These drugs are habit-forming and lose their effectiveness over time as the brain builds up tolerance, so that you need more and more to get the same effect. I've seen many older women who were prescribed Valium for anxiety and insomnia during their perimenopausal years and who were still addicted to it twenty years later.

Other medications that can initially help sleep problems include the SSRI antidepressants such as fluoxetine (Prozac), venlafaxine (Efexor), and sertraline (Lustral). Like the benzodiazepines, these can also lose their effectiveness over time.

There are newer hypnotics available now, which are likely to be addictive and which are said to affect the sleep pattern less, enabling you to wake more refreshed. However, it is wise to avoid any hypnotic medication if possible.

Over-the-counter sleep remedies such as diphenhydramine (Nytol or Dreemon) interefere with the production of the brain chemical acetylcholine, which is very important for memory. Over time, the use of these drugs can cause serious memory problems and confusion.

Natural Sleep Aids

NATURAL PROGESTERONE

Try 1/4–1/2 teaspoon 1.5–3 per cent natural progesterone skin cream at bedtime. Natural progesterone also binds to the GABA receptors in the brain and has a calming effect. Addiction to its brain effects is very rare but has been reported; I've only seen it in one patient in more than twenty years of practice.

KAVA KAVA

The herb kava kava is known to induce relaxation and natural sleep within thirty minutes. It is available in health food shops or pharmacies. Look for a standardised product that lists the amount of kavalactones in each capsule. The dosage for insomnia is 150–210mg of kavalactones one hour before bedtime.

VALERIAN

If kava kava doesn't provide enough relief, add valerian. Studies comparing it to small doses of the benzodiazepines and barbiturates have shown that it is just as effective in inducing sleep and preventing night-time awakening, but without inducing morning sleepiness.[4] Valerian has a very bad taste, so I recommend taking it in capsule form. Dosage is 150–300mg of a product standardised to 0.8 per cent valerenic acid at bedtime.

MELATONIN

The hormone melatonin is secreted by the brain's pineal gland in response to cycles of light and darkness. It produces drowsiness. Our natural melatonin secretion is affected by depression, shift work, seasonal affective disorder, and jet lag, and supplemental melatonin can often help the sleep problems associated with these conditions. Usual dose is 0.5 to 3.0mg taken an hour before bedtime. If you are a shift worker, you can maintain a normal sleep pattern by taking melatonin about an hour before going to bed – even if bedtime occurs in the middle of the day. Melatonin also helps reset your biological clock if you have to go on a new sleep/wake cycle.

Melatonin is only available on prescription in the UK at present, but may be ordered from abroad in small quantities for your own personal use.

5-HTP

Melatonin is made from the precursor molecule 5-HTP (5-hydroxy-tryptophan), which has also been found to be very effective for treating sleep disorders, as well as PMS and seasonal affective disorder. It is safe and several brands are now available in the UK (see Resources). The starting dose is usually 100mg three times per day. This can be very gradually increased over several months' time to a dose of 200mg three times per day.[5]

Note: Even natural substances such as valerian, natural progesterone, and kava kava may eventually lose their effectiveness over time, because they bind to the same place in the brain as prescription sleep drugs. It's best to use them sparingly, and only after you've tried other routes to a good night's sleep.[6]

Depression: An Opportunity for Growth

Twenty-five per cent of women will suffer from at least one major depression in their lifetimes. Women receive the vast majority of prescriptions for drugs like Seroxat and Prozac.

But contrary to popular myth and medical opinion of the past, depression is *less* common among middle-aged women compared to women of other ages.[7] Having said that, there are still a significant number of women who experience midlife depression or an exacerbation of underlying depression when they enter midlife. Dr Gladys McGarey, a family doctor and friend of mine who has been in practice for over forty years, told me that before hormone replacement therapy and antidepressant medication, she sometimes saw women who negotiated the change by closing the door and taking to their beds, leaving their families to care for all the details of daily life.

Months later, many emerged from the chrysalis of depression rejuvenated and ready to face the second half of their lives. By then, of course, their families' expectations about their roles and duties had also been transformed.

Fortunately, there's now a great deal more that can be done to support women's bodies through midlife depression. If you are depressed, it is crucial that you take action to get help. Depression can rob you of the pleasure of your achievements or the initiative to make changes for the better. It is also an independent and highly significant risk factor for both coronary artery disease and osteoporosis.[8]

Remember that depression, sadness, or anger often accompanies the emotional growth spurt that our psyches are undergoing. Just knowing this is sometimes all that is necessary to get you past the dark days. Sometimes outside help in the form of diet, herbs, or even antidepressant medication is needed. Before you can decide what action to take, you need to ask yourself the following questions:

- Am I depressed? (Depression often is masked as unexplained symptoms such as chronic pain, constipation, headache, mood swings, or backache.)

- What is my depression related to?

- Would medication help me?

The discussion below may help you to answer them.

The Anatomy of Depression

Depression exists on a spectrum, from the blues, which go away on their own, to the normal grief following a loss, to a more persistent and dangerous disorder. In major depression, as defined by psychiatric handbooks, a person not only suffers from depressed mood, but also has changes in appearance, behaviour, speech, perception, and thoughts. When you are depressed, your insight and judgement can be affected, as can your ability to work, take care of yourself, and function in society. Depressed people may appear sad or have an expressionless face. Poor posture and grooming are sometimes evident. If you are depressed, you may derive very little enjoyment from normal daily activities, and you may begin to complain about numerous physical aches and pains that never bothered you before. (Statistics gathered at centres for chronic pain show that up to 90 per cent of those with chronic pain have emotional stress factors such as depression that contribute significantly to their pain syndromes.[9]) Depression is often accompanied by sleep disturbances: you may be unable to get out of bed, or you may suffer from insomnia or early morning awakening. Appetite disturbances – either overeating or loss of appetite – can result in significant weight gain or loss. Your thoughts can be affected by depression, and you may have difficulty concentrating and remembering things. (Many midlife women blame their memory loss on ageing when it's really caused by depression.[10]) Your mind can go around and around in circles, and you may dwell on thoughts of guilt, self-blame, hopelessness, helplessness, and worthlessness. As depression deepens, thoughts of death and suicide can occur.

If you recognise yourself in this description, I urge you to consult your doctor without delay. You and your doctor will be able to evaluate whether or not you are suffering from a major depressive disorder and whether or not you need medication and professional assistance to work through the backlog of unfinished emotional business that may be contributing to it. Now is the time to address your unmet needs. Treatment can be life-saving.

Depression and Hormone Replacement

All sex hormones, including progesterone, oestrogens, and androgens, can affect mood, memory, and cognition in complex and interrelated ways. Receptor sites for these hormones are found throughout the brain and nervous system, and nerve tissue itself has been found to produce them. Oestrogen, the hormone that predominates during the first half of the menstrual cycle, has been shown, for example, to increase mood-enhancing beta-endorphins in menopausal women as well as in menstruating women.[11] It has also been shown to boost levels of serotonin and acetylcholine, neurohormones that are associated with positive mood and normal memory.[12] Though androgens such as testosterone have not been as well studied as oestrogen, they, too, appear to be associated with improvements in mood and vitality.[13] Given this, it's not surprising that many women report they feel better when they take some kind of hormone replacement therapy. When the dosage of oestrogen or androgen is too high, however, women often report adverse effects such as headache and increased anxiety. Synthetic progesterone is frequently associated with depression in women. Bioidentical progesterone only rarely has this effect.

IRIS: A CLOUD DESCENDS AT MIDLIFE

Iris first came to see me when she was fifty-one. She had not had a period in six months. Iris was a very slim, attractive, healthy woman who exercised regularly, took nutritional supplements, and had a fulfilling career. She told me that starting about a year previously, a cloud had come over her mood, and she couldn't shake it. She couldn't pinpoint any particular life crises or other changes that might have precipitated her dark mood. Since her oestrogen and progesterone levels were low, we decided to give oestrogen replacement with natural progesterone a try.

When Iris came back two months later, she looked like a different person. She told me, 'Within a few days of taking the oestrogen and progesterone I felt like the lights went back on in my head.'

Iris continued to feel better for the next two years. But then her depression returned despite the hormone therapy. Iris told me that she had begun to have flashbacks and memories of sexual abuse from early childhood. In retrospect, she realised that these memories had begun to surface during perimenopause. Though she had tried to ignore them and get on with her life, she felt that they had finally culminated in depression, which she was initially able to quell with oestrogen and progesterone. When even that stopped working, she realised that 'the only way out was through'. She had to be willing to allow her body to feel and her brain to know what had happened to her as a child so that she could finally release the pain she'd been holding on to for a lifetime.

Iris consulted a skilled art therapist, who helped her work actively with her dreams and the creative process. She also signed up for a series of weekly full-body massages, which helped her release muscle tension. She later told me, 'I was so surprised when the tears came the first time the massage therapist touched me. But I felt safe and secure, and she intuitively knew enough to simply let me do what my body needed to do. I just lay there and let myself feel everything. I let myself sob.'

Within six months, Iris's depression lifted completely and has not returned. She continues with her hormone replacement because it feels right for her.

Many women at midlife finally have enough ego strength, life skills, and support systems in place to feel and release the unacknowledged pain of their pasts safely. For those who are finally willing to do this kind of work, depression and other symptoms may be alleviated rather quickly.

Treating Depression: The Conventional Approach

Today, antidepressant drugs are usually the first treatment offered if you are suffering from depression. The popular drugs fluoxetine (Prozac), paroxetine (Seroxat), and sertraline (Lustral) work, in part, by increasing the availability of the neurotransmitter serotonin in your brain. (Together with a number of related drugs, they are classed as selective serotonin reuptake inhibitors, or SSRIs.) Another commonly prescribed group of drugs, the tricyclic antidepressants, have been used successfully for many years. Tricyclics include imipramine (Tofranil) and amitriptyline (Triptafen).

Despite their helpfulness, however, you need to know that antidepressant medications, like any drug that alters brain chemistry, may have side effects that can be quite troublesome. Prozac and other SSRIs can cause nausea, loss of appetite, headache, nervousness, insomnia, restless leg syndrome, and difficulties with libido and sexual dysfunction. The tricyclic antidepressants can cause blurred vision, dizziness, dry mouth, heart rate disturbances, constipation, and difficulties with memory. You may have to try a different drug or dosage level in order to find the one that works best for you.

Despite these difficulties, a six-month trial of antidepressant medication is worth considering if you feel miserable and stuck. Optimally, the medicine will result in a gradual lifting of your depression. This will give you the energy to mobilise your own resources to make positive changes in your life.

To support your treatment, I recommend the following:

• *Stop drinking.* Alcohol consumption can make depression particularly persistent. This is partly because alcohol is itself a depressant, and partly because women too often use alcohol as a way to suppress their feelings.

• *Engage in regular exercise.* Exercise changes brain chemistry (by increasing beta-endorphins, lowering catecholamines, and increasing monoamines, and both aerobic and non-aerobic forms have been shown to be helpful in individuals with mild to moderate depression. (In some studies, 50 per cent of people with depression were cured with exercise alone.[14]) Exercising twenty to thirty minutes per day four to five times per week can have a significant positive effect on your mood. It doesn't matter what you do – even dancing around the house to the radio will help.

• *Get outside in the natural light as much as you can.* This helps combat seasonal affective disorder (SAD) and raises your brain levels of serotonin naturally. In the winter, you may need a light box or full-spectrum light bulbs to get enough light. (See Resources.)

• *Take a good multivitamin that supports your body and brain, and make an effort to eat well.* If you are to function optimally, it is important that your brain gets balanced levels of serotonin, essential fatty acids, and glucose. Avoid refined carbohydrates, eat protein at least three times a day, and be sure to include a source of healthy fat in your diet regularly. Eating balanced amounts of complex carbohydrates (with protein) provides the body with appropriate amounts of tryptophan, a building block of serotonin.

• *Avoid frequent consumption of caffeinated drinks and refined sugar.* There is evidence to suggest that they may play a role in recurring depression.

• *Be sure to give your medication a chance to work.* Half of those who stop their medication within three months of starting get depressed again. To avoid this, it's a good idea to stay on your medication for a minimum of six months, if your depression is severe enough to warrant this approach in the first place.

Antidepressants Do Not Cure Depression

Many experts believe that depression is a recurrent disease. Of the patients who experience a major depression, 50–85 per cent have additional episodes after they are successfully treated. Studies have shown that about 80 per cent of people on antidepressants have a recurrence within three years after stopping medication.[15] Though these statistics seem grim, they would be much less so if all of us were willing to take a good look at what depression really is.

All too often antidepressants are given in a vacuum, as though depression were just a 'Prozac deficiency'. But depression is not a simple chemical disorder that lands on you when you least expect it. And depression is not a natural human condition. Studies have shown that depression is virtually non-existent among many indigenous peoples. Depression is a consequence of how we live our lives. To get over it, we must be willing to make some changes that will support healthy brain biochemistry. Otherwise, depression is likely to recur. I have never prescribed antidepressants of any kind unless my patient was also willing to enter some kind of therapeutic relationship with a counsellor to help her sort out the aspects of her life that needed improvement. In other words, we, as a society and as individuals, need to understand that getting on the right medication does not guarantee a cure for depression.

Like all symptoms, depression is one way your body's inner wisdom tells you that something in your life is out of balance. Often its message is that a part of you has ceased to grow or has stagnated, or that you have lost the passion for living that is a natural part of being alive. It may also be a hint that you are angry with someone but do not feel free to express that anger directly. Depression may result from unresolved loss and grief over the loss of a loved one through separation or death.

The best cure for depression that I know is to be completely honest with yourself about everything you are feeling – even, and especially, those feelings you've been told you shouldn't have, such as jealousy, anger, guilt, sorrow, and rage. All of these feelings are part of being human. They will never hurt you if you simply acknowledge them, express them safely, and, ultimately, accept yourself for having them. Then you must take action. I've never seen depression lift without the sufferer taking some kind of positive action to help herself. This could be as simple as volunteering at an animal shelter.

In my experience, staying in dead-end jobs and/or relationships is a major factor associated with unremitting, chronic depression in women. If you feel depressed and 'dead', and this has been going on for six months or more, it is probable that either you have unresolved grief about an important loss in your life or you continue to partici-pate in relationships or jobs that do not replenish you at the deepest levels. There is no medication, supplement, exercise, or herb that will cure this problem. However, they *can* be a valuable support as you work on the problems that are preventing you from moving forward in your life.

I'd suggest that you consider an antidepressant medication if:

- You've had three or more episodes of depression.

- You have suffered from low-level depression your whole life and have also had a major depressive episode (called double depression).

- You have leftover symptoms after going off an earlier course of antidepressants.

- You are having your first depression at midlife or later.

Are Antidepressants Safe?

There are apt to be side effects from the long-term use of any drug that alters brain chemistry, and many of the popular psychotropic drugs on the market today are too new for anybody to say with authority that they are safe in the long run. Candace Pert, the scientist who discovered the receptor sites for many important chemicals in the brain associated with mood, commented:

> I am alarmed at the monster that Johns Hopkins' neuroscientist Solomon Snyder and I created when we discovered the simple binding assay for drug receptors 25 years ago. Prozac and other antidepressant serotonin-receptor-active compounds may also cause cardiovascular problems in some susceptible people after long-term use, which has become common practice despite the lack of safety studies.
>
> The public is being misinformed about the precision of the SSRIs [Prozac, fenfluramine (part of fen-phen), Lustral, Seroxat, Faverin, etc.] when the medical profession oversimplifies their action in the brain and ignores the body as if it exists merely to carry the head around.[16]

I couldn't agree more, especially in light of a new 'breakthrough' PMS drug now being heavily marketed to women in the US. This so-called 'new' drug, Serafem, *is simply Prozac under a new guise* and with a new indication – an indication guaranteed to support women's continued mistrust of their body's wisdom.

Think of psychotropic drugs as a bridge to help you cross a particularly rough stream in your life. But don't plan to live on that bridge for good. The true cure for depression lies in learning the skills associated with full emotional expression and then taking positive action.

Supplements to Combat Depression

If you prefer to try alternatives to prescription medications, the following vitamins, herbs and other supplements have demonstrated clinical effectiveness. (Remember to follow the lifestyle suggestions on pages 307–309, as well.) Do not combine them with prescription medications without consulting your doctor.

VITAMINS AND OTHER NUTRIENTS

Deficiencies of biotin, folic acid, vitamin B_6 (pyridoxine), vitamin B_{12}, and vitamin C have all been linked to depression. Vitamin B_6 deficiency, for example, has been shown to lower levels of serotonin. Vitamin B_6 has a role in the production of the monoamine neurotransmitters, which are important for mood stabilisation. Deficiencies of calcium, copper, magnesium, and the omega-6 fatty acids may also relate to depression. For preventive and/or therapeutic benefits, consider adding the following nutritional supplements to your programme:[17]

- *Pyridoxine (B_6)*: recommended dose, 50–500mg per day (Pyridoxine should be taken with the other B-complex vitamins listed on page 219.)

- *Vitamin C*: recommended dose, 1,000mg per day

- *DHA (docosahexaenoic acid)*: 100–200mg twice per day

ST JOHN'S WORT

This herb, which contains the active ingredient hypericin, has been very well researched, with some studies indicating that it is as effective as Prozac in treating mild to moderate depression. The usual dose is 300mg of herb standardised to 0.3 per cent hypericin, three times per day. As products vary, check the dosage on the bottle.

VALERIAN

If you have an anxiety component with your depression, add valerian to your St John's wort. The usual dose is 100–300mg standardised extract containing 0.8 per cent valerenic acid.

GINKGO

If your depression is associated with attention and memory problems and you are aged fifty or older, consider *Ginkgo biloba* in addition to St John's wort. The usual dose is 40–80mg three times per day.

INOSITOL

Inositol is an effective over-the-counter alternative to many commonly prescribed antidepressants.[18] The exact mechanism of action is unknown, but it appears to be linked with the serotonin system, affecting the same pathways of brain chemistry as do the tricyclic and SSRI antidepressants, but without the side effects. I've prescribed the product Effervescent Inositol, which also contains vitamins B_3 and B_6 and magnesium, for several patients, who have tolerated it well. One, a person with a very significant family history of depression, used it following the loss of a loved one. She reported, 'In the past, before Inositol, I would have gone through my grief and then fallen into a black hole. This time I could still feel all of my feelings deeply, but I was able to move through them without a depression hangover.' Effervescent Inositol is well tolerated in doses as large as 18–20g per day. (See Resources.)

5-HTP

5-hydroxytryptophan is a compound naturally produced in the body from the amino acid tryptophan, which is an important precursor to serotonin. Although tryptophan is found in many foods, it can be difficult to consume enough tryptophan in the diet to overcome serotonin deficiency. (Tryptophan supplements were once widely used as sleep aids, but they were taken off the market after some products were found to be contaminated.) 5-HTP can be extracted from plants and is now available as a nutritional supplement. It has been used for decades in Europe as an approved treatment for both depression and sleep problems. The side effect of nausea is sometimes reported, but an enteric-coated formulation should help avoid this. The usual dose is 100–200mg three times per day. (See Resources.)

If mild depression is your primary problem, I'd recommend that you start with St John's wort first. It has a history of hundreds of years of safe use. If after two months you've not noticed any difference, switch to 5-HTP. Reports on 5-HTP use have been particularly positive from people suffering from weight problems and insomnia in addition to depression. Be sure to get it from a reliable source, because of the possibility of contamination. If you also suffer from symptoms of panic disorder, obsessive-compulsive disorder, or anxiety plus depression, then I'd recommend a trial of Effervescent Inositol.

Remember, each of the suggestions above works well in some people but not in others. This is true whether you opt for medication, exercise, psychotherapy, nutritional supplements, or another approach. You need to be willing to experiment in order to find the approach that seems to beckon to you.

Memory Loss at Menopause: Is This Alzheimer's?

Many women experience 'fuzzy thinking' or 'woolly head' during perimenopause. They complain of forgetting names or misplacing objects or having difficulty understanding their bank statements. This is not the beginning of Alzheimer's disease. It is a fairly normal state that many women go through as our hormones change and our brains rewire. Some become terrified of this fuzzy-headed feeling because of their need for a high degree of intellectual control. Others find themselves willing to trust the process once they're reassured that it's normal – part of the wisdom of perimenopause that focuses our attention inwards. The same thing often happens both premenstrually and during the postpartum period.

Memory problems at midlife are also due to temporary overload from the many external demands on your limited time. It's like trying to make a phone call to Australia from the UK on Christmas Day: you can't get through because all the lines are busy. If you can't remember something instantly, just relax, do something else for a while, and give yourself the time, space, and respect that allows your brain to retrieve stored information. Getting anxious and putting yourself down for forgetting only makes the problem worse.

But Aren't We Losing Brain Cells?

A woman's brain reaches its peak size at about the age of twenty, followed by a gradual decline in size throughout the rest of her life. If bigger is better, that would mean that we also reach peak wisdom and intelligence by the age of twenty. That this is a completely ridiculous notion is made immediately obvious if you watch much MTV.

In fact, studies have shown that throughout our lifetime, as we move from naïveté to wisdom, our brain function becomes moulded by our experience. Think of your brain as a tree that requires regular pruning if it is to acquire its optimal shape, size, and function. Brain cell loss with ageing is akin to pruning the non-essential branches. In addition, while the number of neurons may decline, the interconnections among them continue to grow. These connections – created by dendritic and axonal branching – actually increase with age, as our capacity to make complex associations increases. In short, the older and more experienced you become, the more efficient and sophisticated your brain.

Preventing Alzheimer's: Some Lessons from the Nun Study

Even with reassurance that it's normal to go through some transient changes in thinking and focus during perimenopause, many women still fear becoming demented and unable to live independently as they get older. Alzheimer's disease currently affects about four million Americans and four hundred thousand people in the UK. It is the leading cause of dependence and institutionalisation in the elderly. It appears at an earlier age in women than in men, and up to two-thirds of cases reported have been in women – in part simply because women live longer. Currently about 5 per cent of women have dementia of some type at sixty. This climbs to 12 per cent after seventy-five. After eighty-five, between 28 and 50 per cent of all people suffer from some form of dementia, depending on what studies you believe. (This 50 per cent figure is felt by many authorities to be an exaggeration.[19]) Given these numbers, each of us will want to do everything we can to care for and enhance our brain function at perimenopause – long before memory problems or dementia have a chance to develop.

Alzheimer's disease was named after Alois Alzheimer, a German neuropathologist who, in 1906, looked under a microscope at the brain tissue of a fifty-five-year-old woman who had spent the last years of her life in a mental institution, where she was prone to paranoia and fits of anger. Alzheimer identified two substances in her brain that have come to be associated with the disease: dense *plaques* formed by the protein beta-amyloid outside the brain cells, and stringy *tangles* within the nerve cells themselves. Whether these plaques and tangles are the cause of Alzheimer's dementia is controversial. We do know, however, that there's a great deal of overlap between the senile dementia caused by cerebrovascular insufficiency and stroke and that which is associated with the plaques and tangles of Alzheimer's disease.

Alzheimer's also has a genetic component.[20] But even if Alzheimer's runs in your family, that does not mean you will inevitably get it. Brain function is multifactorial, meaning that it is affected by many different aspects of our lives, from the amount of antioxidant-rich vegetables we eat to the level of education we've attained. It is also shaped by events and behaviours that begin in childhood and continue into old age. That's why there will never be a hormone or magic pill that can guarantee brain protection for life. However, you can affect your brain health by the lifestyle choices you make.

Nowhere has this been more convincingly demonstrated than in the famous study of a group of hundreds of nuns belonging to the School of Sisters of Notre Dame, who have donated their brains for study after death.[21] Because these women have spent much of their lives in the order, there is a wealth of data about each woman, often spanning many decades. One surprising finding was that a greater or lesser capacity for complex thought – known as 'idea density' – in early life was correlated with the likelihood of developing Alzheimer's disease in later life. Upon entering the convent (usually in her early twenties) each of the nuns was required to write an autobiography. When linguistics experts analysed these years later, they found a startling correlation between the nuns' language skills and the eventual occurrence of Alzheimer's. The lower their idea density, the higher their risk.

Another fascinating finding from the Nun Study is that the presence of plaques and tangles in the brain does not always predict the mental status of an individual. One of the nuns had strikingly good mental status and attitude before her death in her late eighties; researchers were startled to find severe loss of neurons and multiple amyloid tangles in her brain at autopsy. This evidence supports a great truth: that the physical body and the spirit are inextricably linked. For people who are optimistic, lively, and engaged, as this particular nun was, anatomical limitations often seem not to result in disability.

On the other hand, the Nun Study has shown that small-vessel disease, in the form of mini-strokes, is strongly predictive of dementia. Chronic depression also seems to be correlated with Alzheimer's. When we shut off the circulation of blood to an area of our body, we are shutting off life force. Similarly, depression is a shutting down of the life force within us.

Oestrogen and Alzheimer's

An impressive number of studies have shown an association between oestrogen use and the delay or even prevention of Alzheimer's.[22] This link makes biological sense because oestrogen (as well as progesterone and testosterone) has been shown to stimulate the regeneration of damaged neurons. Oestrogen also appears to increase the production of the neurotransmitter acetylcholine, which regulates memory, learning, and other cognitive functions. In fact, oestradiol (a type of natural oestrogen) binds to the areas in the brain that are associated with memory: the cortex, the hippocampus, and the basal forebrain. Oestrogen has also been shown to enhance nerve cell branching.[23] Some studies, but certainly not all, suggest that hormone replacement may decrease the risk of stroke in perimenopausal women.[24] Research also shows that women with the highest endogenous levels of oestradiol have the lowest risk of Alzheimer's disease.[25]

This certainly sounds like good news for those of you who are worried about Alzheimer's. Many doctors prescribe oestrogen to prevent Alzheimer's, a practice that I feel is reasonable in some situations.[26] But the Alzheimer's/oestrogen data need to be put into perspective. Alzheimer's, after all, is not simply the result of oestrogen deficiency. And there's clearly a difference between the bodies of women who are able to make small amounts of oestradiol after menopause and those who aren't, differences that cannot be duplicated simply by taking oestrogen.

Dementia of all types, including Alzheimer's, is probably also associated with free-radical damage to brain tissue, which results from the overproduction of series 2 eicosanoids and inflammation, eventually leading to the damage or death of brain cells. Free-radical damage and the resulting tissue inflammation are the final common pathway by which emotional, physical, and environmental stressors of all kinds adversely affect every tissue in our bodies, including our brains.[27]

Studies also show that those who are well educated, in good health, and financially secure, with above-average intelligence and social status, and who actively pursue their interests as they age, have a very good chance of preserving their memory as they grow older. In fact, they may even improve it, whether or not they're on oestrogen.[28]

The input of all these factors makes it very difficult to prove a cause-and-effect relationship between oestrogen and Alzheimer's prevention. When compared to women who are not taking oestrogen, women on oestrogen are much more apt to match the profile for those most likely to maintain healthy brain function. This is an inherent weakness in epidemiological studies: they can identify associations and trends, but the conclusions drawn from them may turn out to be completely erroneous. (I'm reminded of the joke about the village drunk, whose favourite drink was Scotch and soda, suggesting to local authorities, 'I'm going to have to cut down on that soda – it's affecting my judgement.') Only a controlled, truly randomised, double-blind, prospective, case-controlled study with a large number of women will be able to tell us definitively whether oestrogen is the key factor in prevention of Alzheimer's dementia, or whether other factors are more prominent and oestrogen is only 'along for the ride'.

The data on oestrogen and brain function right now mirror the link between oestrogen and heart disease as we understood it in the early 1990s. At that time many doctors and researchers were absolutely convinced that oestrogen could prevent heart attacks, and could cite many retrospective and epidemiological studies to 'prove' it. So when two very large long-term studies of oestrogen replacement (the US HERS study and the Women's Health Initiative) failed to show a decrease in heart attack from conventional oestrogen replacement, they were shocked. (See chapters 5 and 14.) It is entirely possible that the same kind of long-term study on oestrogen and Alzheimer's might not show any firm benefit, either. We simply do not know.

Still, even though further confirmation is needed, there is some rather convincing evidence of the beneficial effect of hormones – not just oestrogen – on brain function.[29] Women who have undergone premature menopause have a slightly higher risk of early dementia.

And there is evidence that small baseline amounts of oestrogen are essential for certain memory functions. Many women's bodies produce enough throughout life, while some do not. The research of Dr Barbara Sherwin has shown that women's verbal memory decreases following hysterectomy with removal of the ovaries, but then returns to normal following hormone replacement.[30] Sherwin used only oestrogen replacement, but other studies support a role for progesterone and probably androgens as well.[31]

Ovarian hormones also bind to areas of the brain that are important for mood regulation. This helps to explain research findings indicating that oestrogen has significant antidepressant effects and that progesterone decreases anxiety and promotes restful sleep. While the research on oestrogen and memory is not conclusive, a small amount of bioidentical oestrogen (and/or progesterone or testosterone) may be a logical choice, depending upon your own hormone levels, family history, and other lifestyle factors.

Non-hormonal Ways to Protect Your Brain

Consider the following brain-health-enhancing practices:

• *Feed your brain with nutrients.* A diet high in refined sugars and including partially hydrogenated fats is associated with depletion of many nutrients necessary for optimal brain function. For brain function as for every other aspect of your health, I recommend a relatively low-fat diet that contains lots of fruits, vegetables, and whole grains. Studies have shown that demented and depressed patients often have inadequate levels of zinc, B vitamins (especially vitamin B_1, or thiamine), selenium, and antioxidants such as vitamins E and C, compared to patients with normal mental function.

Zinc, for example, is necessary for optimal transport of the B vitamins into the cerebrospinal fluid. This fluid bathes and nourishes the brain and spinal cord. Many women do not get adequate levels of zinc in their daily diets.[32] In one study of severely demented patients, ten patients were given vitamin supplements for two months, while a control group was not. After one month, the patients who received the supplements showed clinical memory improvement.[33] Some authorities also feel that Alzheimer's is associated with the inability of some elderly people to absorb enough minerals, vitamins, and essential trace elements from their food.[34] They may also have problems with transporting these nutrients from the blood to the brain. Since nutritional supplementation improves memory in people who are already demented, imagine the preventive potential of feeding your brain properly!

• *Quell potential free-radical damage to your brain tissue.* A great deal of brain health is affected by free-radical damage. Get serious about antioxidants. Make sure your diet is rich in vitamins C and E, the B vitamins (including folic acid), and selenium.[35] Another class of powerful antioxidants is the proanthocyanidins found in pine bark and grape pips (one brand name is Pycnogenol). (The dosage ranges for these are given in chapter 14.) Studies have shown that the risk of stroke is very low in those women who eat at least five servings of fruits and vegetables per day. Clearly, brain protection is yet another reason to eat plenty of these nutrient-rich foods.

• *Avoid smoking and excessive alcohol intake.* Cigarettes are well-known factors in causing cardiovascular disease and small blood vessel changes that decrease oxygen to your brain, among other areas. And excessive alcohol intake affects the basal forebrain, an area associated with memory.

• *Enhance your brain's acetylcholine levels.* Many factors can affect your acetylcholine levels and, subsequently, your memory. If you're already on oestrogen or other hormones to treat other symptoms, stick with them – though I wouldn't recommend hormones solely for Alzheimer's prevention, be reassured that they are probably helping your acetylcholine levels. And avoid drugs that are known to decrease acetylcholine levels.[36] You'd be amazed by how many of these there are and by how few doctors realise their adverse affect on brain function. Check the label of any medication used for sleep, colds, or allergies to see if it contains diphenhydramine. Examples of such medications include Benalyn, Uniflu, Panadol Night, Dreemon, Medinex and Nytol. The cough suppressant dextromethorphan also affects acetylcholine and has other anticholinergic effects that can impair memory. It is found in a wide range of cough and cold remedies.

- *Try pregnenolone, progesterone, or DHEA.* Studies suggest that pregnenolone, progesterone, and DHEA – related hormones that act as neurotransmitters in the brain – can promote the same dendritic and axonal branching between brain cells that is seen with oestrogen. Pregnenolone, which is available over the counter, is particularly promising. It is a precursor to DHEA and many other hormones, and it is better tolerated than DHEA in many women. Because it is a non-patentable hormone, we don't see nearly as much research on it as we do with oestrogen, but I consider it an excellent choice for those who cannot take oestrogen. The recommended starting dose is 25–50mg per day; it has been safely used in doses as high as 100–200mg per day. Start low and gradually increase. If you are already taking natural progesterone, this will probably give you a similar benefit, since preg-nenolone is also a precursor for progesterone. DHEA, too, has been shown to play a crucial role in the preservation of brain function.[37] The usual dose of DHEA for women is 5–25mg per day. (See pages 120–123.) Get your level of DHEA checked first and supplement only if it is too low.

Other Brain Food Choices

The food supplements listed below have been shown to help memory in many people. Try just one at a time, so that you know if it works for you. Use your intuition to pick one to start with. Your first impulse will usually be the right one.

GINKGO

Ginkgo biloba is the number-one prescription herb in Europe, with more than forty double-blind studies demonstrating its benefits. It appears to work by increasing blood flow to the brain, and it is widely used to treat arteriosclerotic blockage of the small arteries in the brain. The usual dosage is 40–80mg three times per day.

GOTU KOLA

Widely known as a 'memory herb', gotu kola *(Hydrocotyle asiatica)* also increases circulation to the brain. The usual dosage is 90mg per day. *Note:* Gotu kola is a stimulant and should not be taken at bedtime.

GOOD FATS

Nerve fibres throughout your body are coated with a fat called myelin. For good brain and nerve function, you need small amounts of high-quality (not partially hydrogenated) fat in your daily diet. I recommend consuming olive oil, sesame oil, or fatty fish such as salmon or sardines. DHA (docosahexaenoic acid), made from algae, at a dose of 100–200mg per day, is my first choice for taking oil in supplement form. (See Resources.)

SOYA

In Japan, where consumption of soya is far higher than it is in the West, the incidence of Alzheimer's and other dementias is much lower than in the West. The Bowman Gray School of Medicine at Wake Forest University in the US was recently awarded a patent for the use of soya to prevent Alzheimer's disease.[38] Preliminary research has shown that soya phyto-oestrogens affect the brain like oestradiol, but not as strongly.[39] And since it definitely helps the cardiovascular system, soya may help prevent the strokes that are so common in dementia.

Substances Your Brain Doesn't Need

ALUMINIUM

Aluminium has been found in the brains of Alzheimer's patients, and this disease has been associated with increased tissue levels of aluminium along with decreased levels of zinc and selenium. Although the nature of the link is not clear, there is evidence to suggest that aluminium is, indeed, a brain toxin in individuals who are genetically predisposed to Alzheimer's. If you have any Alzheimer's sufferers in your family, I'd recommend that you avoid aluminium cookware, antiperspirants containing aluminium, fizzy drinks from aluminium cans, and baking powder containing aluminium.[40]

ASPARTAME

Aspartame, with the proprietary names Canderel and NutraSweet, is an excitotoxin, which means that it causes nerve cells to overfire. In susceptible people this can lead to the death of brain cells. This is one of the reasons aspartame has been associated with a multiple-sclerosis-like syndrome in some women.[41] The aspartame in diet colas seems to cause the worst problems in susceptible women.

Some women are addicted to diet cola, drinking several litres per day without taking in much else in the way of other nutrients. This is a set-up for a wide range of neurological symptoms in susceptible individuals, including headache, dizziness, anxiety attacks, memory loss, slurred speech, numbness, muscle spasms, mood swings, severe depression, personality changes, PMS, insomnia, fatigue, hyperactivity, heart palpitations, arrhythmia, chest pain, hearing loss, ringing in the ears, blurred vision, decreased sense of taste, skin lesions, nausea, digestive disturbances, water retention, and seizures. If you have a history of such problems, avoid this artificial sweetener, especially in the form of diet colas. (Aspartame-induced symptoms go away when consumption is stopped.) Other, safer sweeteners include the herb stevia (Not available in the UK, but see Resources.).

SERMs (SELECTIVE OESTROGEN RECEPTOR MODULATORS)

Given the role of ovarian hormones in brain function, the anti-oestrogen drugs tamoxifen (to prevent breast cancer) and raloxifene (to prevent osteoporosis) stir up some legitimate concerns about the whole-body effects of oestrogen deprivation over time. Just as tamoxifen blocks the effects of oestrogen on the breasts, there is also compelling evidence that it blocks some of the effects of oestrogen on the brain.[42] Raloxifene (Evista), a drug prescribed to women to prevent osteoporosis, also affects the brain. This is one of the reasons hot flushes (which are mediated in the hypothalamus) are listed as one of the side effects of SERMs. Depression is also among a host of other side effects. Though these drugs have their place and may be appropriate for some women who are truly at very high risk, the very real potential drawbacks of these drugs are not getting enough attention.

If you're currently taking tamoxifen or raloxifene, it's doubly important for you to follow some of the suggestions outlined above to protect your brain function. Many women report alleviation of their tamoxifen-associated depression, for example, when they take high doses of soya. This may be because of soya's hormonal effects. (For a fuller discussion of SERMs, see chapters 5 and 13.)

Maximising Midlife Wisdom

Your brain is like your muscles. If you want it to stay in peak form, you have to use it regularly. Brain function is also profoundly affected by our expectations and attitudes about life. While there is no formula – hormonal or otherwise – to 'cure' ageing, there are many things you can do to preserve your mental vitality.

Step one: Stop yourself indulging in any stereotypical thinking about the ageing process. Start viewing yourself as a younger person, unfettered by the age-related problems the media tells us all to expect. Don't ever allow yourself to make comments such as 'I'm too old for this!' I've seen this kind of thinking in women who are only in their early thirties! My mother told me that when she reached sixty, her post was suddenly full of advertisements for all kinds of health aids, ranging from incontinence pads to hearing aids. She simply 'recycles' this information in the waste-paper basket.

Step two: Stay mentally active and socially connected. Continuing to expose yourself to new ideas, new people, and new environments is as necessary to staying mentally healthy as physical exercise is to maintaining the health of your heart, muscles, and bones.[43] Remember that learning causes actual growth of new neurons, even in an older brain.[44] Step outside the comfort of familiar territory. Cultivate a wide social network of individuals from diverse age groups. Take classes, get together with friends, learn a new sport or activity, start a new career or business, engage in volunteer work. Tone your brain cells and neural pathways with new ideas, new connections, and new thoughts every day.

I've noticed that some of my older friends tend to get a vacant look on their faces when they are with a group of new people or in an unfamiliar setting. Although they seem fine in their own homes, they can't seem to keep up with the conversation when challenged with a new situation. They've spent so much time screening out any newness from their environment, digging themselves deeper into the safety of their day-to-day ruts, they've lost the ability to adapt to change. It's tragic to witness what happens to the faces, bodies, and minds of these formerly vital people as they begin this downhill slide.

The famous brain researcher Marian Diamond says, 'There's a very simple principle when it comes to the brain. Use it or lose it.' When our nervous system no longer receives new input, it atrophies, a phenomenon that has been demonstrated clearly in the laboratory. In one study of ageing rats, Diamond added new toys and other novel items to enhance the environments of some rats, while leaving the other rats in their familiar surroundings. At the end of the study, the rats in the enriched environments had more cortical brain tissue than those with the standard environments. Interestingly, this change in brain structure occurred even in old rats that were 75 per cent of the way through their life spans.[45]

Step three: Develop an optimistic attitude towards life. Optimism – the ability to perceive the glass as half full instead of half empty – is a natural protectant against depression. Also, an impressive body of research has documented that optimists are healthier and live longer. In one study of individuals with no risk factors for heart disease, for example, depressed people were four times more likely to suffer from heart attacks than their optimistic, non-depressed counterparts; since heart disease is also associated with dementia, you can see the connection between a healthy attitude and a healthy brain.

Step four: Actively work with your thoughts and behaviours to modify those personality traits – such as hostility, pessimistic thoughts, and the tendency to isolate yourself socially – that are known to be associated with premature death and disability. If necessary, seek help from a therapist. Cognitive behavioural therapy (CBT) can make you more aware of your negative, self-limiting thoughts and help you find ways to redirect them in a more positive, empowering direction. This does not mean denial of life's difficulties. CBT also teaches you how to accept your situation and validate it, but at the same time deal with it more constructively. As a result, you learn to worry less.

Step five: Develop and express a healthy sense of humour. Read writers who make you laugh. Or watch reruns of comedy programmes you loved years ago.

Step six: Eat healthily and exercise regularly. A large body of research has demonstrated that almost all dementia is due, in part, to small-blood-vessel disease in our brains. The number-one reason why so many of us get these blood vessel changes is because we eat poorly and avoid exercise. Get moving, every day. This includes walking, aerobics, sports, swimming, or lifting weights. Movement keeps the blood flowing to all your organs, including your brain, and brings more nutrients and oxygen to your tissues. If you want, you can get your movement and social needs met at the same time by taking up a sport with a group of people who are non-competitive and just enjoy the fun of moving.

Step seven: Practise full emotional expression and heal your life as you go along. The emotional pattern associated with heart disease, including hardening of the arteries in the brain, is a tendency to avoid feeling your emotions fully – whether those emotions are positive or negative. One of my perimenopausal patients once told me:

> I grew up in a household in which we were taught to be afraid of strong emotions. You weren't allowed to feel too good – or too bad – about anything. If we needed to cry, we were told to go and bury our face in a pillow so that we wouldn't disturb the rest of the family. If we shouted with joy about a good mark or winning a game, we were told not to 'blow your own trumpet'. So I learned to distrust an entire range of feelings – basically anything except bland and boring pleasantness. Not surprisingly, dementia, depression, and heart disease run very strongly in my family on both sides. At midlife I feel as though I have to completely relearn how to feel. Often I have to tune in to symptoms in my body and just sit with them until I start to feel the emotion associated with them.

If you find yourself feeling sad, for example, just allow yourself the fullness of your feeling. What you will find is that it dissipates. But if you try instead to make yourself feel something else, and put yourself down for having an 'unpleasant' emotion, then that emotion will get locked in your body and may be expressed later as a disease.

Hostility, on the other hand, is a stuck chronic emotional pattern. It can be self-destructive to loiter in this space for very long, and the best way to get out is to find something to appreciate about every situation you are in, no matter how small it is, until appreciation begins to replace hostility as a mental and emotional pattern.

Step eight: Never retire. Don't allow yourself to start thinking about 'retirement' at midlife, the way so many people do. Instead, do what Dolly Parton does: find out what you love to do for work, and you'll never work a day in your life! You may wish to retire from working for a company or for another individual, but you need to have something that you're interested in doing – for pay or not – every day of your life.

In conclusion, consider the following experiment. In a recent study at Boston's Beth Israel Deaconess Hospital in the US, researchers Dr Jeffrey Hausdorff, a geriatrician, and Harvard graduate student Becca Levy tested the effect of subconscious beliefs on walking speed. Walking speed often declines with age, and that in combination with balance and coordination problems as well as other factors, such as medication, produces the stereotypical elderly 'shuffle'. The researchers tested healthy individuals aged between sixty-three and eighty-two by first getting them to walk down a hall the length of a football field. They measured both speed and 'swing time' – the time the foot spends off the ground. After that, the participants played a brief computer game. On half of the computers, upbeat words like *accomplished, wise,* and *astute* flashed across the screen just long enough to register subconsciously. The other group had negative words like *senile, dependent,* and *diseased* flashed across their screens. The participants then walked down the same hallway again. This time, the positively influenced group walked 9 per cent faster and had much more 'swing time' and much less shuffling. The negatively influenced group didn't get any worse, perhaps because they, like most of us, had already been saturated by society's negative ageing stereotypes.[46]

This study is clearly a wake-up call for becoming conscious of our own beliefs about ageing and the physical effects of those beliefs. I've seen far too many women talk themselves into physical deterioration starting as young as thirty! And who hasn't witnessed the black balloons and jokes about being 'over the hill' at birthday parties for friends turning forty?

Dr Ellen Langer, a Harvard psychologist who wrote the classic book *Mindfulness,* observed: 'The regular and "irreversible" cycles of ageing that we witness in the later stages of human life may be a product of certain assumptions about how one is supposed to grow old. If we didn't feel compelled to carry out these limiting mind-sets, we might have a greater chance of replacing years of decline with years of growth and purpose.'[47]

Amen.

ELEVEN

From Rosebud to Rose Hip: Cultivating Midlife Beauty

A few weeks ago my former harp teacher, Miss Alice Chalifoux, came to borrow my harp for her students to use at the summer harp school, where she has been teaching for over sixty years, and where I myself first took lessons when I was fourteen.

Though she's never paid much attention to diet, exercise, or supplements, her skin is pink, fresh, and smooth, her eyes are bright, she's never sick, and her irreverent and earthy sense of humour is utterly delightful. With a twinkle in her eye, Miss Chalifoux told me that she has cut her schedule right down this summer. She's only teaching thirty-six hours a week – about half time by her standards. She is a perfect example of a woman who is beautifully attuned to the power of what I call the rose hip stage of life, sowing her seeds of wisdom and inspiring others wherever she goes. Her impish soul shines out through every pore, its youthful effects written all over her face. Miss Chalifoux is ninety-two years old.

No one would deny that every season of the year is imbued with its own special beauty and wisdom. The same is true of the seasons of our lives. Most of us know or have seen at least one woman like Miss Alice Chalifoux, who is living proof that beauty is possible at every season of our lives, depending upon how we live them.

Perimenopausal women can be likened to the full-blown rose of late summer and autumn, as it begins to transform itself into a bright, juicy rose hip – the part of the rose that contains the seeds from which hundreds of other potential roses can grow. Unfortunately, our culture worships only the rosebud stage of development, thereby rendering relatively invisible the beauty of the other stages. In fact, not so long ago, the dewy rosebud was often used as a prominent symbol for ads selling conventional hormone replacement drugs to women. The subliminal message is clear: if you use hormone replacement therapy, you can stay at the rosebud stage of beauty for the rest of your life and never have to go through the process of maturing and ripening into the resilient and potent rose hip. But it's not true.

Once you're on the way to becoming a rose hip, you can't go backwards to being a rosebud, though our culture certainly entices us to try. Only very recently, for example, have we seen any fashion or make-up models older than twenty-five in the mainstream media! Losing the allure of the rosebud stage of life and learning how to replace it with the strength and resilience of a rose hip is not always easy, but it is absolutely necessary if you are to look and feel your very best as a woman in the full bloom of midlife. Just remember that when you're becoming a rose hip, any attempt to remain in the rosebud stage tends to look desperate and ridiculous. It's like trying to glue the autumn leaves back onto the tree and then paint them all green to simulate the spring. It simply doesn't work. Instead, our task is to come to appreciate the beauty and power of the season we are in, instead of longing for what can no longer be.

This is a particularly difficult task if, before menopause, you were the type of woman accustomed to using the power of your looks and body to attract the attention of men whenever you so much as walked into a room. If this has been true for you, then you're viscerally familiar with the power of external feminine beauty and have, perhaps, capitalised on it since adolescence. If your looks have charmed people for years, it is quite likely that you will have a harder time with becoming a rose hip than someone who didn't have this experience and therefore had to turn inwards at an earlier age to find her sense of worth and beauty. I had an acquaintance like this once. When she reached forty-five, she bemoaned the fact that men no longer turned to look at her when she walked into a room. Since all of her influence and money had always come to her by virtue of her appearance and its effect on powerful men, becoming a rose hip was truly a harsh wake-up call, letting her know that her former wiles would no longer serve her in the second half of life. Those of you who've never had that experience in the first place will probably have a much easier time settling into the rose hip stage.

But whether or not we were ever raving beauties, all of us want to look our best at every age. During perimenopause, we may never be rosebuds again, but we can still remain as attractive as possible by paying attention to good skin and body care. And we may even want to avail ourselves of plastic surgery or other cosmetic procedures. More choices are available to budding rose hips than ever before.

Making Peace with Your Changing Skin

One of the most distressing parts of midlife for many women is watching our skin begin to sag and get 'crepey'. I began to notice changes in my skin – a tendency toward more dryness and some fine wrinkles around my eyes – starting in my late thirties. When these first became noticeable, I decided to like them, since they reminded me of my father's eyes, which were always surrounded by the crinkles of lots of laughter and smiles. But I also wanted to do everything possible to keep those lines from getting deeper and more unattractive as time went on.

One of my newsletter subscribers eloquently shared the common dilemma of midlife skin changes and their potential emotional impact:

I am forty-eight years old, at my ideal weight, and extremely fit. I work out on a regular basis and lift weights as part of my exercise programme. I hike whenever I get the chance. However, it seems like almost overnight, the skin on my legs has become extremely slack. As I look down when I walk, I can see the skin on my thighs shake with each step. I'm sure it's the result of cumulative sun damage along with many years of putting on and losing those stubborn 10lb. Is there anything that can be done? I now use sunscreen whenever I am outdoors, never sunbathe, and try to keep my weight stable. Must I resign myself to wearing long dresses? Are there any supplements I can take? Is there anything that would rebuild the collagen? Any surgery that would help? I'm in the process of a divorce after twenty-seven years of marriage and am, naturally, concerned about my appearance. I'd be very grateful for any suggestions.

Fortunately there's a great deal that we can do to both preserve the health of our midlife skin and even heal some of the damage that has already been done. While we're doing this, however, we still have to go through midlife with the courage to live our lives joyfully and fully, despite such things as ageing skin and changing bodies. I know both from my practice and from my own life experience that this feels much harder when you're going through a divorce or loss of a life partner.

Nevertheless, it's important to remember that many women find love and happiness at midlife and beyond, regardless of a little sun damage or sagging here and there. This point was brought home to me rather dramatically recently during an event at which I spent time talking to two different women. One, a stunning woman in her late thirties with flawless skin and an almost perfect figure who was also a very successful businesswoman, was bemoaning the fact that there simply weren't any good men around with whom she could find happiness.

About half an hour later I met another woman. About fifty-five years old, she had a plain but lively face, unadorned by any make-up, and she was at least 3 stone overweight. Since we were discussing medical topics, she told me about a mastectomy she'd had years before that had left her chest quite disfigured. In the course of the conversation, she said, 'I think we underestimate men, don't you? They can be so sweet.' It turned out that she was going out with three different men, one of whom she felt was the one she was destined to marry! This woman's inner beauty and sense of humour made me feel happy just being near her. When I compared her energy and attitude to that of the show-stoppingly beautiful woman I'd met earlier, I realised how transient the impression of mere physical beauty can be when it's not lit from within by a beautiful soul.

I'm very comforted by what I learned that day from those women and their experiences, and I return to it whenever I begin to succumb to the cultural and media-driven notion that after thirty-five it's all downhill for women, our best years are behind us, and no one will ever love us again because we are no longer twenty-five. I've come to see that nothing could be further from the truth.

A Primer on Skin: Our External Nervous System

To prevent unnecessary ageing of the skin – which manifests as dullness, sallowness, uneven pigmentation, dryness, and wrinkles – you first need to understand what your skin does for you and how it does it.

The skin is derived from the embryonic layer known as the neuroectoderm, the same tissue layer that becomes the brain and the peripheral nervous system. It functions as a kind of external brain, gathering information about our outer environment through its ability to sense pressure, temperature, pleasure, and pain.

The research of Dr Tiffany Field on the striking immune-system-enhancing benefits of massage is compelling evidence of just how intimately our skin is connected with and affected by every aspect of our health, from our emotions to our nutrient intake. Our skin is, quite literally, the boundary between us and our environment. As our first line of defence against the vagaries of that environment, including bacteria, viruses, excessive ultraviolet radiation from the sun, wind, air pollution, and secondhand smoke, it is not only vulnerable to what's going on outside of us, it's also affected by our internal environment, both emotional and nutritional.

The condition of your skin says a great deal about how well you're fitting into and feeling supported by your current environment. If, for any reason, you feel as though you cannot be safe or true to yourself in your environment, and you are not particularly aware of this, then your skin may react for you. That's why it is well known in dermatology that patients may need simultaneous treatment of their skin and their mind and emotions for best results. Dermatitis and hives, for example, are two of the conditions known to be caused by a mixture of psychological and physical factors, while disorders such as psoriasis, hair loss, and eczema may also be affected by psychological factors. Almost everyone has had the experience of developing a large pimple in a prominent area of her face just when she was most concerned about looking her best for some big social event, or breaking out in oral herpes (cold sores) just before going out on a date, or getting itchy hives on taking a new job or moving to a new city. Sooner or later all of who we are and have been shows up on our faces.

The Anatomy of the Skin

The skin consists of three layers: the outer epidermis, the middle dermis, and a fat layer underlying both of those. The paper-thin epidermis is a protective layer of dead skin cells that holds in moisture and oil. It is constantly being shed and replaced as fresh cells push their way up to the surface, get flattened, and then die. As we age, the sloughing process tends to slow down, which is one of the reasons why skin tends to lose its 'freshness'.

FIGURE 15: THE ANATOMY OF THE SKIN

© 2001 by Northrup and Schulz

At the base of the epidermis are the basal cells, which contain the melanin-generating cells known as melanocytes. The amount and type of melanin determines the tone of your skin – a trait that is inherited from your parents.

The dermis layer, which makes up about 90 per cent of the skin, is where the nerve receptors and blood vessels are located. It also contains sweat glands and sebaceous glands; the latter produce oil and are attached to hair follicles. Blackheads and pimples inevitably arise from clogged sebaceous ducts at the root of hair follicles. The sweat and oil secretions from the dermal layer help protect the skin from infection by creating a protective acid mantle, but this mantle is easily disrupted by using harsh detergent and non-pH-balanced soaps.

Two proteins known as collagen and elastin, which give skin its elasticity and flexibility, are also located in the dermis layer. On average, collagen production starts to diminish at a rate of 1 per cent per year starting in our twenties. By midlife we may have lost up to 20 per cent of our collagen layer, though there is enormous variation among different individuals. The darker your skin tone, however, the more collagen and elastin it has – which is why the skin and bones of dark-skinned women tend to be more resistant to the wear and tear of ageing compared to those of Caucasian descent, and also why black- and brown-skinned women are less apt to have wrinkled skin compared to white-skinned women. Those with yellow skin tend to fall somewhere in between.

In addition to the thinning of the collagen layer of our skin with age, our oil glands tend to decrease their secretions, resulting in a greater tendency towards dryness. By about the age of fifty, the capacity of the skin to repair itself also slows down, for reasons that aren't entirely clear but may be related to free-radical damage (see the next section).

Free Radicals and Skin Ageing

If you take a look at the skin on your buttocks and lower back, you'll notice something important. Skin that has been protected from environmental pollutants and excessive sunlight is smoother and more wrinkle-free than elsewhere on our bodies. That means that skin ageing is related to more than simply chronological age. It's also related to our environment – both inside and outside our bodies.

Premature ageing of the skin – and of every other cell in our body – is related to the production of what are known as free radicals, oxygen molecules that have become unstable because they have lost an electron in the course of interacting with other molecules in our body during such basic metabolic processes as breathing and digestion. Free radicals are also produced when sunlight hits the skin, and by toxins of all kinds, including cigarette smoke and air pollutants. In the body, these unstable free radicals bounce around, attaching themselves to the cell membranes of virtually any tissue that is available in order to stabilise themselves with an electron from that tissue. If they take an extra electron from collagen in our skin, for example, this can damage the collagen. Over time the skin becomes stiff and discoloured and loses its elasticity. It's much like the process by which iron rusts when left out in the open air.

Wrinkles result from the breakdown of elastin and collagen fibres in the deeper layers of the skin. Collagen and elastin are responsible for the resilience of the skin, allowing it to stretch and contract. When collagen gets broken down, skin tends to sag and wrinkle.

Free-radical damage can also harm and break down the fats within our cells and cell membranes, and the DNA of the cells, where the genetic code resides. In fact, many scientists have now come to the conclusion that free-radical damage is one of the primary causes of ageing, including skin wrinkling, and age-related diseases such as heart disease, Alzheimer's, arthritis, and so on.

Since some free radicals are produced as an unavoidable part of daily living, it's not surprising that our bodies have developed defence systems for dealing with them. This defence system is based on the effects of molecules known as antioxidants. These include vitamins C and E found in foods, and others produced in the body, such as glutathione, catalase, and superoxidedismutase. Antioxidants work by donating electrons to the unstable free radicals, thus rendering them harmless by preventing them from combining with other molecules and damaging our tissues.

Given this defence system, one might wonder why we age at all. As with all things, it's a question of balance. Though our bodies manufacture antioxidants and we ingest them in foods and as supplements, sometimes our antioxidant systems become overwhelmed by the sheer number of free radicals produced by such things as cigarette smoke, air pollution, sun exposure, diets that are heavy in trans fats or other suboptimal ingredients, and emotional stress of all kinds. The resulting free-radical damage in our bodies is known as oxidative stress. Hundreds of research studies suggest that we can keep the oxidative stress in our bodies to a minimum by ingesting antioxidants, avoiding environmental toxins, and maintaining emotional equilibrium.

How Smoking Damages the Skin

Midlife is the time when the ill effects of smoking become as plain as the nose on your face. Women who smoke heavily have a paler skin tone and more lines and wrinkles than non-smokers. Some of this effect is from the decrease in circulation to the skin caused by nicotine. Decreased skin circulation results in fewer nutrients getting to the skin and a decreased ability of the skin to release the toxic waste products of cell metabolism. This results in a slowing of skin growth and rejuvenation.

In addition to this, smoking directly poisons the ovaries, leading to decreased levels of oestrogen, which is necessary to help maintain elastin and collagen fibres.

How Excessive Ultraviolet Radiation Damages the Skin

It is estimated that about 70 per cent of the change we see in our skin as we age is the result of damage done to collagen fibres in the dermis. Sun damage, in particular, causes the skin to lose its resiliency and elasticity.[1] Skin that is chronically overexposed to the sun is in a constant state of mild inflammation. Though we've all been brought up to feel that a tan makes us look more youthful in appearance, this is an illusion. The mild inflammation and swelling of tanned skin plumps the skin up, temporarily minimising wrinkles, and gives the appearance of a more youthful look. But once the tan goes away, the wrinkles reappear, and what you're left with is skin that has lost its normal architecture.

Excessive exposure to ultraviolet radiation results in tissue inflammation that begins with free-radical damage to skin cell membranes followed by the release of harmful inflammatory chemicals (you guessed it – eicosanoids) that ultimately damage collagen and elastin fibres. Eventually collagen and elastin fibres that were originally flexible and fluid become stiff and hard. The ageing process that your skin collagen goes through is much the same as what happens to a flexible and clear egg white when you drop it in a hot frying pan: the fluid protein in the egg white is transformed into denatured protein, a dense, hard, inflexible type of protein. Ultraviolet radiation also damages the blood vessels in the skin, thus decreasing the flow of blood and other nutrients to this organ. This is in part the reason for those dilated blood vessels on the cheeks and nose.

Preventing or Treating Wrinkles

The key to younger-looking skin at perimenopause is to avoid smoking and overexposure to the sun (the earlier the better) and to use antioxidants, both topically and internally. Unfortunately, many women don't see the damage sun does to their skin until they've already spent their teens, twenties, and thirties sunbathing. By then, it's harder to deal with the damage, though still possible. Some women, however, by virtue of their genes, simply seem to have wrinkle-free youthful skin for a lifetime, regardless of how much sun exposure they get. But most of us have to give our skin a helping hand when it comes to midlife preservation or improvement.

Midlife Skin Care Regime

• *Cleanse your skin regularly.* The skin has been called a 'third kidney' because it removes almost as much waste material from the body each day as the kidneys themselves. If your skin is dry, you need to cleanse it thoroughly once per day. If it's oily, then twice per day may be better. Remove all make-up every night. When you care for your face, don't forget your neck – it's the first place you notice the effects of ageing. Cleansing your skin thoroughly will clean out your pores and allow your skin to remove waste products efficiently from your body as you sleep, a time when your body is rejuvenating itself.

Use a cleansing lotion or soap that preserves the acid mantle of the skin, because it's one of your body's natural defences against infection and spots. Look for the term 'pH balanced' when shopping for a soap or cleanser. If your skin is dry, be sure to look for a non-drying, moisturising cleanser. If your skin is oily, you can use a stronger product for cleansing and an oil-free moisturiser. Those with combination skin should use a cleanser specifically formulated for this type of skin. Many good brands are available. (See Resources.)

If your skin is oily, be sure to avoid overuse of astringents, which usually contain alcohol. They can actually make an oil problem worse and also damage your skin over time.

• *Close pores after cleaning.* Use a toner to close the pores after cleansing, especially if your skin is oily. Or simply use cool water to close the pores – it works well for all skin types.

• *Renew skin with exfoliants and topical antioxidants.* One of the reasons that skin starts to look dull and old at midlife is that the rate of skin growth and cell turnover slows down. As a result, the plumper new skin cells that give your complexion a glowing appearance tend to stay below the surface. In order to help remove old dead skin from the surface, open your pores, and speed up new skin growth, you'll need regular exfoliation. This can be done either mechanically, with a flannel, or with products that contain fruit acids, which include alpha hydroxy, beta hydroxy, or glycolic acids. (See below.)

Avoid using abrasive cleansers such as those made from the hulls of nuts, which is like cleaning your skin with sandpaper. This can lead to breakage of capillaries and microabrasions of the skin that raise the risk of infection and even acne.

If your skin is oily, apply a mild cleanser to a flannel, and use that to exfoliate each night. Use a clean flannel each time to decrease the amount of germs that your skin comes into contact with. Follow this with an application of a mild alpha hydroxy, beta hydroxy, or glycolic acid product and/or one of the antioxidant products I recommend below. Many products on the market today contain both antioxidants and fruit acids. If your skin is dry or sensitive, skip the flannel and simply use an alpha hydroxy acid (AHA) or antioxidant preparation to do your exfoliating for you.

• *Use a sunscreen every day on your face, neck, and hands.* Make a habit of putting sunscreen with an SPF of 15 or higher on your face, neck, and hands every morning except during the brief early morning or late afternoon 'sun bath' that I advocate for optimal vitamin D levels (see chapter 12).

• *Moisturise.* If your AHA, antioxidant, or sunscreen formula is not in a moisturising base, then finish off your daily skin care regimen with a light moisturiser for day and a richer formula for the evening. This helps much-needed moisture remain in your skin cells, keeping them plumped up.

Exfoliants and Antioxidants

FRUIT ACIDS: Alpha hydroxy acids and other fruit acids do double duty as exfoliants and antioxidants. As exfoliants, they work in three ways: (1) they help dissolve the 'glue' that holds dead skin cells together, thus resulting in easier removal, so new and plumper cells can rise to the surface; (2) they increase the hydration of the skin; and (3) they encourage the repair of elastin and collagen in the skin and may even help thicken it a bit.

Commercial products usually contain from 5 to 10 per cent fruit acids, concentrations that are low enough and safe enough for all skin types and tones. It's always best, however, to test any product first, either on the inner part of your elbow or just under your jawline. If your skin is sensitive, start with a 5 per cent product. If you can tolerate that, gradually work up to a 10–12 per cent product. You may experience a slight stinging with some products until you get used to them. Higher-strength AHAs (up to 70 per cent) are used to lighten the skin or cause a deeper peel and should be used only by professional beauticians or doctors.

Fruit acids help normalise your skin whether it's dry or oily. If it's oily, they remove the top dead layer of cells, thus allowing oil to flow out of the follicle more easily so that it can be removed without stripping away essential moisture. If your skin is dry, fruit acids remove the dry dead layer and stimulate cell renewal.

It usually takes about two weeks before you'll notice a difference in your skin with regular use of a fruit acid. Most people start by using AHAs only at night, but once you know they work for you, you can apply them twice per day.

As antioxidants, fruit acids can also alleviate some of the free-radical damage that results from exposure to sunlight and pollutants in the air.

ANTIOXIDANT VITAMINS AND HERBS: Research has shown that vitamin C, green tea extract, vitamin E, and vitamin A can be applied topically to help the skin resist damage from ultraviolet light and repair it if it occurs.[2] These are available in a variety of products. However, in order for a topical antioxidant to deliver effective results, it must be in a form that is maximally absorbed by the skin. Dr Nicholas Perricone, an assistant clinical professor of dermatology at Yale in the US, has done extensive and pioneering work in the use of antioxidants.[3] He has found that topical vitamin C ester (which is fat soluble), alpha-lipoic acid (which is both water and fat soluble), and a substance known as DMAE are particularly effective, often producing visible results within a few days.[4]

VITAMIN C ESTER: Research has shown that in the proper form, vitamin C, a powerful and ubiquitous antioxidant, can restore a smooth surface and youthful glow to ageing skin. This is but one aspect of the very well-documented role it plays in protecting virtually every organ in our bodies from the effects of ageing. In the skin, vitamin C is essential for the production of collagen. It also helps heal inflammation because it blocks the production of some of the inflammatory eicosanoids.

The problem with using natural vitamin C topically is that it's very acidic, which is irritating to the skin. It is also water soluble and breaks down rapidly, losing its potency within twenty-four hours. That's why most products containing conventional vitamin C aren't effective. But when vitamin C is combined with palm oil to create what is known as an ester, it becomes non-acidic while maintaining its antioxidant and collagen-enhancing properties. Because vitamin C ester is fat soluble and can penetrate the thin membrane that encases a cell, it offers maximum protection against free radicals in the place they do the most damage – the outer membrane of the cell. Studies have shown that vitamin C ester (also known as ascorbyl palmitate) is absorbed much more quickly and achieves levels in the skin that are ten times higher than natural vitamin C (ascorbic acid). Vitamin C ester is also stable and can be added to creams and lotions, where it will keep its potency for months.

Dr Perricone's research has shown that vitamin C ester cream helps heal sunburn and even seems to help psoriasis. And because vitamin C ester helps stimulate the growth of fibroblasts, the cells that help produce collagen and elastin in human skin, it has been shown to help reduce fine lines and wrinkles, firm skin that is sagging because of damaged collagen, and heal inflamed or irritated skin. (See Resources.)

TOCOTRIENOLS, A HIGH-POTENCY FORM OF VITAMIN E: Up until very recently, scientists felt that the tocopherols, particularly d-alpha tocopherol, were the most potent part of the vitamin E complex, and the alpha tocopherols have been widely used in cosmetics and other products for over thirty years. Newer research has demonstrated that the tocotrienols, another part of the vitamin E complex, are more effective. They inhibit peroxide formation – a measure of free-radical damage – much more efficiently than alpha tocopherol, and they're better at increasing the levels of the various skin enzymes that help protect the skin from ultraviolet damage. In fact, research suggests that the tocotrienols are forty to fifty times more powerful than other forms of vitamin E.[5] This new type of high-potency vitamin E is made using a special extraction process on rice bran oil or palm fruit oil. The resulting liquid can easily be mixed into creams, lotions, shampoos, or other cosmetics. Dr Perricone's research shows that these products can help dry, damaged hair, severely dry skin, and brittle fingernails. Look for the words 'high-potency E' or 'HPE' on the label to be sure you're getting the right products.

ALPHA-LIPOIC ACID: Alpha-lipoic acid (ALA) is a completely natural antioxidant molecule that is present in every cell of our bodies. ALA is both water and fat soluble, which enables it to work both on the surface of cells and deep within them, as opposed to ordinary vitamin C (water soluble) and vitamin E (fat soluble). As a result of this universal solubility, ALA can increase the positive effects of other antioxidants. It is also the only antioxidant that can increase a cell's metabolism, which tends to slow down with ageing. This enhances the cell's capacity to heal.

ALA plays a very special role when it comes to quelling inflammation – the condition that precedes lines and wrinkles. It prevents the cell from producing the types of eicosanoids (cytokines) that damage the cell in the first place. But it also activates a factor within the cell that turns on enzymes that actually digest collagen already damaged by free radicals. That is why the topical application of ALA results in remarkable improvement in wrinkles and fading of facial scars.

Alpha-lipoic acid also helps prevent the toxic effects of too much sugar in the cell. Excess cellular sugar attaches to just about every protein in the body; when it attaches to collagen, the collagen becomes stiff and inflexible – like the cooked egg white I mentioned earlier. In addition, ALA promotes healthy levels of nitric oxide, a substance that helps control blood flow to the skin (and is the basis for the effects of the drug Viagra). This increased circulation decreases swelling and oedema, thus reducing under-eye puffiness. It also gives the skin a healthy glow. Finally, ALA helps decrease ruddiness and shrink large pores for reasons that aren't yet clearly understood.

DMAE (Dimethylaminoethanol): An antioxidant found in abundance in fish, DMAE can be mixed with nutrients and other antioxidants and applied topically. Because it prevents free-radical damage not only to collagen but also to the nerves and muscles underneath the skin, it can be very effective at improving the appearance of ageing, sagging skin.

Topically applied DMAE works within minutes of application, and its firming effect lasts for nearly twenty-four hours. Continued use results in firmer skin virtually wherever it's applied. DMAE also boosts the effects of other antioxidants and results in increased smoothness and reduction of fine wrinkles. DMAE works in part by becoming part of the cell membrane, where its antioxidant properties help the membrane to resist stress more effectively.

DMAE preparations are typically available at cosmetics counters in better department stores (see Resources).

Skincare by Prescription Only

If you follow the insulin-normalising diet I recommend in chapter 7 and institute the skin care regimen I've outlined above, including a good antioxidant product with either alpha-lipoic acid, vitamin C ester, or tocotrienols, then you probably won't need anything else for your skin. Nevertheless, it's worth knowing about the popular prescription skin care medications that are available. There are two basic kinds: retinoic acid derivatives and hormone-containing products.

RETINOIC ACID DERIVATIVES (RETINOIDS):   Retin-A, Isotrex, Roac-cutane, and Acticin are all prescription medications derived from retinoic acid, a form of vitamin A that helps prevent or reduce fine lines and wrinkles, reverse sun damage, and heal acne.

These substances are powerful antioxidants, and regular use of retinoic acid as prescribed by a doctor can result in reduction of fine lines and wrinkles, stimulate blood flow to the skin, even out pigmentation, and help prevent wrinkles and lines from forming in the first place.

But retinoic acid is not for everyone. Side effects include redness, dryness, itchiness, and increased sun sensitivity. It takes anything from two to six months to notice a real difference if you're not taking any other steps to improve your complexion, and you must be absolutely committed to rigorous sunscreen use.

I personally used a form of Retin-A prescribed for many women before I discovered Dr Perricone's research and products. Though the Retin-A worked and was non-irritating, it resulted in excessive flakiness of my skin, which I'd sometimes notice on my cheeks and jawline at the worst possible time – usually looking into the mirror just before leaving for a speaking engagement! Not all women have this problem, but I find I get much better results with the topical and systemic antioxidant programme I now use.

TOPICAL APPLICATION OF HORMONE REPLACEMENT THERAPY: Skin contains receptor sites for hormones, and it is well documented that oestrogen, which also has antioxidant effects, helps preserve the collagen layer of the skin. Declining hormone levels are one of the reasons for the thinning of the collagen layer during the peri-menopausal years. Many women who've undergone surgical or medical menopause notice skin changes within a few months of the loss of their hormonal support unless they take steps to replace those hormones or take phytohormones.

Research has shown that topical application of oestrogen can increase collagen thickness, decrease pore size, and help the skin hold moisture. In Europe, oestrogen is often prescribed to help beautify the skin. You can get these same benefits by using hormones topically.

If you are already on bioidentical hormone replacement (see pages 138–41), ask your doctor to prescribe your hormones via a formulary pharmacist (Boots the Chemists) so that they can be put into skin lotion. A formula developed by Joel Hargrove, MD, head of the Menopause Center at Vanderbilt University Medical Center in the US, contains 150mg of oestradiol and 1,500mg of natural progesterone per 10oz bottle of fragrance-free Jergens lotion. This equals 2.5mg oestradiol and 25mg progesterone per tsp (5cc). The usual dose is 1tsp on the skin daily after bathing. (Clearly, it's easy to vary this amount according to your individual needs.) All blood levels tested using these amounts were in the therapeutic range for hormone replacement with no adverse effects.[6] Research has also shown that this oestrogen–progesterone balance protects the endometrial lining from overstimulation by oestrogen.[7]

In my experience, most women are delighted with this method of using hormone replacement. It improves the skin, enhances moisture, and provides the benefits of hormone replacement, all at the same time. As with any type of hormone replacement, it's always best to use the lowest dose that does the job. Levels that are too high can result in excessive oil secretion, acne, and even excessive growth of facial hair.

TOPICAL OESTROGEN: If you are not on hormone replacement already but want to try oestrogen for its skin benefits, ask your doctor to prescribe a small amount of oestrogen just for this purpose. A formulary pharmacist (Boots the Chemists) can put a small amount of oestradiol or oestriol in an ointment or cream. Use of the cream is safe and effective, without the adverse side effects of too much oestrogen. A 1996 study found that the use of dilute topical oestrogen produced marked improvement of elasticity and firmness of the skin along with increased skin moisture, decreased pore size, and decreased wrinkle depth. The dose used in the study was 1g of an ointment containing 0.01 per cent oestradiol and 0.3 per cent oestriol, applied daily to neck and face. Monthly determinations of blood hormone levels of oestradiol, follicle-stimulating hormone (FSH), and prolactin failed to show any significant systemic hormonal changes using these dilute amounts on the skin.[8]

TOPICAL PROGESTERONE: Many of my patients have seen skin improvement, including decreased midlife acne, greater moisture, and fading of age spots, by using a 1.5–3 per cent natural progesterone cream on their skin. This may be all you need without resorting to a prescription for oestrogen cream.

Beautiful Skin from the Inside Out:
The Right Foods and Supplements

Good skin isn't just an 'outside' job. The skin is a mirror for the health of your insides as well as your outsides. Take antioxidant vitamins (more about that below) and eat at least five servings of fruits and vegetables daily. Many of the hundreds of substances present in these foods, such as lycopene in tomatoes and lutein in dark green and yellow vegetables, have been clinically proven to help prevent and heal sun damage to the skin. Since antioxidants work in concert with each other, the greater the variety of fruits and vegetables you eat, the better.

The insulin-normalising diet I recommend for balancing hormones at midlife also helps keep your skin in good shape. Limit caffeine, and cut down as much as possible on high-glycaemic-index foods such as biscuits, sweets, pies, cakes, and non-whole-grain breads, all of which can cause fluid retention from excess insulin secretion. They are devoid of skin-nourishing vitamins and minerals, and quickly break down into sugar, which, as I explained above, causes collagen to lose its flexibility. (This is one of the reasons why diabetic individuals whose blood sugar is not tightly controlled often develop cataracts in the collagen-rich lenses of their eyes and have difficulty with wound healing. It is also why oral supplementation with alpha-lipoic acid has been shown to alleviate some of the side effects of diabetes.)

FIBRE: Make sure that you're getting enough fibre. Nothing shows up on the skin faster than chronic constipation! I've seen many cases of acne clear beautifully once bowel function is normalised. One of the most effective ways to do this is simply by eating 1/4 cup of ground golden flaxseed (linseed) each day. In addition to the 11-plus grams of fibre you'll get, linseeds are also loaded with skin-beautifying omega-3 fatty acids and phyto-oestrogens. Fruits and vegetables are also rich in fibre in addition to their antioxidants.

WATER: You may also see a dramatic improvement in your skin if you drink eight glasses of water per day.

FISH: Fish, especially salmon, sardines, and swordfish, is rich in both the omega-3 fats, which are important for building healthy cell membranes everywhere in the body, and DMAE, the antioxidant cell stabiliser I mentioned earlier.

SOYA: One of the most common benefits women notice after several months of supplementing their diets with significant amounts of soya protein (100–160mg of soya isoflavones per day) is improvement in their skin tone, hair, and nails. One woman who takes the soya supplement Revival wrote, 'Within two months of beginning this soya drink, my nails became stronger and more resilient than ever, my hair has taken on more body, and my skin has never looked more radiant. I'm thrilled.' Soya's phyto-oestrogen content helps strengthen collagen everywhere in the body, whether in facial skin, vaginal tissue, or bone.

SKIN-AIDING SUPPLEMENTS: Though all of the various supplements that I recommend at midlife help the skin (see chapter 7), the antioxidants, such as coenzyme Q_{10}, vitamin C, vitamin E, proanthocyanidins, and alpha-lipoic acid, are particularly important.

Research has shown, for example, that proanthocyanidins from pine bark or grape pips help protect skin from the damaging effects of too much ultraviolet radiation. In one study, this powerful antioxidant was shown to prevent ultraviolet activation of a certain area in the nucleus of skin cells, reducing the inflammation that occurs after sunburn.[9] Many individuals have reported healthy changes in their skin, nails, and hair as a result. The usual dose is 40–120mg per day; I personally take 60–80mg per day.

Coenzyme Q_{10}, which is found in every cell of the body, is fat soluble and concentrates in the plasma membrane of cells, where it protects against free-radical damage. This antioxidant is used up when skin is exposed to ultraviolet radiation and other environmental insults, so it makes sense to supplement your diet with it or apply it topically. It is also found in red meat, salmon, and nuts. Coenzyme Q_{10}, like alpha-lipoic acid, assists in cellular metabolism, and it works well when used along with alpha-lipoic acid. The usual dose in supplement form is 30–100mg per day. In one German study there was a 23 per cent reduction in fine lines on the face when a cream containing coenzyme Q_{10} was used topically.[10] Creams with coenzyme Q_{10} (PharmaNord) are readily available in health shops.

Vitamins E and C taken as supplements have also been shown to help protect against the UV-generated free-radical damage that can lead to skin changes. The dose of vitamin C used was only 200mg; for vitamin E, it was 1,000IU.[11] The results are apt to be even more impressive with the newer, more potent forms of vitamin E – the tocotrienols. The supplement regimen recommended in chapter 7 will give you all the skin-nourishing nutrients you need.

Skin Care from Your Refrigerator

Once or twice per week, if you have the time, you can give your face a healthy dose of antioxidants, fruit acids, and plant hormones by using ingredients that you can find in your refrigerator. Choose the food that most appeals to your sense of smell; you'll be getting aromatherapy benefits as well as direct benefits to your skin. Plain yogurt applied to your face makes a nourishing mask that gives your skin the benefits of lactic acid and also the hydrating effects of milk proteins. You can add pureed fresh fruit to it. (Don't use sweetened yogurt. The sugar is harmful to the skin.)

I love thinly sliced cucumber applied to my eyelids and cheeks to help me relax and get ready for evening. Green-tea bags, moistened and applied to the eyelids, also give your eyes a soothing antioxidant lift. And mashed-up fresh fruits such as peaches, strawberries, or apples can all be mixed with finely ground oatmeal to form a nourishing facial mask. You can also use parsley or even fresh basil, rosemary, or thyme. Remember, the skin will absorb the nutrients from these foods in about fifteen minutes, so you don't need to lie down any longer than that to benefit from a rejuvenating facial mask.

Midlife Acne

Anything that compromises the immune system, whether emotional stress or nutritional deficiency, will tend to exacerbate the underlying conditions that lead to acne. So will hormonal imbalances in which the body produces too much androgen. Any time you are under stress, your cortisol and insulin balance is likely to be upset; this, too, can affect your skin – and the rest of you as well. At perimenopause, the same stormy emotions that were present at adolescence often arise again, along with the hormonal swings that exacerbate the situation. It's no wonder that spots are so common during this life stage.

Are You Thin-skinned and in Need of Individuation?

Both adolescence and midlife are key developmental periods of our lives when we go through the process of individuating and defining who we are in relationship to others. The skin is the first contact surface between the mother and the infant, and for our entire lives it represents a boundary between us and other people. Some researchers believe that skin disease may be thought of as an attempt to define who we are in relation to other people and what a healthy boundary between us should be.[12] I agree.

When I was in my early thirties, a time in life when hormones are relatively stable and skin is usually at its best, I developed a very troubling case of acne. It took me a while to understand what was going on. I'd never had much in the way of skin problems in my teenage years, and since I was exercising regularly, taking vitamins, and eating a whole-food diet, it seemed strange to me that I should suddenly be experiencing acne at my age. However, I was working at the time in a surgery where my ideas on nutrition, emotions, and the mind–body connection were not well accepted, a fact I dealt with by way of a lot of self-deprecating humour, hoping this would enable me to stay safe and fit in as best I could. I desperately wanted the approval of my colleagues and was so thin-skinned that I was constantly trying to forestall any criticism of my ideas and beliefs. Finally, at the age of thirty-five, I realised that I couldn't continue using so much of my energy to try to blend in, and so after a good deal of soul-searching, I took a leap of faith and left to co-found Women to Women. My four-year-long skin problem cleared up within three months and has never returned, even though I'm now smack in the middle of midlife hormonal changes!

The Anatomy of Acne

1. Androgenic hormones such as DHEA and testosterone increase production of sebum by the sebaceous glands.

2. Sebum makes the hardened outer layer of skin (the keratin-rich cells known as the horny layer) turn over faster. This results in pores and hair follicles that are clogged with dead skin cells and oil.

3. Skin bacteria of the type known as *Propionibacterium acnes* feed off the sebum and break it down into free fatty acids.

4. Free fatty acids attract white blood cells and other inflammatory molecules (eicosanoids) from the immune system.

5. An acne pimple or a blackhead is the result.

Hormones and Midlife Acne

There are numerous studies showing that sebaceous gland activity is heightened by androgens such as DHEA and testosterone and reduced by oestrogen or removal of the ovaries, which reduces androgen levels.[13] This is the reason why contraceptive pills often help clear up acne. But whether or not higher levels of hormones result in acne is an individual matter. Women with the most severe forms of acne generally have a genetic predisposition to androgen sensitivity in their skin, even at hormone levels that are normal.

When sebaceous glands are small, as in children and the elderly, acne does not occur. It is usually first seen in adolescence, when sebaceous gland development begins to take place. It occurs primarily on the face, back, and chest. Endocrinologists have long theorised that acne is an endocrine disease resulting from abnormal androgen production. Hair follicles and attached sebaceous glands contain a specific enzyme known as 5-alpha-reductase, which can convert oestrogen into the androgen testosterone. That's why some women experience an increase in acne when their oestrogen levels rise, due either to perimenopause or to being put on overly high levels of hormone replacement therapy. But two women who are on identical hormone replacement regimens, eat exactly the same diet, and have the same amount of stress in their lives may have skin reactions that are entirely different. That's why all treatments, including prescription medications, have their place and can be useful.

Natural Treatments for Acne

If your acne is mild to moderate, I'd recommend that you use the natural treatment programme I outline below. If your acne is severe, you may also want to add one of the medications I discuss below, or follow the advice of a skin care specialist.

• *Eat a good diet.* Follow the high-fibre, insulin-lowering diet outlined in chapter 7, because a diet too high in high-glycaemic-index carbohydrates, as I've already stated, is associated with excessively high levels of insulin, which in turn can cause higher than normal production of androgens. For many women, this is all that is necessary to clear up acne completely.

• *Take supplements.* Take a comprehensive vitamin and mineral supplement daily (see chapter 7). It is well documented that zinc, vitamin C, and the B vitamins are essential for healthy skin functioning. Many women notice that their hair and skin improve dramatically when they start on a good supplementation regimen.

• *Lose excess body fat.* Get your body fat percentage into the healthy range. Excess body fat is associated with higher than normal androgen levels. Even a small fat loss of 5 to 10lb can make a significant difference in insulin and androgen as it affects the sebaceous glands.

• *Follow the skin care regimen for the general care of midlife skin (pages 336–8).* Remember that the fruit acids alone often work very well for acne. Alpha-lipoic acid also can be effective against acne, and may in addition help reduce or completely eliminate acne scars.

• *Try home remedies for pimples.* When you notice a pimple that hasn't come to a head yet, apply tea tree oil at night. The antibacterial properties in the oil will often result in significant regression of the pimple by morning. Some women use tea tree oil daily.

Another effective treatment is to make a paste of baking soda and lemon juice and apply it to the pimple. Baking soda also makes an excellent exfoliating agent unless your skin is sensitive.

• *Remove blackheads.* For blackheads, get a professional facial with blackhead removal about once per month until your skin has cleared. After that, you can use one of the readily available blackhead removal strips such as Bioré. Limit use to once per week to avoid overdrying the skin.

Acne Medications

VITAMIN A DERIVATIVES: Tretinoin (in Retin-A) is a prescription medication that increases skin cell turnover and allows sebum to be released more easily so that it doesn't get trapped. Isotretinoin (Roaccutane) is an oral vitamin A derivative that powerfully inhibits both sebum production and growth of acne-causing bacteria. It is the single most effective treatment for severe acne that doesn't respond to other measures. However, it is very irritating and should never be used by anyone who is pregnant or trying to get pregnant, because it can cause birth defects.[14] It is only available for hospital use in the UK.

BENZOYL PEROXIDE AND SULFUR-CONTAINING PRODUCTS: Various lotions, creams, or gels containing benzoyl peroxide or sulfur are often used for their antibacterial and drying properties. Benzoyl peroxide penetrates the hair follicle and produces oxygen, thus suppressing the growth of acne-causing bacteria, which thrive in an anaerobic (oxygen-free) environment. Although often effective, these treatments can be very irritating to the skin.

ANTIBIOTICS: Tetracycline or erythromycin work by preventing the acne bacteria from breaking down the sebum into the free fatty acids that result in pimples. I do not recommend the use of antibiotics because they kill off the healthy bacteria in the bowel, which can lead to suboptimal absorption of nutrients, diarrhoea, and repeated yeast infections. It can also lead to antibiotic resistance.

CONTRACEPTIVE PILLS: Oral contraceptives are often used to reduce sebum production. They do this by decreasing the brain's signal to make hormones from the ovaries. I'd avoid these synthetic hormones unless you feel you have no other choice and are unable or unwilling to follow a healthier diet or use one or more of the topical treatments recommended above.

Rosacea

Rosacea is a common condition at midlife (forties and fifties) and occurs much more often in women than in men. It is characterised by blood vessel dilatation on the blush areas of the face and upper chest, often accompanied by red, raised bumps (papules) and pustules. When the skin of rosacea patients is looked at under the microscope, it shows oedema (swelling), dilated blood vessels, and collections of white blood cells in the little red bumps. Rosacea clearly demonstrates the seamless connection between emotions and skin, for it always gets worse when women are under significant emotional stress. Psychological studies have linked rosacea with a disordered blushing reaction. Though blushing is a normal response to the emotions of excitement, shame, or embarrassment, in those with rosacea the body's normal response goes too far because the emotion is held too frequently or too long. Studies have shown, for instance, that people prone to this disorder are likely to be perfectionistic and have a strong need to please others. They also have a predisposition to excessive feelings of guilt and shame.[15] Given our culture, it's not surprising that more women than men have rosacea.

CHERYL: ROSACEA AND SHAME

Cheryl first came to see me when she was forty-two and having problems with irregular periods. She also had persistent reddening of the skin around her nose and cheeks, which her dermatologist had diagnosed as rosacea. Though she was on various topical antibiotics for the problem, they didn't help much. Her problem always seemed to be exacerbated premenstrually, but with such irregular periods, which sometimes came every two weeks, she never knew when her skin would look good and when it would flare up.

As I worked with Cheryl over the next year, we both noticed what a barometer her skin reddening was for emotional turmoil. And Cheryl had plenty. During the year that her rosacea first appeared, she was in the middle of an affair with a married professional – an affair that took place in his office. Over time she discovered that she wasn't the only woman with whom this man was sexually involved. When she discovered this, she felt deeply ashamed. Her childhood history revealed that she had been the victim of incest by her father, something she had also kept secret for years. But Cheryl had a great deal of courage. She began to go to groups for incest survivors and also started individual therapy. At the same time she committed herself to improving her diet and lifestyle on all levels. Over the next few years Cheryl became stronger and more independent. Eventually she even had the courage to forgive herself for becoming involved with an unscrupulous man in the first place. As Cheryl connected with her inner wisdom and supported herself physically through diet and exercise, her rosacea cleared up, slowly but surely. She now notices flare-ups only occasionally, and only when she reverts to old emotional patterns of shame and neediness, feelings that she now has the skills and self-esteem to work through effectively.

Treatment Options

Standard conventional treatment for rosacea includes intermittent antibiotics such as metronidazole (Flagyl) and topical steroids to reduce inflammation and white cell accumulation in the papules. Though these treatments are somewhat effective, they won't help the reddened skin. Topical steroids and antibiotics also have side effects, such as an increased risk of infection and thinner skin in the long run.

Conventional treatment to reduce the blushing reaction includes the use of anti-anxiety drugs such as Valium. Though these drugs can certainly reduce feelings of anxiety, they are highly addictive.

Dr Nicholas Perricone, the dermatology researcher mentioned earlier, has reported that alpha-lipoic acid preparations also work beautifully for rosacea. I now suggest alpha-lipoic-acid-containing preparations for all patients with rosacea. I've also seen rosacea disappear in women who follow the type of insulin-lowering diet I recommend in chapter 7.

Some women report that supplementing their diets with betaine hydrochloride, which increases stomach acidity, helps rosacea, for reasons that aren't entirely clear. If you decide to take this supplement, which is available in health food shops, make sure you take it with food. Otherwise it creates a sensation like heartburn. Usual dose is 500–1,000mg with meals.

Mind–Body Approach to Skin Problems

Did my description of the psychological profile of a rosacea patient or someone suffering from midlife acne strike home? If it did, then next time you feel yourself becoming overwhelmed by emotions of shame, anxiety, or anger, try the following:

1. Take a full, deep breath – all the way down into your belly. (We often stop breathing when we feel a strong emotion, as a way to stop feeling it.) Exhale and continue to breathe fully.

2. Close your eyes.

3. Identify where in your body you are feeling the emotion.

4. Describe what you are feeling. Does it have a shape or a colour or a sound?

5. Don't try to change your feeling. Allow yourself to feel it fully, exactly as it is.

6. Keep breathing and moving around while doing this – breathing and moving will help you move the emotion right through.

Here's what you're apt to notice: the minute you give your emotion a chance to be felt fully, it goes away. You can use this technique any time you feel any difficult emotion. And guess what? You'll find that you have the ability to deal with it without outside help.

Hair in the Wrong Places

Many women notice an increase in coarse or dark hair on their chins and upper lips starting at midlife. Although this can be quite distressing, it is perfectly natural and is the result of the higher androgen to oestrogen ratio that prevails beginning in perimenopause. Androgen can transform fine peach-fuzz-type hair (known as vellus hair) into coarser hair (known as terminal hair). Sometimes, however, excessive facial hair can be a sign of an underlying hormonal imbalance, such as in the condition known as polycystic ovary disease. Coarse facial hair is also common in women whose diets are too high in refined carbohydrates, which shifts the hormones in the direction of androgens. But usually the growth of facial hair at midlife is not a sign of hormonal or nutritional problems, but simply the normal result of proportionally higher levels of androgens.

The same androgenic hormones that are associated with thickening and darkening of hair on your upper lip and your chin may cause hair loss on other areas, like the head. Androgenic hormones affect the hair follicles of the scalp by shortening what is known as anagen (the growth phase of the hair growth cycle), which causes the hair to regress to a finer, thinner texture. But how androgen affects the hair depends in part on where the hair is located. The androgen receptors in the hair follicles of other areas of the body vary in terms of numbers and sensitivity. That's the reason why excessive androgen can thin out the hair on your head while increasing the amount and thickness of the hair on your face. Of course, not only are there differences in androgen sensitivity in different bodily sites within the individual, but there are differences between individuals. Thus a relatively low level of androgen may result in facial hair growth in some women and not in others. Amount of body and facial hair also varies among different racial groups. Dark-haired, darkly pigmented Caucasians of either sex tend to be hairier than blondes or fair-skinned individuals.

Hair Removal Techniques

As normal as it may be, excess facial (or body) hair may be something you wish to deal with cosmetically. In general, I don't recommend plucking, waxing, or shaving, because over time this can distort the hair follicle, making permanent hair removal more difficult if you decide on that later. But before opting for permanent removal, you may want to try the insulin-balancing diet suggested in chapter 7. As an interim cosmetic intervention, it's best to simply cut the hair as close to the skin as possible or bleach it. If you do decide on permanent hair removal, keep in mind that fine, non-androgenised hair (the peach-fuzz type of hair that is present everywhere on the body) may undergo androgenisation at any time during perimenopause or beyond. So even though you may have had your existing coarse hair removed, you may be producing new hair regularly, especially during times of stress, when androgenic hormone levels increase. Sometimes hair growth will also be encouraged by the hormones you're using or your diet and stress levels.

ELECTROLYSIS: Electrolysis is a procedure done by a trained professional that involves sending an electric current into the hair follicle via a carefully placed needle. It can take several treatments per hair follicle to truly destroy that hair follicle and prevent the hair from regrowing. Electrolysis is uncomfortable, so you may want your doctor to give you a prescription for a topical anaesthetic known as EMLA (lidocaine and prilocaine), which must be put on the skin an hour before the treatment. Over time – usually a few weeks to a few months – regular electrolysis sessions will result in far fewer dark hairs. But you'll probably have to continue to go for treatments every month or so, as new vellus hairs are transformed into terminal hairs. Make sure that your electrolysis professional is well trained and qualified.

LASER HAIR REMOVAL: Laser technology for hair removal is improving all the time and can be very effective. Like electrolysis, it is painful, so a topical anaesthetic (EMLA) is used before the procedure. Make sure you go to a doctor who is well trained in laser technology, because it is a rapidly evolving field.

PRESCRIPTION MEDICATIONS: The medications mentioned on page 359 for the treatment of hair loss on the head may also, ironically, be effective for treating hair growth on the face, since both may be a result of the hormonal shifts that occur at menopause.

Alopecia Androgenica:
Midlife Hair Loss from Hormonal Imbalance

Though some women begin to experience some hair loss at menopause secondary to hormonal shifts in the body, most do not. Saying that significant hair loss is secondary to menopause would be like saying that dementia is a normal part of ageing. Nevertheless, hair loss at perimenopause is a relatively common problem that erodes self-confidence and self-esteem and makes it difficult to enjoy yourself fully in a social situation.

Alopecia androgenica, which results in what we call male pattern baldness, is by far the most common cause of hair thinning and loss in women at midlife. Typically, the hair becomes finer and thinner and may eventually recede, though in women usually the front hairline is preserved. Up to 13 per cent of premenopausal women and 37 per cent of postmenopausal women suffer from hormone-associated hair loss to some degree.

I recently received the following illustrative letter from Evelyn, one of my newsletter subscribers.

I am writing in an attempt to get some clarification on natural hormone replacement. I had a complete hysterectomy last July at the age of forty-four – fibroids. My doctor started me out on Premarin, and I had no problems that I was aware of. However, I had read many books on natural hormone replacements and decided to go with Dr Hargrove's regimen [see page 343], which my doctor prescribed for me. I have been using four drops of the hormone lotion to control hot flushes. I noticed after a while that my skin became oily and I am having problems with acne. Also, and what concerns me the most, is that my hair is thinning quite rapidly.

I have had a blood test for hormones and thyroid – everything was within normal limits. The saliva test showed that my hormone levels were higher than in a young, healthy female. I am trying to lower my dose to see if it will have an effect on my hair. I understand that too much oestrogen can cause hair loss. My doctor encourages me to go back on the pharmaceutical alternatives, which he tells me he has used successfully for more than twenty years. At this time I am very confused and would do almost anything to stop my hair from falling out. Please, give me some advice on how to pursue this problem.

Clearly Evelyn is converting oestrogen to androgen, and the androgens are having an effect at the level of her hair follicles. That's why her skin is getting oily, she's getting acne, and her hair is thinning.

Although the hormone regimen she is on works well for many women, transdermal hormones go right into the bloodstream and as such can give higher levels with lower doses than when the hormone is given orally. I suggested that Evelyn either switch to an oral oestrogen–progesterone preparation or cut right down on her topical oestrogen and progesterone. For reasons that aren't entirely clear, some women simply do better with oral hormones. I also suggested to Evelyn that she make sure she is following an insulin-lowering diet so that excess insulin from refined carbohydrates isn't pushing her body towards higher androgen production. She could also use a high-dose soya supplement to help her hot flushes and to keep her bones healthy. This infusion of phytohormones might allow her to cut her dose of oestrogen, so there would be less of it around for her body to convert into androgen.

If you have hair follicles that are particularly sensitive to androgen, like Evelyn, any hormone replacement regimen that has too much androgen for your body can result in hair loss. The problem goes away once you stop the drug. Most hormonally associated hair loss is not caused by hormone replacement regimens, however; it is the result of an imbalance in your own body's hormonal production.

Androgen-associated hair loss can be likened to the canary in the mine. It is a symptom that often signals a much more pervasive hormone imbalance that affects many women to one degree or another. Though, as I mentioned, up to 37 per cent of menopausal women will have some hair thinning from increased androgen production at menopause, about 10 to 15 per cent of women have full-blown androgen-excess syndrome, characterised by facial acne, male pattern hair loss, upper-body obesity (apple-shaped figure), insulin resistance, increased facial hair, and adverse changes in lipid profile.

This syndrome, which overlaps with syndrome X, outlined in chapter 7, is associated with polycystic ovary syndrome, adrenal hypersecretion, genetic factors, excessive body fat, or unknown causes. Because all of these factors set the scene for early onset cardiovascular disease and diabetes, your hormone-associated hair loss needs to be seen as only one aspect of a much larger systemic imbalance that you can do a great deal to help alleviate.

How to Get Your Hair Back – and Improve Your Health at the Same Time

First get your doctor to test you to see if there is a systemic cause for your hair loss. Diagnosing the type of hair loss you have will help clarify which options are most likely to work.

Make sure your hormone levels are normal. Even though the vast majority of women with hair loss will be found to have normal androgen levels, it's important to rule out the occasional rare abnormality, and also to remember that it's usually not your body's absolute level of androgen that's the problem, but your hair follicles' heightened sensitivity to androgen. Ask your doctor to check your thyroid and hormone levels. Arrange yourself to get salivary tests for DHEA, free testosterone, and androstenedione levels. If you do fit the description of someone with full-blown androgen-excess syndrome, have your lipid profile, blood pressure, and blood sugar checked as well, which your doctor may agree to do.

Even if your hormone levels come out as normal, do the following:

- Follow the hormone-balancing diet outlined in chapter 7.

- Lose any excess body fat. If your body fat percentage is above 30 per cent, as measured in your doctor's surgery or fitness centre, the excess fat is a factory for androgen and could drive your insulin levels, blood pressure, and blood lipids into unhealthy ranges. Excess body fat caused by a sedentary lifestyle and a diet too high in refined carbohydrates and trans fats is probably the key issue in combating not only androgen-associated hair loss, but also the health problems often associated with it.

- Take a good vitamin and mineral supplement (see chapter 7) to help your new hair grow in fully.

- Try Chinese herbs. Shou Wu Pian is a Chinese herbal medicine that often works very well to help restore hair growth. My acupuncturist has used it for years, and I have seen wonderful results, including a reduction in grey hair. (See Resources.)

TREATING THE SURFACE – MINOXIDIL (REGAINE) LIQUID: Minoxidil is currently the only drug approved by the MCA for its beneficial effect on hair growth, but it is only available on private prescription, not on the NHS. Minoxidil is a potent anti-hypertensive medication that when taken by mouth lowers blood pressure by dilating blood vessels. It was discovered by accident that it increases hair growth. Though it is not clear how it enhances hair growth when applied topically, it may increase the size of the hair follicle, prolong the growth phase of a hair follicle, increase blood flow to the skin, or enhance DNA synthesis. Side effects are rare but may include skin irritation and a short-lived increase in heart rate. In one study, a 2 per cent solution of minoxidil increased the total weight of hair by over 40 per cent over a forty-week period of use.[16] When researchers combined a 2 per cent solution of minoxidil with 0.025 per cent tretinoin (Retin-A) and used it four times per day as a scalp spray, 90 per cent of the women in the study showed visible and cosmetically significant improvement in hair quality after six months.[17]

PRESCRIPTION MEDICATIONS FOR HORMONAL HAIR LOSS: The drugs doctors prescribe to rebalance systemic hormonal imbalances work well for some, though not all, women with hormone-associated hair loss. However, too often they help the symptoms without really addressing the underlying cause – too much body fat, unhealthy diet, sedentary lifestyle, and so on – or helping you learn how to heal yourself by using the body's own internal wisdom. If you use any of the following medications, complement them with appropriate diet and lifestyle changes.

• *Birth control pills* with ethinyl oestradiol, 30–35mcg, for twenty days of the cycle. Birth control pills sometimes work to stop androgenic hair loss for the same reason they help acne – they reduce the body's susceptibility to the effects of androgen on the hair follicle and its attached sebaceous gland.

• *Dexamethasone,* 0.125–0.375mg at bedtime. Dexamethasone is a powerful steroid that suppresses the production of androgens, thereby increasing the amount of hair on the head. It also treats the acne that accompanies male pattern hair loss in many women. Unfortunately, it has all the potential side effects of too much cortisol, such as an increase in insulin, thinning of the skin and bones, and an increased susceptibility to infection.

• *Spironolactone* is an anti-androgen which, taken orally, decreases total and free testosterone. It is available in some countries, but is not licensed to be used in this way in the UK.

In some women, an individualised hormone replacement prescription, such as the ones described in chapter 5 and above for skin, can help balance hormone levels and help alleviate androgen excess.

Making the Most of the Hair You've Got

While you're working from the inside out – or the outside in – you'll still want to look your best. Make the most of what you've got . . . and enhance it.

Consult a professional who specialises in hairpieces, hair extensions, weaves, and body perms. You might even want to enquire about hair transplantation for women by a dermatologist or plastic surgeon.[18]

Here are some more tips for making thin hair appear its best:

• Use gentle shampoos, and don't shampoo more than every other day.

• Don't brush your hair when it's wet – this stretches out the hair.

• Avoid teasing – it can break your hair.

• Chlorine damages hair. Shower with pure water. If your water is chlorinated, use a shower filter that removes it.

• Ask your hairdresser to recommend professional products for fine hair that will give you extra volume.

When Good Skin Care Isn't Enough: Deciding on Cosmetic Procedures

Sometimes the results you're looking for will be unattainable with diet and good skin care alone. If you have a 'fixable' aspect of your face that bothers you every time you look in the mirror, it may be time to consider getting outside help. Whether you want to enhance your smile with cosmetic dentistry or get rid of the bags under your eyes that always make you look tired even when you're not, there's no doubt that fixing an energy-draining aspect of your appearance can improve the quality of life. That's why so many women get teeth braces at midlife, or have skin peels to give them a fresher look that simply can't be achieved any other way. Cosmetic surgery of all kinds is growing by leaps and bounds because of vast improvements in technology and increasing demand.

It seems to me that it is almost impossible to go through the normal process of facial ageing in this culture and not wish that something could be done about certain parts of your face, especially the eyelids and jawline. If you're one of the lucky ones who really aren't at all bothered by sagging eyelids or jowls, bless you. If, however, you want an appearance-enhancing face lift, eyelid surgery, skin peel, liposuction, laser surgery, or other cosmetic polishing of your exterior, then bless you, too. Through the years I've referred many patients for various plastic surgery or dermatological procedures. Nearly all of them have been thrilled with the results.

In addition to giving referrals for plastic surgery, while I was still at Women to Women I even took a course in how to do deep facial skin peels. We did the procedure at the surgery and then cared for the women at a private home for four days thereafter. I always thought of this service as a kind of 'cocoon' experience in which the newly peeled and vulnerable women were kept safe, warm, and healthy while they shed their old skins and prepared to face the world with a renewed countenance. I must admit that the results were spectacular for the women (and one man) who went through with the procedure. I was always thrilled on the last day to witness the 'unveiling' as we helped our patients remove their masks of powder and apply make-up to cover their renewed but very red skin. This was especially true for those whose difficult and painful past histories had lined their faces with expressions of anger and depression they had since worked through. Virtually all of the women I treated had done lots of inner work. Now they simply wanted their outsides to match their insides.

One of my patients had her eyes done at the age of forty-one, about one year after a mastectomy. With the bags under her eyes surgically corrected, she looked brighter and fresher than she had in years. And her new look helped her outlook and possibly her immune system as well.

If you decide to consult a plastic surgeon or if you already have an appointment booked, I'd recommend the following:

• Be sure that you're having a cosmetic procedure because it makes you feel better. Don't do it for your husband, boyfriend, or mother. Over the years I've seen that the results of surgeries are always much better when our motivation for having them is clear.

• Choose the right doctor. When it comes to cosmetic surgery, especially laser techniques, there is a great deal of crossover between the profession of dermatology and plastic surgery. For example, laser skin peels that include the eyelid area (which may be done in a doctor's consulting rooms) give a result that is often as good as a face lift obtained with a surgeon's knife. Look for a consultant plastic surgeon or, in the case of laser procedures, a dermatologist or other practitioner with extensive training in laser technology.

• Don't choose a private doctor or clinic just because they offer the lowest prices. All surgical and laser procedures carry a certain amount of risk. This risk increases if doctors or clinics cut corners on care and safety to keep prices low.

• Make sure you go to someone with whom you feel completely comfortable. (This same criterion goes for body workers or anyone else who will be working with your body in any way – including a dentist.) Ask yourself: 'Does this person have the kind of clinical, objective, and healing touch that will allow me to feel comfortable even if I have to stand in my underwear and have him or her look at my body and take pictures as part of my care?' A good doctor will put you at ease even in this kind of situation. If there's any feeling of discomfort, go elsewhere. That's what happened with a friend of mine who went to see a plastic surgeon in order to have both her nose and her deviated septum fixed. (She had had a broken nose since childhood.) The surgeon kept staring at her breasts, which are relatively small, while she kept trying to get his attention back on her nose. She had no desire to have breast implants. Though this man had all the right credentials, had trained at all the best places, and is perfectly competent technically, he also had what I've come to call the sleaze factor. His attitude made her uncomfortable. So she chose someone else to do her surgery. Her feeling of unease was confirmed when she later heard via the grapevine that he had told his wife, also a doctor, about some of the surgeries he had done and upon whom. This information had made its way around the community. Such a breach of confidentiality is completely unacceptable, but it happens. You can avoid this kind of situation by trusting your gut reaction as well as a surgeon's credentials.

• Keep your surgery decision to yourself as much as possible. You'd be amazed at the number of judgements your friends may make concerning cosmetic surgery, depending upon where you live. Some of your friends won't think you're very spiritually evolved, for instance, if you want to remove the bags under your eyes. Frankly, how you look is none of their business.

• If at all possible, go away to have your procedure done. Too many of my patients have had the experience of being at home with a bruised face after plastic surgery, looking like battered women, and then having to answer the door for the plumber, the postal worker, and everyone else who comes along.

• Give yourself enough time. Recovery from eyelid or facial surgery usually takes a minimum of two weeks before you look presentable. So use this time for reading or taking a much-deserved retreat from your usual routine. It will speed your healing process and help the inside of you as much as the outside.

• Make arrangements to be waited on for at least the first three days post-op. Though you may feel fine, you're apt to be more tired than usual and perhaps a bit weepy and emotional during this vulnerable time. Give yourself the space you deserve.

• Stock up on the Chinese patent herb Yannan Pei Yan and begin taking it, one tablet four times a day, as soon as you possibly can after surgery. This herb speeds healing and cuts right down on post-operative bruising. I also recommend taking at least 2,000mg of vitamin C for two weeks pre-op and four weeks post-op to help build up collagen in your skin. You can also use skin cream containing vitamin C ester to speed up healing.

• Use guided-imagery tapes before and during surgery, and ask your surgeon and anaesthetist to work with you. (See Resources.)

• Be realistic. Cosmetic surgery won't change your life, despite what our culture would lead you to believe. If you are beautiful on the outside but ugly, depressed, or unhappy on the inside, your appeal will begin to fade within thirty seconds of walking into a room. I'm sure you've all had the experience of meeting people who become more and more attractive right in front of your eyes as you begin to know and appreciate the humour, joy, or fun they bring to every situation.

Varicose Veins

The chances are you don't like the look of prominent blue varicose veins and want to do whatever you can to prevent them or, if you already have a few, minimise them. Appearance isn't the only problem with varicose veins, however. If they get bad enough, they are often associated with a painful, heavy feeling in the legs, especially at the end of the day. Happily, there are a number of strategies to help you prevent varicose veins in the first place, or keep them from getting worse if you already have a few.

Let's start by going over what varicose veins are and why they develop. The term *varicose* refers to a vein that is dilated, tortuous, and located just beneath the skin. Quite often the valves of these veins, which are designed to keep the blood from flowing backwards, no longer work as they should. When a surface vein stretches and loses its elasticity, and the valves don't shut properly, blood flows backwards, pooling in the affected vein, which then enlarges into a mass of blue tissue beneath the skin. Varicose veins can be large, having the appearance of blue worms, or they can be very small and purplish blue in colour. These small 'spider' veins often occur in a fanlike pattern in the thigh area. Varicose veins, whether large or small, are the end result of poor circulation.

Diet and Varicose Veins

It is very clear that the fundamental cause of varicose veins is a diet high in refined carbohydrates and low in fibre – the same kind that is also associated with heart disease, breast cancer, and bad skin. Such a diet often results in subtle nutritional deficiencies, excess weight, and constipation, all of which increase intra-abdominal pressure, which over the years puts too much pressure on the veins in our legs.[19] Chronic coughing does the same thing – and so does excess fat in the abdomen.

Varicose veins are virtually non-existent in rural Africa, where the diet tends to be high in fibre-rich whole foods and very low in refined foods. But thanks to our own very different diet, almost all of us in the West are at an increased risk for developing at least a few dilated veins in our legs. Varicose veins can also be aggravated by the hormonal changes that women experience during three specific times in our lives: at the onset of our menstrual periods, during pregnancy, and at the beginning of menopause. These are the times when we are most susceptible to subtle changes in our blood flow that put us at increased risk for damage to our vein walls. Because of these hormonal changes, varicose veins can show up as early as the age of twenty. In men, by contrast, varicose veins develop evenly throughout the lifespan up until the age of seventy and don't appear to be hormonally related.

Programme for Preventing or Treating Varicose Veins

Now that you know what you're dealing with, let's get down to the business of keeping your veins in top shape.

• *Give your legs the support they deserve.* If you already have varicose veins or if you have a family history of varicose veins, make sure that you wear compression or support stockings of some kind whenever you know you will be on your feet for a long time. And elevate your legs as much as possible. I have a family history of varicose veins, so when I was a trainee doctor, I always wore compression stockings when I was on call at night. Putting those stockings on always gave me a new lease of life. Though I was only in my twenties at the time, I found that when I didn't wear them, my legs ached and my ankles got swollen after being on my feet all night. These are available at your chemist and may be prescribed by your doctor. Avoid standard knee-highs and thigh-high stockings if you have varicose veins, because the elastic at the tops of these impedes venous blood flow and increases the pooling of blood in the veins that is the cause of the problem in the first place.

• *If you take oestrogen, make sure you're taking the right dose.* Low-dose oestrogen replacement therapy does not appear to cause varicose veins in women, but occasionally a woman will notice that her legs ache and seem to swell more when she is on oestrogen replacement, and existing varicose veins may seem to get worse. If you've noticed that your veins seem to be worse on oestrogen replacement, consider lowering your dose.

• *Avoid constipation by following a diet that has adequate fibre, plenty of water, and very few refined carbohydrates.*

• *Use your muscles to keep your blood moving.* Rhythmic exercise such as walking, biking, running, or swimming keeps your blood moving and uses the mechanical action of your muscles to get the blood out of your veins and back to your heart. I've seen many women cure their symptomatic varicose veins and improve the cosmetic appearance of their legs by starting and staying with a regular exercise programme.

• *Nourish and protect your vein linings.* The herb bilberry *(Vaccinium myrtillus)* contains flavonoid compounds known as anthocyanosides, which are potent antioxidants that improve microcirculation and protect vein linings. These same substances also increase blood levels of a hormone known as prostacyclin (an eicosanoid) that prevents platelet aggregation, so blood flows more smoothly through the vessels. This herb has been successfully used to help prevent and treat varicose veins in pregnancy.[20] The usual dose is 160mg per day for general prevention of varicose veins, and up to 480mg per day to treat varicose veins that already exist. The flavonoid compounds in berries, particularly blueberries, blackberries, and raspberries, are also very helpful for keeping veins healthy.

• *Keep your vein walls slippery.* Research has shown that individuals with varicose veins have a decreased ability to break down fibrin in their vein walls. Fibrin is a protein in blood that is involved in clotting. When it isn't metabolised properly by an enzyme known as plasminogen activator, it coats the inside of the vein, causing it and the surrounding skin to become hard and lumpy. Normally veins have enough plasminogen activator already in their walls to keep fibrin from building up. But when they become varicose, the levels of plasminogen activator decrease.[21] So you have to import your own.

A substance known as bromelain, found in pineapple, has been shown to act in a manner similar to plasminogen activator to cause fibrin breakdown.[22] In supplement form, it can be used to improve varicose veins that already exist or, in smaller amounts, to prevent them.

The usual dose of bromelain is 125–450mg three times per day on an empty stomach. Use the smallest amount as general prevention, and the larger amount to treat veins that are already present. Bromelain is readily available at health food shops. You can also get bromelain by eating pineapple.

• *Make sure you're getting adequate amounts of vitamin E.* Since vitamin E deficiency has been associated with the exacerbation of varicose veins, you'll need to get enough of this vitamin every day. An adequate dosage is 100–400IU per day, the amount I've already recommended for your daily multivitamin/mineral combination.

When to Consider Treatment – Either Surgery or Sclerotherapy

If your varicose veins are causing you pain of any kind that doesn't respond to the measures I've outlined (and that includes feeling too embarrassed to wear shorts or a bathing suit), I'd recommend that you look into sclerotherapy or vein-stripping surgery. Sclerotherapy is an outpatient procedure that involves injecting your unsightly veins with a solution that irritates the inside of the vein wall, causing it to seal shut. Sclerotherapy has been safely used in Europe for the last fifty years. The surgeon may also do an initial evaluation of your veins using Doppler ultrasound to determine whether or not you need surgical vein stripping in addition to the sclerotherapy.

The vast majority of cases can be treated by injection alone.[23] But large varicose veins with poor valves that run from your groin all the way down to your knee or below may not be treatable with injection alone. Vein stripping is a process in which the dilated, tortuous veins just at the surface of the legs (the saphenous veins) are tied off (ligated) and surgically removed. Most vascular and general surgeons are experts in this procedure. Vein stripping is done under general anaesthesia and will require a hospital stay.

Should you decide to go through with sclerotherapy via injection or laser, I recommend that you follow all my suggestions for maintaining healthy veins before and after your treatment. Doing so will lower your chances of having any recurrent problems.

Despite our best efforts to appear youthful, life is full of challenges that sooner or later etch themselves on our faces and bodies. Happily, at midlife most of us are far better equipped to handle this than we were when we were twenty and still believed that our lives would be perfect if we could just lose that final 5–10lb or if our noses looked different. The crucible of perimenopause removes some of our self-consciousness. We've had enough life experience to be happy that our legs still work, even if they don't look perfect, happy that there are amusing things to laugh at, even if doing so creates crinkles around our eyes. What a relief!

TWELVE

Standing Tall for Life: Building Healthy Bones

*L*ast summer I had the privilege of seeing rock-and-roll legend Tina Turner live in concert. At an age (sixty plus) when the majority of women have resigned themselves to slowing down and taking it easy, Tina tore up the stage in her towering heels (an athletic feat in itself), belting out her signature high-energy music for two solid hours while outshining dancers less than half her age. Her awe-inspiring performance laid to rest any notion about the inherent limitations in physical stamina that are supposed to come with growing older. I was thrilled that my teenage daughters were with me, so that they, too, could internalise this icon of female power and health. Watching Tina Turner that night, I was reminded anew that we perimenopausal women can hone our physical strength and skills for years to come if we are willing to continue to move, to work our muscles regularly – and, of course, to unload any Ikes who are holding us back.

Tina Turner – and thousands of other older women who stand tall in their lives – offer a clear alternative to the realities of osteoporosis. You don't have to look very far to see women who are bent over or otherwise crippled by this devastating disease. Osteoporosis begins in earnest at perimenopause, but its effects may not appear until twenty or more years later, often when it is too late to do much about it. When it comes to bone health, prevention is absolutely essential. And that prevention must begin in perimenopause.

Osteoporosis: The Scope of the Problem

Bone loss starts silently, asymptomatically. In the early stages it is called osteopenia. As it progresses to osteoporosis, the bones become increasingly porous, brittle, and subject to fracture. Make no mistake: this is a potentially fatal disease. It is estimated that by the year 2020 anywhere between 18 and 33 per cent of all Western women over the age of sixty-five will suffer from a hip fracture by the time they reach the age of ninety. Of those who sustain hip fractures, 12–20 per cent will die of related complications. (The lifetime risk of death from a hip fracture for a fifty-year-old woman is equal to the lifetime risk of death due to breast cancer.) Of those who don't die from complications, 50 per cent will never regain their ability to walk and therefore will not be able to return to independent living.

Osteoporosis also increases the risk for wrist and vertebral crush fractures, which can result in pain, disability, and disfigurement. It is the vertebral crush fractures, in which the bone in the spine collapses, that result in the shrunken, hunched-over posture – complete with dowager's hump and pot belly – that is so common in older women. If your mother or grandmother looks like this, you may be seeing your future – unless you act now.

A study showed by the age of eighty-five a large number of Caucasian women in the US will have at least one partial deformity in their spine.[1] The risk for African-American women is less, while the risk for Asian-American women falls somewhere in between. This difference is related, in part, to the fact that women with more pigment in their skin also have a thicker collagen matrix upon which their bones are built. The same applies to British women of different ethnic origins. Men also have thicker, stronger bones than women, partly for genetic reasons and partly because of their higher levels of bone-building testosterone. Though men, too, may get osteoporosis, it's often related to alcohol intake or steroid use and shows up at a later age than in women. Osteoporosis currently costs the health service millions of pounds per year, with hip fractures representing 80 per cent of the total expense.

Given these discouraging statistics, it is little wonder that so many doctors are quick to prescribe either oestrogen or one of the new bone-building drugs such as raloxifene (Evista) or alendronate (Fosamax). Please remember, however, that statistics are derived from

FIGURE 16: FEMALE VERTEBRAE

(Bone cross-sections)

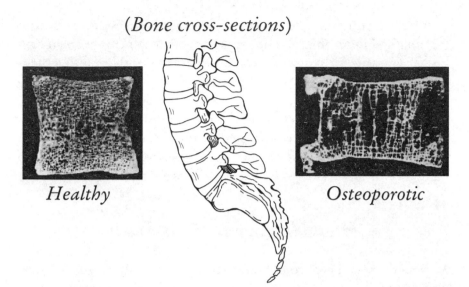

Healthy   Osteoporotic

entire populations and may not have anything to do with you personally. In my practice I have seen eighty-year-old women with the bone
density measurements of an average twenty-five-year-old. I have also
seen twenty-five-year-olds with the bones of an average eighty-year-
old. And today there are many safe and natural options available to
help you either maintain the bone you have or build it to new,
healthier levels.

We're Designed for Lifetime Sturdiness

There is nothing inherent in the human condition in general, or the
postmenopausal woman in particular, that causes our bones to
weaken and break as we age. We were designed to live on this planet
well supported by sturdy bones from youth to old age. Like other
degenerative diseases so common in Western civilisation, such as
coronary artery disease, hypertension, and obesity, osteoporosis is
either unknown or very rare among indigenous peoples living time-
honoured lifestyles characterised by a strong connection with the
wisdom of the earth. A deep sense of connection to the earth shores
up the health of our first emotional centre – the part of our emotional
anatomy that is associated with a sense of belonging, and with our

basic sense of safety and security in the world. This sense of safety affects our bones, blood, and immune systems.

When an entire culture teaches us to regard our bodies as uncontrollable and unreliable, it is not surprising that so many women have lost their sense of connection and support – with resulting first-emotional-centre disease such as osteoporosis. It is also not surprising that so many are beginning to lose bone at earlier and earlier ages, a side effect of becoming overly thin – an endeavour fuelled by our drive to be accepted by a culture maniacally focused on appearance.

The gravity of the earth itself (weight-bearing exercise) and sunlight are two of the keys to bone health, as we will see in this chapter.

How Healthy Bone Is Made

If you want to keep your bones strong and healthy, you need to understand the dynamic and effortless way in which your body is designed to build and remodel bone throughout your life. The process that results in osteoporosis is actually a survival mechanism created over millions of years of evolution to help your body maintain biochemical balance. Once you begin to work with that essential body wisdom, even bones that have already weakened can regain strength.

Bone metabolism is a complex process in which construction and demolition crews work side by side. Each of our 206 bones harbours cells that continually deposit a protein framework made from collagen. Minerals from the blood then attach to this matrix and harden into bone. Those same bones also contain cells that can break down that structure. In childhood, as we grow, the bone builders keep ahead of the bone destroyers. But the balance can shift as we get older. A wide variety of conditions – including depression, deficiencies of vitamin D and bone-building minerals, and steroid use – can allow the osteoblasts, the cells that make bone, to be outpaced by the osteoclasts, the cells that break down bone. The result is weakened bones.

Bones Are Storehouses for Essential Minerals

Bones are the major storehouse for calcium, phosphorus, and magnesium as well as other minerals, all of which are necessary for the healthy functioning of every cell in the body. Calcium, for example, regulates processes ranging from the beating of the heart and the clotting of blood to the firing of nerve cells. When blood calcium levels become low, a series of complex and interrelated biological reactions is activated:

- The parathyroid gland (in the neck) releases parathyroid hormone (PTH).

- PTH stimulates the kidneys to convert the body's stores of vitamin D into an active form and release calcium from the surface of the bone. It also slows down the mineralisation of bone, which uses calcium.

- Activated vitamin D acts on the intestine to increase the absorption of calcium from food, encourages the kidneys to retain calcium that would otherwise be lost in the urine, and facilitates the release of more calcium from the bone.

As soon as calcium levels in the blood are restored to an acceptable level, all of these feedback mechanisms are reversed. Similarly complex feedback loops are involved in the metabolism of the other essential minerals.[2]

It is the job of the osteoclasts to break down microscopic bits of bone, thus releasing minerals into the blood. Each day over 300mg of calcium is dissolved from our bones. Over a year's time 20 per cent of our adult bone mass is recycled and replaced as our bones continually undergo breakdown and renewal in response to the overall needs of our bodies. If more minerals are taken out than are replaced, the end result is low bone mass.

Bones Constantly Remodel Themselves to Adapt to Physical Stress and Strain

Among the amazing properties of the basic bone cell, the osteocyte, is its ability to act like a strain sensor, evaluating the amount of stress placed on a bone. Though the exact mechanism by which this happens isn't entirely understood, stress on a bone sets up a tiny electrical current that attracts calcium and other minerals to the site. This is known as a piezoelectric effect and is similar to the mechanism by which quartz crystals operate in electronics and clocks.

What is fascinating about this process is that it takes into account precisely where bone is needed and where it needs to be reduced. The old song about how 'the hip bone's connected to the thigh bone' is about more than mere anatomical proximity. All of our bones, like every other cell in our bodies, are functionally connected to each other. A strain on a bone in our leg not only helps build that bone, but also helps determine the bone density in our spine and shoulders.[3] Regular stress on bones is absolutely essential to maintain strong bone. It's a case of use it or lose it. It's well documented, for example, that the weightlessness experienced by astronauts results in significant bone loss, as does prolonged bed rest.

One more piece of the puzzle falls into place when you know that osteoblasts and osteoclasts, the builders and the destroyers, communicate via proteins known as osteoprotegerine (OPG) and OPG-ligand. As one researcher explains it, 'OPG-ligand is like the accelerator of your car. If you step on OPG-ligand, you lose bone. OPG is the brake of the system. If you step on OPG, then you have more bone. The balance between the two determines how much bone we have.'[4] Scientists are now finding that almost all of the substances that stimulate bone loss do so by slashing production of OPG, boosting creation of OPG-ligand, or both. For example, the drug prednisone can set off quick and dramatic bone loss. In the lab, treating osteoblasts (bone builders) with prednisone inhibits their ability to make OPG but heightens their OPG-ligand production. In contrast, oestrogen stimulates osteoblasts to produce OPG.

Immune status and bone health are also closely connected – which is not surprising, given that both are under the influence of the first chakra. Osteoclasts (the bone destroyers) are derived from the same bone marrow cells that make white blood cells. This helps explain why individuals with such seemingly unrelated diseases as rheumatoid arthritis, lupus, diabetes, multiple sclerosis, hepatitis, depression, and lymphoma have osteoporosis in addition to their other symptoms. Scientists have found that anything that stirs quiescent T cells, a ubiquitous part of our immune systems, into action also triggers them to make OPG-ligand. And any time you turn on T cells (as in chronic infections and autoimmune disorders), you get bone loss.

The function of both osteoclasts and osteoblasts is influenced by many other factors as well, including levels of oestrogen, testosterone, thyroid hormone, and insulin, nutritional status, and hormones (such as noradrenaline and cortisol) produced by emotional stress.[5] There is also some evidence to suggest that OPG-ligand may stimulate osteoclasts or other substances, such as the 'bad' eicosanoids, to degrade cartilage. This translates over time into joint destruction and arthritis.

FIGURE 17: BONE REMODELLING

Bone Building
OSTEOBLAST
(*increases bone density*)

Stimulated by:
- Progesterone
- Oestrogen
- Testosterone
- Isoflavones
- SERMs
- Vitamin D
- Exercise

Bone Demineralising
OSTEOCLAST
(*decreases bone density*)

Stimulated by:
- Immune System Disorders
- Depression
- Inactivity
- Nutrient-Poor Diet
- Steroid Drugs
- Depleted Hormones

© 2001 by Northrup and Schulz

Clinical trials are now under way using a type of synthetic long-acting OPG to turn off osteoclasts and thus halt bone loss.

The Ups and Downs of Bone over the Life Cycle

We begin developing our skeleton in utero, and it rapidly increases in size throughout childhood, adolescence, and young adulthood. It reaches its maximum size and density (known as peak bone mass) somewhere between the ages of twenty-five and thirty. Over her lifetime a woman may lose 38 per cent of her peak bone mass, while a man may lose only 23 per cent of his.[6] But some individuals are resistant to bone loss.[7] One study, for example, showed that 38 per cent of men and 2 per cent of women aged fifty-five and sixty-four lost almost no bone over a period of eleven years.[8] Nevertheless, many women begin to lose bone in their late thirties, long before oestrogen levels begin to fall. This loss tends to accelerate perimenopausally. The average Caucasian woman loses 2–4 per cent of her bone mass per year in the first five years after menopause. After that, loss slows down markedly or disappears.[9] In men, accelerated bone loss is more apt to begin in the late sixties.

What is intriguing is that low bone density alone does not necessarily result in fractures. Thousands of people walk around daily with very low bone density – yet only a small percentage of them experience fractures. It has been shown, for example, that in Japan hip bone density is markedly lower than it is in the US, and yet the incidence of hip fractures is two and a half times less than it is in the US. And the Japanese consume less calcium than we do in the West.[10]

What is the difference between bones that fracture and those that don't? The difference concerns two factors: basic bone architecture and the repair capability of bone. It appears that even those with osteoporosis still have enough bone mass to withstand the stresses and strains of daily life. Research has shown, for example, that a vertebra that has lost 50 per cent of its bone mass is still strong enough to withstand five times the strain load that it would normally be subjected to. If the bone were otherwise normal, in other words, it shouldn't fracture. This means that many women who are diagnosed with low bone density will never go on to get fractures.

Still, we all know that bone fractures do occur in women with osteoporosis, even at very low strain levels – in fact, it has been documented that some women spontaneously fracture their hips and then fall as a result, not the other way around. So osteoporotic fractures must involve more than decreased bone mineral density. There must be something else wrong with the quality of the bone and its self-repair process.[11] Poor bone quality results from factors such as nutritional deficiencies, lack of exercise, and too much insulin.[12]

The Anatomy of Bone

Bone comes in two types: trabecular and cortical bone. Cortical bone is the tough, protective outer layer of bone. It is more calcified than inner trabecular bone, which is spongy and includes the marrow, where blood cells are made. About 80 per cent of all bone in our bodies is cortical and 20 per cent is trabecular. The arms and legs are mostly cortical bone; hips are a mixture of half and half; while the spine, ribs, jaw, and lower two-thirds of the wrist are mainly trabecular bone. Because trabecular bone is more loosely packed and porous and has more surface area than cortical bone, it is more susceptible to bone loss, which is one reason why fractures from osteoporosis tend to occur earlier in the spine and wrist, while hip fractures occur later.

Bones have to be strong enough to withstand hundreds of pounds of pressure, but flexible enough to withstand twisting and turning without breaking. This flexibility is provided by the living protein collagen, which makes up about 23 per cent of all bone. (This is the same substance that gives skin its elasticity and thickness. Thin skin is also associated with thin bones.) The minerals attached to the collagen matrix are arranged in a crystalline structure that gives bone its rigidity and strength.

We were designed to maintain strong, heavy bones throughout our lives, as are all animals. If we have reached peak bone mass in our twenties, then we can stand a certain amount of bone loss as we age without being at risk of fractures. But because of the vagaries of our modern lifestyle, including lack of exercise or over-exercise, smoking, poor diet, or anorexia and bulimia, many women never reach their peak bone mass by the age of thirty. And it appears that the matrix of the bone that *is* present may not be normal. So many women begin perimenopause with a deficit in their bone banks.

Medical anthropologist Dr Susan Brown, director of the US Osteoporosis Education Project and author of the ground-breaking book *Better Bones, Better Body: Beyond Estrogen and Calcium,* points out that the bones of people who are living in Westernised countries are growing ever weaker, and that we now face a virtual epidemic of poor bone health.[13] Research shows that women living several centuries ago had stronger bones than modern women and that Near Eastern populations of some twelve thousand years ago had a bone mass that was nearly 20 per cent higher than it is today.[14]

Are You at Risk of Osteoporosis?

To determine your personal risk of thinning, poor-quality bones, review the following list. If none of the risk factors applies to you, chances are good that your bones are just fine. You can simply continue the healthy lifestyle you are following. If, on the other hand, you can identify with several of them, you need to take steps right now to ensure that you'll be able to take steps literally in the future! Note that some of the risk factors for osteoporosis overlap those for heart disease.[15] As you improve your bone health, you'll also be helping your heart.

• Your mother has been diagnosed with osteoporosis or has had a hip or other osteoporotic fracture. Osteoporosis tends to run in families, but there's still a lot you can do to prevent it.

• You are fair-skinned and blue-eyed. Because of genetic factors, blue-eyed blondes and those with red hair have less collagen in both their bones and skin than do those with brown, black, or yellow skin tones. This gives them less bony matrix on which to lay down minerals. Black women have the least risk of osteoporosis because they tend to have thicker bones and more robust collagen stores than Caucasian women.

• You are quite thin or tall, or have a slight build and/or less than 18 per cent body fat. Tall women, especially those with small bones, may be at risk for purely mathematical reasons: they enter menopause with less bone to lose. In addition, body fat is where much of a woman's natural oestrogen during and after perimenopause is manufactured. The less fat she has, the less oestrogen her body will produce to support her bones.

• You smoke. Chemicals in cigarette smoke poison the ovaries and decrease your hormone levels prematurely. Oestrogen, testosterone, and progesterone all have bone-protective effects.

• You spend most of your time indoors. Women who are exposed to very little natural sunlight may be deficient in the natural vitamin D normally produced in sun-drenched skin. Vitamin D is necessary for healthy bone mineralisation. The sunlight–bone health link is so important that I've devoted an entire section to it later in this chapter.

• You are sedentary and spend less than four hours per day on your feet. Bones stay healthy only when they have vertical vectors of force placed on them regularly. A sedentary lifestyle provides insufficient weight-bearing exercise to stimulate bone growth. Many studies have shown that bed rest is associated with osteoporosis. In contrast, weight training has been shown to build bone density even in post-menopausal women who aren't on oestrogen.

• You are (or were) a 'fitness fanatic', that is, you become irritable and unreasonable if you are unable to get in your daily run or other exercise. The lifestyle of the fitness fanatic includes dieting for weight loss and/or engaging regularly in strenuous exercise such as marathon training. Dietary restrictions and the chronic stress of overtraining can impair mineral intake and absorption. It also messes up what is known as the hypothalamic–pituitary axis – the exquisite feedback loop between the brain, the body, and our hormone levels. Chronic overexercise without adequate calorific or mineral intake results in stress fractures in ballet dancers, gymnasts, footballers, and competitive runners, among others. Such fractures are currently on the rise in young athletes and can set the stage for later osteoporosis.

• You have a history of amenorrhoea (no periods) associated with excessive exercise and/or anorexia nervosa.[16] Amenorrhoea results in a derangement of the hypothalamic–pituitary axis similar to that seen in depression. The end result is lower oestrogen, androgen, and progesterone, and an eicosanoid profile that favours osteoporosis and other diseases.[17]

• You drink more than 25g of alcohol per day. (The following servings each contain about 10g of alcohol: ½ pint of beer, a small glass of wine, and 1 measure of spirits.)[18] Alcohol interferes with the function of both osteoblasts and osteoclasts, thus inhibiting your body's ability to lay down new bone and to remodel old bone.[19]

• Your liver is overstressed. The liver's ability to produce and metabolise oestrogen is essential for the growth and maintenance of strong bones at any age. Drinking more than two alcoholic drinks per day, taking medication known to be hard on the liver (such as certain cholesterol-lowering drugs), and infection with viral hepatitis are among the significant liver stressors that can harm bone health.

• You drink more than two units of caffeine per day (1 cup of coffee = 1 unit; 1 can of cola = 0.4 units). Caffeine results in increased urinary excretion of calcium; the more you consume, the more calcium you lose. If your calcium intake is relatively low to begin with, regular caffeine consumption could result in significant loss of bone over time. If, on the other hand, your calcium and mineral intake is high, a couple of cups of coffee a day probably won't matter much. *Note:* Even though tea contains caffeine, both green and black tea have been shown to build bone mass – probably because of their phyto-oestrogen content.

• You are or have been clinically depressed for a significant period of time. Numerous studies have shown that depression is an independent risk factor for osteoporosis. Depressed people have high levels of the immune system chemical known as IL-6, which overstimulates the osteoclasts (cells responsible for breaking down bone). Depression is also associated with abnormalities in the hypothalamic-pituitary-adrenal axis and with elevated cortisol secretion, which predispose one to bone loss.[20]

• Your diet is poor – little fresh food, few leafy green vegetables, and lots of junk food. Such a diet doesn't provide minerals and other nutrients necessary to support the growth and maintenance of a solid bone foundation.[21]

• You went through premature menopause (before the age of forty), have had your ovaries removed surgically, went through menopause as a result of radiation or chemotherapy, and/or have prematurely grey hair. A woman who enters menopause prematurely for any reason is at increased risk for osteoporosis unless she gets adequate hormone replacement during the years when her body would normally have been producing higher levels of hormones. Non-surgical premature menopause, and the premature greying of the hair that often accompanies it, are the result of an autoimmune reaction affecting the ovaries and hair follicles. The cause of these reactions isn't clear.

• You take steroid drugs regularly for conditions such as asthma or lupus. Steroid drugs result in accelerated breakdown of tissue in the body – including the collagen matrix for both skin and bone.[22] Steroids also diminish the sensitivity of the bowel to vitamin D, which in turn reduces calcium absorption.[23] Prolonged steroid use may also significantly decrease oestrogen and androgen levels.[24]

• You use anticonvulsant medication regularly or benzodiazepines such as diazepam (Valium), chlordiazepoxide (Librium), or lorazepam (Ativan).[25] These drugs have also been found to interfere with bone metabolism.

• You've had at least two consecutive bone density tests at least six months apart, done on the same machine, that reported below-normal scores for your age.

• You have a thyroid disorder. Women who suffer from hyperthyroidism are at risk because the excess thyroid hormone (thyroxine) that their bodies make stimulates the osteoclasts to break down bone. Those with hypothyroidism may also be at risk if their dose of thyroid medication is too high. If you have thyroid disease, make sure you are on the lowest dose of thyroid replacement possible for your condition, and follow a sound programme for maintaining bone health.[26] (For a holistic approach to thyroid disease, see *The Thyroid Solution: A Mind–Body Program for Beating Depression and Regaining Your Emotional and Physical Health,* by Dr Ridha Arem.)

Whether or not you are at high risk of osteoporosis, understand that, like the rest of your body, bone is a living work in progress. That means that there is always something you can do – ranging from drugs to dietary change – to help yourself build bone.

Measuring Bone Density

It's very important to get a baseline bone density screening either before or during perimenopause. Although fractures aren't likely to show up until a woman is in her seventies and eighties, now is the best time to do something about any potential problems. Unfortunately, many doctors' practices won't pay for bone density screening unless you've already had documented osteoporotic fractures. This is typical of the Western crisis approach to medicine, which too often neglects prevention. However, I urge you to make this investment in your health.

Because doctors have to be very careful about what they spend their practice budget on, your doctor may not feel that there is sufficient indication to order a bone density test on the NHS. You can, however, arrange to have this test done privately.

Heel Bone Density

When I was forty-eight years old, I had my first bone density test via a machine known as an OsteoAnalyser. This measures the density of the heel bone by running a very low dose of X-rays through the heel bone while it is bathed in warm water. (Other heel bone tests use ultrasound – see Resources.) I found the entire experience very empowering. My bone density was fine, but as a result of seeing my personal number on a standard graph, I found myself more motivated to take my calcium and magnesium supplement consistently – twice per day instead of only at night. I also became more determined not to skip taking my minerals when I'm travelling, which is when my routine tends to fall apart.

Heel bone density testing is gaining increasing recognition as an accurate and cheap method of screening for women of all ages. For example, it is being used to do baseline screening on teenage girls who are at risk of not achieving maximum bone density because of dieting. Heel density tests do not require a doctor's prescription and may even be offered at your local pharmacy. They are not as accurate as a full-scale DEXA test (see below) because they measure only one area of your body. But they are a valuable early warning system.

DEXA Testing

Dual energy bone densitometry (DEXA) is the current gold standard. It uses a very low dose of X-rays to measure bone density both in the spine and in the hips. A woman's bone density is then charted on a graph to see how it compares to normal bone densities for a given age. The US National Osteoporosis Foundation (NOF) and World Health Organisation (WHO) both rate bone density according to a standard curve on which 0 equals the norm. Severity of bone loss is then determined by how far a given measurement falls below that mean. As you can see from the chart below, WHO and NOF differ slightly in their classifications of osteopenia and osteoporosis.

Like heel bone density, DEXA is a static test – a snapshot in time. One reading won't tell you whether your bone density is increasing, decreasing, or remaining the same. You need at least two successive tests at least six months apart to determine what the trend is and whether or not you need to make adjustments in your bone health

Bone Density Classification

	WHO	NOF
NORMAL	0 to −1.0	0 to −1.0
OSTEOPENIA	−1.0 to −2.5	−1.0 to −2.0
OSTEOPOROSIS	Less than −2.5	Less than −2.0

Source: World Health Organisation, *Assessment of Fracture Risk and Its Application to Screening for Postmenopausal Osteoporosis*, Technical Report, Series 843 (Geneva: WHO, 1994).

routine. For example, small-boned women may register on the low end of a DEXA test even if their bones are not at risk.

DEXA testing is available at a number of hospitals. You may be able to arrange a test privately by phoning your local X-ray department. This test is about three times as expensive as heel density tests. Because readings vary from machine to machine, try to have your consecutive measurements taken on the same machine.

Skin Thickness Testing

A number of studies have shown that ultrasound measurement of skin thickness (which is dependent upon healthy collagen) predicts fracture risk as accurately as conventional bone density testing.[27] The accuracy increases when both skin thickness and bone density are combined. Unfortunately, this test has not caught on widely in the UK.

Urine Test for Bone Breakdown Products

As bone breaks down, it releases minute collagen fragments into the urine that can be measured. Because a certain amount of bone breakdown is normal, everyone's urine contains some collagen fragments. But when the breakdown products in the urine are unusually high, you may well be losing bone faster than is healthy.[28] This can be measured as Deoxypyridinoline (Dpd). Unlike the static measurement of the scans, these tests can give you a day-by-day reading of the metabolic state of your bones long before a bone density test will register a problem. They also give you a way to monitor your progress once treatment is initiated. Tests used to be ordered by a doctor, but postal packs can be sent to your home and then returned directly to the laboratory. (See Resources.)

The Bottom Line

Bone density screening and urine testing are a marriage made in heaven. A simple bone density test (either heel density or fully fledged DEXA test) will give you a baseline. Normally you have to wait six months to a year to know if you are gaining bone, losing bone, or staying the same. But sometimes the subsequent tests continue to read on the low side, even though you have stemmed the bone loss or begun building new bone.[29] That's where the urine test comes in. It can tell you immediately whether or not you are losing bone, and if you are, you can repeat it every month or so to make sure that the bone-building programme you're on is working. Your test will show you when you are no longer peeing out your bones! Once your tests indicate that your bones are stable, I suggest that you retest your urine for bone loss every year or two.

These tests can let midlife women know how they're doing in time to prevent further bone loss and even increase bone density years before osteoporosis becomes evident. They allow you to create health daily, not wait until symptoms start!

HELGA: EXERCISE DAILY, BONE LOSS DAILY

Helga first consulted me when she was fifty-seven, five years after her periods had stopped. Active and healthy, she rode horses nearly every day, spent long periods of time outside, and did much of the heavy stable work herself. She had never smoked, and drank only an occasional glass of wine. She wanted to avoid oestrogen and wasn't really having any symptoms that bothered her. She simply wanted to be sure that her overall health was good and that her bones were in good shape.

Helga was blonde, blue-eyed, and fair-skinned and had always been trim and small-boned, weighing only 7½ stone (48kg) at her 5 foot 4 inches height. When her initial bone density test showed that her bones were a bit more than two standard deviations below the mean, I wasn't too concerned, given that her slight build, not significant bone loss, was apt to be the reason for this low reading. I put her on a good supplement regimen (see below) and suggested that we repeat her screening test in six months. When that result came back, it was a bit lower than the first time but not significantly so. To be on the safe side, however, I suggested a urine test. I was very surprised when this test showed that she was losing bone rather quickly.

Given her reluctance to take oestrogen or other bone-building medications, I suggested a whole-soya product that delivers 180mg of soya isoflavones per day, a dose that has definitely been shown to help preserve and build bone density. I also recommended 30mg of natural progesterone per day in the form of a skin cream.

I wondered if Helga's ongoing bone loss in the face of a healthy lifestyle could be related to depression or some other loss. Helga had emigrated to the US from Sweden when she was thirty years old and married an American with whom she had three children. She and her family had always enjoyed regular visits to Sweden to visit her mother. But her mother had recently died, leaving Helga without any remaining family in Sweden. Her youngest child had also recently left home. I told Helga that our bone health is often at risk during times when the very foundations of our lives undergo dramatic and irrevocable change. Though emotionally stoic by nature, Helga acknowledged that she had been feeling a great deal of grief in the past year.

Though we can never replace our families or go back to 'the way it was', it is possible for all of us to re-create sustaining relationships in our lives. So in addition to adding the soya oestrogens and progesterone cream to her regular exercise and supplement programme, I suggested to Helga that she seek out some new social ties with other friends of Swedish descent in order to reconnect with her heritage. Within two months, her urine tests returned to normal and she stopped losing bone.

Bone-building Programme

No matter how many risk factors you identified, it's never too late (nor too early) to build your bones – even if you are ninety or already have significant bone loss. As long as you're alive, your bones are dynamic, living organs that respond daily to every aspect of your life – from your emotions to your diet. First, address the risk factors that are under your control:

- *Cut back on or eliminate alcohol and caffeine.*

- *Stop smoking.* Acupuncture can help you a great deal with this.

- *Follow the perimenopausal diet plan outlined in chapter 7.* Eat five servings of low-sugar fruits and vegetables per day. These are all high in potassium and boron, which help protect your bones by reversing urinary calcium loss.[30]

- *Eat phyto-oestrogens.* Soya and ground linseed are particularly potent in this regard. Several recent studies suggest that regular intake of soya protein has a bone-protective effect that is equivalent to that provided by oestrogen. A six-month double-blind study at the University of Illinois in the US found that postmenopausal women on a diet that was high in soya isoflavones were protected from spinal bone loss.[31] Another recent study followed fifty postmenopausal women who consumed three servings of soya milk a day (about 7.5oz each) or three handfuls of roasted soya nuts, for a total daily dose of

60–70mg of isoflavones. In twelve weeks the study noted a 13 per cent increase in osteocalcin, a marker of bone formation, and a 14.5 per cent decrease in markers for osteoclasts, cells that cause bone loss. The benefits of soya were not compared side by side with hormone replacement therapy, but soya protein revealed a bone-forming benefit that oestrogen does not provide.[32]

• *Drink green tea.* Green tea is especially rich in phytohormones and antioxidants. Research has shown that women who drink either green or black tea regularly have stronger bones than those in a control group.[33] I keep a jug of naturally decaffeinated green tea in my refrigerator and drink it regularly throughout the day.

• *If you are depressed, get proper treatment.* Regular exercise and exposure to natural light are sometimes all that is necessary. If you work under fluorescent fixtures, replace them with full-spectrum light bulbs. Though most full-spectrum lights don't provide the UVB light necessary to stimulate vitamin D and calcium uptake, they definitely can help relieve depression and seasonal affective disorder. Interestingly, the nutritional supplement St John's wort, which has proven antidepressant effects, also lowers a cytokine ('bad' eicosanoid) known as IL-6 that is involved with immune system activation. When its levels are normalised, bone density may be positively affected. It is unclear whether standard antidepressant medications also have this effect.

• *Get your hormone levels checked.* Many postmenopausal women have testosterone levels that are normal even for a premenopausal woman, making them much more resistant to osteoporosis without additional hormones. Some women also have oestrogen levels that remain in the low–normal premenopausal range long after menopause. If this is the case, you won't need hormone supplements to support your bone mass.

Hormones That Help Build Bone

Supplementing with oestrogen (which is far more common than supplementing with DHEA or testosterone) has been shown to help prevent bone loss.[34] In fact, the first FDA-approved indication for oestrogen replacement was the prevention of osteoporosis. Some studies have demonstrated a nearly 50 per cent decrease in risk of fractures with conventional HRT.[35] But that doesn't mean all women need oestrogen therapy to maintain healthy bone mass. Those women whose bodies continue to make even a small amount of oestradiol or testosterone naturally have been found to have a significantly decreased risk of osteoporosis compared to those whose bodies no longer are able to make these hormones.[36]

Keep in mind, however, that bone mass is affected by far more than just oestrogen. For example, it has been demonstrated that half of the total vertebral bone loss that a woman in the US will experience during her lifetime occurs before she goes through menopause.[37] In addition, some studies have failed to find any significant differences between the spine and hip bone densities between pre- and peri-menopausal women and their postmenopausal counterparts. For example, research at the USDA Human Nutrition Research Center on Aging failed to show any accelerated rate of bone loss in the hip or wrist among women close to menopause. Nor did they find any significant change in bone mineral density in the group of women as a whole, a finding that has been duplicated in a Swedish study.[38] Some authorities even hypothesise that only 10–15 per cent of a woman's skeletal mass is affected by oestrogen.[39] And some women on oestrogen replacement still lose bone mass over time.[40] While it is clear that oestrogen plays an important role in bone health, it's just one factor. I recommend taking the lowest dose of oestrogen possible, since bone protection has been demonstrated even at very low doses.

Consider hormone replacement therapy if you've had any of the following conditions associated with decreased hormone levels:

- History of amenorrhoea lasting for six months to a year or more

- Premature, surgical, or medical menopause

- History of steroid use

- Strong family history of osteoporosis (mother or grandmother with obvious osteoporosis)

- A diagnosis of osteopenia or osteoporosis

Remember, hormone replacement helps preserve bone density only as long as you take it. Once you stop, you begin losing bone. The same is true for the effect of exercise on bone.

If you can't use oestrogen or androgen, consider natural progesterone, as either a 1.5–3 per cent transdermal cream or as a prescription pill. Synthetic progestogen has been shown to stimulate osteoblasts (bone builders). The same may be true for natural progesterone in either skin cream or pill form.[41] An ongoing study of 2 per cent progesterone cream for hot flush relief found that the perimenopausal study participants (who would ordinarily be losing bone) didn't show any bone loss in the first year of the study. But their bone mass didn't increase, either. The longer term effects are still being studied.[42]

Bone-building Nutrients

Currently many Western women do not get adequate calcium every day – not to mention all the other nutrients that are needed to build healthy bone. Even if your diet is good, make sure your daily supplement programme includes the following:

Magnesium	600–800mg (because of farming practices, many foods are low in this key mineral, so it must be supplemented)[43]
Calcium	600–1,200mg[44]
Vitamin D	200–1,200IU (dosage requirement increases with age)
Vitamin C	1,000–3,000mg
Boron	4–12mg[45]
Zinc	15mg
Manganese	2–5mg
Copper	2–3mg
Vitamin K	70–140mcg

Calcium Supplements

Studies have clearly demonstrated that calcium supplementation helps build bone mass and prevent fractures.[46] It also helps to make other modalities such as exercise, vitamin D supplementation, and hormone replacement more effective in those who are already being treated for osteoporosis.

I prefer calcium supplements that are chelated with amino acids for maximum absorption – calcium citrate, calcium citrate-malate, or a mixture of any of the following: calcium ascorbate, calcium fumarate, calcium succinate, or calcium tartrate. Microcrystalline hydroxyapatite is also a good source of bone-building calcium. Make sure that

FIGURE 18: SOURCES OF CALCIUM

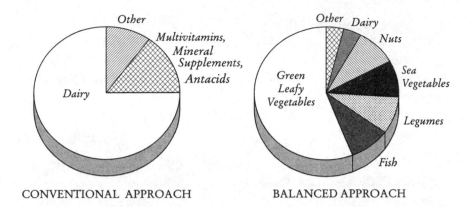

CONVENTIONAL APPROACH   BALANCED APPROACH

Conventional Approach labels: Other; Multivitamins, Mineral Supplements, Antacids; Dairy

Balanced Approach labels: Other; Dairy; Nuts; Sea Vegetables; Legumes; Fish; Green Leafy Vegetables

you take magnesium along with the calcium. A 1:1 ratio of calcium to magnesium is ideal, but 2:1 is also acceptable. (See Resources.)

Magnesium deficiency is as much a problem in bone health as inadequate calcium, and because calcium and magnesium work in critical balance, they should be supplemented together. In fact, too much unbalanced calcium can actually decrease the body's ability to absorb magnesium from food. Dietary surveys have shown that a high proportion of Western women consume less than the RDA for magnesium already. High, unbalanced calcium intake can also block the uptake of manganese, decrease iron absorption, interfere with vitamin K synthesis, and increase faecal phosphorus excretion. Finally, very high doses of calcium carbonate (4–5g per day), which is the type of calcium in antacids, can cause a serious, kidney-damaging disorder known as milk alkali syndrome.[47]

The Protein–Calcium Connection

Rachel, one of my newsletter subscribers, had a query about protein that I've heard from many women.

I am fifty years old and perimenopausal. I have recently been diagnosed with osteoporosis from a DEXA scan, although my gynaecologist would not yet classify me there, since I score –2.0 in my spine and –2.4 in my hips. The point remains [that I feel] I

HIGH-CALCIUM FOODS[48]

There are many good sources of dietary calcium. Yogurt is one of the most easily digestible. A pot of yogurt contains about 300mg of calcium. However, Britons have been culturally conditioned to focus on dairy products as the key to healthy bones. Consider that a 3.5oz can of sardines also contains 300mg of calcium and is loaded with health-enhancing omega-3 fats.

Food	Amount	Calcium (mg)
Green Leafy Vegetables (cooked, unless specified)		
broccoli	1 cup	150
kale	1 cup	179
spinach	1 cup	278
pak choi	1 cup	200
rhubarb	1 cup	348
watercress (raw)	1 cup	53
parsley (raw)	1 cup	122
Sea Vegetables (cooked, unless specified)		
hijiki	1 cup	610
wakame	1 cup	520
kombu (kelp)	1 cup	305
agar-agar (Kanten flakes) used as a thickener for sauces, etc.	1 cup (dry flakes) (16tbsp)	400
dulse	1 cup (dry)	567
Fish (bones: the major source of calcium in fish)		
sardines (with bones)	3½oz (99g) can (drained)	300
salmon (canned)	1 cup	431
oysters, raw	1 cup	226

Food	Amount	Calcium (mg)
Beans and Legumes		
tofu, firm	4oz (113g)	80–150
tempeh	4oz (113g)	172
chickpeas	1 cup (cooked)	150
black beans	1 cup (cooked)	135
pinto beans	1 cup (cooked)	128
tortillas, corn	2	120
Nuts and Seeds		
sesame seeds (must be ground for absorption)	3 tablespoons	300
almonds	1 cup	300
sunflower seeds	1 cup (hulled)	174
brazil nuts	1 cup	260
hazelnuts	1 cup	282
Other Sources		
blackstrap molasses	1 tbsp	137
orange juice calcium fortified	1 cup	210
Mineral Waters		
Perrier	1 litre	140
Mendocino	1 litre	380
San Pellegrino	1 litre	200
Apollinaris	1 litre	91
Contexeville	1 litre	451
Dairy		
milk		
skimmed	1 cup	300
whole	1 cup	288
cheese (Swiss, cheddar)	1½oz (43g)	300
non-fat yogurt	1 cup	294
cottage cheese (low fat)	1 cup	150

am in dangerous territory and I am not yet in menopause. My risk factors are that I recently stopped smoking (in fact, this news is what finally did it), my father has osteoporosis, and I have a small frame.

I am determined to try to reverse this through nutrition, supplements, and exercise, rather than take HRT.

Here's my programme so far: I exercise at least five times a week doing fast walking, free weights, and t'ai chi. I am having a difficult time finding a nutritionist who has expertise with osteoporosis. All the research I've read has said that a high-protein diet leaches calcium out of the body through urine. However, I recently read in *Women's Bodies, Women's Wisdom* that some recent research disputes this. Can you give me more information on your findings? How much protein should I be taking in daily? Does it matter if it's animal protein or not?

Many nutritionists blame too much protein for osteoporosis and kidney disease, and there is research that supports this view.[49] However, Dr Larrian Gillespie, a urological surgeon and the author of *The Menopause Diet*, points out that much of the relevant research has been conducted in hospitals on patients with insulin-dependent diabetes or otherwise compromised health.[50] Though some research has shown that even in healthy people, excess protein, especially in the form of red meat, may cause calcium loss in the urine, this effect is minuscule in comparison to the adverse bone effects of the imbalanced eicosanoids produced by too much stress, alcohol, and refined carbohydrates.

The fact is that for the vast majority of time that humans have been on this planet – about one million years – our main source of food has been nuts, seeds, and fruits foraged in season, plus animal protein. Agriculture, and the grain- and dairy-rich diets that it made possible, has existed for a mere ten thousand years. And recent research into Paleolithic nutrition has found that hunter–gatherer societies – even those in existence today – are healthier on all levels than those whose food sources are primarily grain-based. Plus they don't have osteoporosis.[51]

Here's the bottom line: the same amount of protein that supports overall health supports healthy bones. For a 5 foot 4 inches, 10 stone (63kg) female, that means about 27g of protein at each of three meals per day (about 81g per day total). One ounce of meat or fish contains about 7g of protein; a serving of 4oz meets the requirement. Eggs contain 6g of protein each. An egg white has 4g. Hard cheese contains 6–7g per ounce. Soft cheese has 3–4g per ounce. Curd cheese such as cottage cheese or cheese curd has 7g per 1/4 cup, and tofu has 10g per 1/4 cup. Check the nutrition labels at the supermarket; they almost always include this information.

People who are physically active need more protein than those who are sedentary. Larger women also need more. The fact is that because of dieting and misinformation, far too many women don't get enough protein.

What About Bone-building Drugs?

Far too many doctors prescribe one of the newer bone-building drugs as the first line of treatment for any woman who shows any sign of decreased bone mass – even those who are very far from having actual osteoporosis or even significant osteopenia. Though I applaud the preventive approach, there are many safe and effective alternatives that work more naturally with the wisdom of the body.

Here's a brief rundown of the most commonly available bone-building prescription drugs. Like hormone replacement therapy, these work only as long as a woman is on them.

FOSAMAX (ALENDRONATE)

This non-hormonal drug appears to interfere with osteoclast function, thus preventing bone breakdown. It has been shown to increase spine and hip bone mass and to reduce the risk of spinal fractures about as well as oestrogen replacement.[52] Clinical trials are ongoing to determine if these increases in bone density actually translate into a decrease in hip fractures. In comparison trials, it appears to be better at building bone mass than salmon calcitonin.[53] Fosamax may cause side effects, including nausea, constipation, and heartburn. In some studies, up to a third of the participants had stomach-acid-related complaints, and one in eight required treatment. Some even developed severe oesophageal ulcers.[54] About 50 per cent of women stop treatment within a year. However, Fosamax may be appropriate for women at risk of osteoporosis who cannot or will not take other medications or other measures to build bone mass.

EVISTA (RALOXIFENE)

This selective oestrogen receptor modulator (SERM), like the related drug tamoxifen, has an oestrogenic effect on bone but anti-oestrogenic effects on breast tissue. Though Evista has been shown to help build bone, and though it decreases spinal fractures, it has not resulted in a decrease in the incidence of hip fractures, for reasons that aren't yet clear.[55] Side effects include hot flushes. I'm also very concerned about the possibility of dementia risk with this drug because, like tamoxifen, it blocks the well-known beneficial effects of oestrogen (including the oestrogen our bodies make on their own) on brain cells.

SALMON CALCITONIN (FORCALTONIN)

This is an injectable or nasal synthetic form of the parathyroid hormone that regulates calcium loss in the urine and reduces fracture risk to some extent. Side effects include nausea and flushing. It is not yet licensed in the UK for use in osteoporosis.

Get Strong

Regardless of your diet, supplements, or any hormones you may be on, the big news is that weight-bearing exercise in general and strength training in particular play a crucial role in creating and maintaining healthy bones. If you don't currently exercise regularly, you're not alone. Sixty per cent of the UK population is sedentary, which is one of the main reasons why osteoporosis has reached such epidemic proportions. Remember, it is not the ageing process per se that causes bones to thin – it's the fact that too many women slow down and stop using their muscles.

Weight-bearing exercise helps build bone by stimulating the mineralisation and remodelling process. Every major muscle in our bodies is attached to underlying bone by tendons. Every time a muscle contracts, it exerts a force on the bone to which it is anchored. Any activity that builds up muscle also puts stress on bone and helps build bone mass. We know, for example, that in tennis players the bone density in the racket arm is significantly greater than in the other arm. Yoga and t'ai chi can also help build bone mass. But the most studied method of strengthening bone is weight lifting.

Miriam Nelson, PhD, of Tufts University in the US, has done

ground-breaking research that shows how weight training can slow down and even reverse bone loss. Dr Nelson studied two groups of postmenopausal women, none of whom were on oestrogen replacement, bone-building drugs, or any special supplements. Both groups were sedentary but healthy at the start of the programme. One group remained sedentary while the other began a simple exercise programme. At the end of one year the women who lifted weights for forty minutes twice a week had turned back the clock in several ways. Their scores on strength tests increased to match those of women in their late thirties or early forties. Without dieting, they trimmed down; muscle is less bulky than fat. Their balance improved greatly, warding off falls. The biggest payoff: while the sedentary control group lost about 2 per cent of their bone density during the year, the women who exercised gained 1 per cent.[56]

But stronger bones aren't the only benefit of getting strong. Nelson noted an unexpected but very exciting change in the women who did weight training – a change that I've also seen repeatedly in my own practice. Within a few weeks the weight-lifting women felt happier, more energetic, and more self-confident. As their muscles began to get stronger they became more active and daring. In order to control the study, they had agreed not to join other fitness programmes. But these former couch potatoes were now going canoeing or in-line skating or dancing because they wanted to. Nelson also confirmed that weight training, like aerobic exercise, lifts depression and helps arthritis.[57]

The joys and benefits of fitness are so numerous that I want to do everything in my power to motivate you to get strong. Of all the ways to stay vital, healthy, and attractive, exercise probably gives the most return for the time spent. Whatever your age and condition right now, physical exercise can improve it and give you a new lease on life – guaranteed. In 1994 researchers proved this by instituting a strength-training programme in frail nursing-home patients with an average age of eighty-seven. The exercise group did 45-minute strength-training sessions for the hips and knees three days per week. Within ten weeks, their strength increased by over 100 per cent. In a non-exercising control group, strength declined by about 1 per cent. The improved muscle strength after exercise was unrelated to the age, sex, medical diagnosis, or functional level of the participant. After the strength-training programme some of the participants who had previously used Zimmer frames required only a cane. Exercise also

What Would It Take to Get You Moving?

- Do you enjoy moving your body? Recall a moment in your life in which you were captivated by the sheer joy of dancing, running, swimming, or jumping. When was the last time you felt this way?

- When was the last time that you felt that pleasurable sense of complete relaxation that comes from spending a day immersed in the pleasures of some activity – skiing, hiking, sailing, dancing, or in-line skating?

- What types of activities did you enjoy as a child? As a teenager?

- If you do not exercise now, why not?

- If you don't exercise now, when did you stop? Why?

- Do you feel that you don't have time to exercise? Why not?

improved stair-climbing ability, speed of walking, and overall level of physical activity.[58]

If these kinds of results are possible in frail octogenarians in nursing homes, think what could happen for a fifty-year-old couch potato. The average midlife woman of today is expected to live until at least the age of eighty-five, if not a hundred. You cannot afford to let your muscles and bones slip into decline at midlife. There are too many potentially high-quality years ahead. And there's not a single drug, technological breakthrough, or genetic development on the horizon that can or ever will come close to providing you with the benefits you can derive yourself from getting and staying strong. Besides, women who exercise regularly live six years longer than non-exercisers. If you think you don't have time to exercise, I suggest that you rethink this belief. Slowly shuffling along on a Zimmer instead of striding confidently takes up a lot of time. And dying six years prematurely is truly a colossal waste of time.

Almost every woman I know is too busy to exercise. There are always more things to get done in a day than you have time for. If you wait to exercise until you get everything else done, you are waiting for a miracle. Like muscles that won't get stronger until you reach down and pick up a heavy weight, exercise won't happen in your life unless you make it as much a priority as brushing your teeth or having a shower. The first thing that must change if you are to exercise regularly is your mind. No excuses.

Healing Your Fitness Past

As I write this, my seventy-four-year-old mother is leading a group of women in their thirties on a hiking expedition. These thirty-somethings felt that they could benefit from her experience and expertise. So at an age when many women have relegated themselves to the sidelines, my mother is not only coaching the game, she is also actively playing it. The day before she left for this trip, she got up at six, mowed the huge lawn on the farm where I grew up, watered all the flowers, then played two sets of tennis. After that, she drove several hours to the nursing home to visit a relative, then went out and played eighteen holes of golf before bedtime.

My mother's physical activity level is very impressive, and I don't see it as a standard to which I or anyone else should aspire unless they find it as satisfying as she does. But my mother's physical condition and prowess have helped me understand that physical decline and weakness need not be part of growing older. In fact, it's a legacy I received before birth: my mother skied and hiked through all her pregnancies and later carried each of us children in a backpack during these same activities.

Despite this legacy, I have my own unfinished business about sports and fitness. In contrast to my mother and siblings, I was not interested in spending every free moment on the ski slopes or hiking up mountains carrying a heavy backpack. I liked to read books – by the fire in winter and sitting up in a tree in summer. As an adolescent, I longed for a Christmas morning in which we could all sit around, relax, talk, and drink cocoa, like they did in films. But invariably, as soon as the presents had been opened, everyone rushed out of the door to get in a couple of runs at the local ski resort before our relatives arrived for dinner. My only chance for having the loving family connection that I longed for was to haul out my gear and join them. So I did. And I learned how to ski pretty well.

But my overall sports skills lagged behind those of my mother and siblings no matter how hard I tried. During the summer of my thirteenth year, for example, I practised my tennis strokes daily against the barn door for six solid weeks. My father's only comment was 'You're swinging that racket as if it were a broom.' This left me with considerable baggage about sports. So at midlife I decided to release this baggage and pick up some barbells – and some insight – instead. When I was forty-five I took tennis lessons, more as therapy to recover from my past than from a desire to play regularly. By the end of the season I realised that I was perfectly capable of playing and enjoying a game of tennis. Later that summer I even played doubles with my mother and brother. What a healing!

Dr John Douillard, a fitness expert and the author of *Body, Mind, and Sports,* points out that 50 per cent of women experience their first personal failure with organised physical activity in school gym classes, and that this sense of being a physical 'loser' can stay with you for the rest of your life. At perimenopause you have to ask yourself, 'Do I really want to continue limiting my health and happiness because of something that happened to me in secondary school gym classes, or with my parents when I was six?'

Get out your diary and write down everything you remember about physical activity and sports from when you were eleven to thirteen years old. What did you love to do? What activities felt good? What are your memories from gym classes? What is your family legacy about fitness? What do you honestly believe about the physical capabilities of a woman your age? Aged seventy-five? Aged ninety? What was the fitness level of your mother? Your grandmother? What happens to you when you walk into a gym?

My colleague Mona Lisa Schulz has been able to transform her fitness legacy several times, finally reaching a balance. When she was growing up, her family's idea of a holiday was to drive to the base of a mountain, eat a sandwich, and then drive back home. She desperately longed to get out of the car and actually climb a peak. But her mother always had a bad back, and her father always had a headache and chest pain. Once, when she was sixteen, she wanted to go skiing. Her mother said, 'Don't go or I'll disown you. You've put your father and me through enough already.' (By then Mona Lisa had already had major surgery for scoliosis.) She went skiing anyway, and eventually a large part of her individuation from her family of origin involved proving herself by becoming a competitive athlete in both running and bike racing – which she tended to do excessively as a way to cope with the stress of her family. Though continuing spinal problems eventually halted these activities, she has worked around her physical challenges and still remains strong and fit through walking, biking, and daily workouts on a variety of fitness equipment. She, too, has reached balance.

Exercise to Please Yourself

I've been able to transform my fitness past by individualising my fitness regime to my own temperament and by realising that my sports skills, strength, and fitness level are about me and my body, not a way to win family approval or measure up to some cultural standard. At midlife I've finally found out what is true for me when it comes to physical activity. Every woman needs to do the same. You need to ask yourself, 'What do I want to be fit for?' I've come to realise that unlike my family of origin, I stay fit to live well; I don't live to stay fit. These motivations are both valid – but they're different.

Ask yourself what activities you want to be able to participate in for as long as you live. Just because tae bo or t'ai chi or some other form of exercise is all the rage doesn't mean it's right for you. I tried for years to enjoy running – it was very 'in' in the 1970s and 1980s. But it never felt good. Though I ran regularly throughout medical school, I never felt that elusive runner's high, no matter how long or hard I ran. In fact, I hated it. I finally gave myself permission to stop.

I now go only for those activities that feel right. I love Pilates, the mind–body fitness approach developed by Joseph Pilates that engages the mind, the muscles, breathing, and stretching all at once. I also love seeing how far I've come in two years. Pilates, like any discipline that uses the mind as fully as the body, ends up transforming both. I also do aerobic workouts with weights. I like the challenge of weights, and I like being able to lift heavy objects – I know I could easily remove the window from an aeroplane exit row if necessary! Strong muscles help you move confidently through the world.

RUTH: COUCH POTATO NO MORE

Ruth, fifty-five, came to see me complaining of aches and pains and not being able to sleep well at night. She told me she had brought up five children and was now looking forward to retirement from her job as a government secretary. She had never done any regular exercise. Her initial bone density test showed a slight bone loss despite the fact that she had been on oestrogen for seven years following a hysterectomy with ovary removal for heavy bleeding. In addition to recommending dietary improvement and a supplement programme, I stressed to Ruth that she needed to begin an exercise programme. Her couch-potato status was putting her at risk of significantly tarnishing her dreams for her golden years.

Ruth decided to start a walking programme every morning with some of her friends. Within three months she had lost 10lb without changing her diet at all, her aches and pains were gone, and she was sleeping better than she had in years. Later that year she and her husband both took up skiing and hiking. Though I'm still trying to convince Ruth to begin a weight-training programme, her bone density has stayed steady even without it. Fitness and outdoor exercise have become a regular part of her life.

Start Somewhere – Anywhere

If you simply can't see yourself doing something like weight training just yet, commit to doing some kind of physical activity for just ten minutes daily for thirty days. Here's what I recommend. Put on some music you love and dance around your house. Even if you're in a wheelchair, you can sit and move your upper body. No excuses. I guarantee that by the end of thirty days or much sooner, you'll be looking forward to your daily dance. Just this simple exercise will wake up the inherent, irresistible desire to move that lies within each of us – albeit more deeply buried in some than others!

Movement is contagious. Today's dancing around your living room will eventually wake up enough of your muscles that you'll want to do more. You can always pick up your cat and dance around with him or her. (This is weight training, after all!) Start very slowly and breathe in and out through your nose – this will expand your lower lungs optimally. It can take a while to create flexibility in your ribcage, so don't get discouraged if nose breathing makes you feel out of breath at first. Don't ever push beyond what is comfortable for your breathing and heart rate. But every day ask your body to move a little faster or bend a little deeper. Simply moving your body begins the bone-building process.

Get Support

After you've done your one month of dancing, you'll have created the movement habit in your life. Now's the time to begin adding some weight training. I suggest that you go to an adult education class, or a gym and get one of the staff members to guide you through a personal strength-training programme. This way you'll be learning proper technique, which you can later adapt for home use.

Whether you exercise at home or in a gym will depend upon your lifestyle and temperament. I've done both and find advantages and disadvantages to each approach. The beauty of the gym is that the phone doesn't ring and no one interrupts you. And the entire environment is dedicated to fitness, so you're more apt to get into the spirit of it. But sometimes taking the extra time to go to the gym is too much. My current personal fitness regime combines one-hour Pilates sessions in a studio with a teacher, thirty-minute Pilates mat sessions on my own at home, and one hour of aerobic weight training with videos, each done twice per week. I also take regular forty-five-minute walks. I haven't always been able to get this amount of exercise in. One of the benefits of being perimenopausal is that my time is more my own than at any other time of my life. And I find that I like exercise more now than I ever have.

Build Strength into Your Day

Here are a few tips for adding some strength training to your day-to-day activities. Try these exercises when you're on the phone or have a few spare moments. They cover all the major muscle groups.

• *Toe stands.* Face a wall and stand 12in (30cm) away from it with your feet shoulder width apart. Rest your fingertips lightly against the wall for balance. (As you improve you can use the wall less and less.) Now raise yourself as high up as you can; remain on your toes for a count of three, breathing normally, then lower yourself slowly. Breathe. Repeat a total of eight times. Gradually hold each toe stand for thirty seconds as you become stronger.

• *Heel stands.* Stand facing a wall so that you can put your hands against it if necessary. Slowly raise the toes and balls of your feet until you are balanced on your heels. Remain on your heels for a count of three. Slowly lower. Breathe. Repeat. Try for a total of eight repetitions, and gradually increase the amount of time you balance on your heels so that eventually you're holding each heel stand for a count of thirty.

Both heel and toe stands use your own body weight to strengthen your legs and to improve balance and flexibility.

- **Push-ups.** Although many women hate them, nothing beats a push-up for strengthening the upper body. You can ease into this exercise with wall push-ups. Stand with your feet about 3ft (1m) from a wall. Lean forward with elbows bent and palms touching the wall. Now push off the wall, keeping your back perfectly aligned with your legs, making sure that your head is aligned with your back and not pitching forward. Repeat this wall push-up eight times. Build up to three sets of eight repetitions.

After this becomes easy, you'll be ready for push-ups on the floor. Start on your hands and knees with arms straight. Now bend your elbows and dip your chest to the floor. Go slowly and keep breathing. Try for four knee push-ups. Gradually build up to two sets of eight.

When you get strong enough, you'll be ready for full-blown regulation push-ups. Start on your hands and knees. Then straighten your legs out behind you so that you are supported by your toes and your arms. Your body should form a perfectly straight line with your head in alignment with your spine. Don't allow your hips to jack-knife up in the centre. Now dip down so that your chest almost touches the floor. Push back up. Hold. Repeat. Do four, working up to eight. Eventually you'll be aiming for two sets of eight push-ups.

- **Weights.** Place a set of graduated dumb-bells (2–20lb, depending upon your strength level) in front of your TV. During the advertisements or even during your favourite shows you can easily do a few sets of biceps curls, overhead presses, bent rows, flat rows, or triceps kickbacks. The point is to keep the weights out where you'll run into them regularly.

Take your time. Your body is very forgiving and very responsive if you approach it with respect and love. Each time you lift weights, ask your body if it is willing to breathe a little deeper and lift a bit more weight. Don't push it. On the days when you feel wonderful, do more. When you feel lousy, cut back. Exercise is a discipline, it is true. But once you've made the commitment to do it regularly, get that abusive coach out of your head. The best motivator is the pleasure, joy, and awareness that come from being in your body.

The Sunlight–Bone Health Connection

Everywhere we turn, we are warned about the dangers of exposure to the sun, from premature skin ageing to fatal skin cancer. Though these risks are well documented, they are overstated, especially for those of us who live in northern climates, where sunlight isn't a glaring issue for most of the year. Women past menopause lose up to 3–4 per cent of their bone mass every winter if they live in northern latitudes, above a line drawn approximately from Boston through Chicago to the Californian border,[59] (equivalent to a line drawn roughly north of Spain). Even on a bright sunny day in December in northern latitudes, you cannot get enough ultraviolet exposure to produce vitamin D unless you expose a great deal of your skin to the sun at midday for thirty to fifty minutes or so, a level of exposure that is uncommon. The problem is compounded if your diet is already low in calcium and vitamin D. Forty per cent of individuals with hip fractures in northern latitudes are vitamin D deficient. In women whose diets are adequate in calcium and other nutrients, however, bone mass can be regained in the summer months with regular sunlight exposure.

The truth is that sunlight can help you become healthier and can literally save your life. That's because ultraviolet rays from the sun help your body manufacture necessary vitamin D. As with just about everything else, the key is moderation.

Vitamin D is a hormone that helps your bones absorb calcium. If you don't have enough vitamin D circulating in your blood, you won't be able to use the calcium from your diet or from supplements. Therefore, it is an important factor in preventing osteoporosis. Right now the RDA for vitamin D is based on the amount you need to prevent rickets. Rickets is a disease where vitamin D levels are too low, resulting in the body's decreased ability to produce new bone. In adults, this is called osteomalacia, a gradual softening or bending of bones secondary to failure of bones to calcify.

To prevent rickets, you need just a minimal level of vitamin D (200–400IU per day). But prevention of rickets isn't the only benefit of optimal vitamin D levels. For example, adequate vitamin D can decrease hypertension, so people with higher vitamin D levels enjoy lower blood pressure.[60] It can slow the progression of osteoarthritis and also decrease the prevalence of multiple sclerosis.[61] Vitamin D also helps prevent some cancers, such as breast, ovarian, prostate, and colorectal cancer. In fact, suboptimal levels of vitamin D may be one of the reasons why breast cancer incidence is higher in northern latitudes than in the south.

But in order to lower your risk of these diseases, especially breast, ovarian, and colorectal cancer, you need much higher serum levels than you can get with a teaspoon of cod liver oil or a vitamin D supplement. Your safest and most effective route for this is routine sun exposure.

Sunlight Versus Vitamin D Supplementation

Our bodies were designed to get vitamin D from the sun. Our ancestors ran around the plains of Africa for millennia with large surfaces of their bodies exposed to sunlight. Exposure to outdoor sunlight is a much more reliable predictor of vitamin D levels in your body than your dietary intake. In fact, vitamin D intake in your diet correlates poorly with the amount of vitamin D in your blood. This is partly because oral vitamin D requirements have been found to vary tremendously between individuals. And while it is possible to take in toxic levels of vitamin D from supplements, it is impossible for sun exposure to result in too much vitamin D. That's because our bodily wisdom contains a built-in mechanism whereby we manufacture exactly what we need from the sun – no more and no less. The vitamin D that your body makes on its own from exposure to the sun's ultraviolet rays (specifically ultraviolet B, or UVB) is superior to oral supplementation for helping your body absorb calcium.[62]

Sunlight alone can bring your vitamin D levels into the healthy range. If you expose your face and hands to sunlight without sunscreen for about twenty minutes three to five times per week for four to five months per year (between April and October in northern latitudes), you probably will get enough UVB rays to keep your bone mass intact, because your body has the ability to stockpile vitamin D for use during low-sunlight times. This is nature's wisdom at work, because not all regions are equal when it comes to ultraviolet exposure. If you have very dark skin, you need to be in the sun longer – even an hour or two hours to get the same result.

The more skin you expose, the quicker you make vitamin D, which is why some experts recommend full-body exposure regularly. In fact, full-body exposure for fifteen minutes is the equivalent of an oral dose of 10,000IU vitamin D. (But UV exposure beyond this does not give you higher vitamin D levels.) However, as we age, our bodies become less efficient at making their own vitamin D. So if you are older than sixty-five, you may need more time in the sun to get the same benefit. Here's a general rule: if there's enough sunlight to cause a reddening of your skin when you're outside for any length of time, then there are enough UVB rays to assist your body in making vitamin D.

How to Have Your Sun and Be Safe, Too

Everyone can get the amount of sunlight they need safely by getting outdoors regularly. The benefits of small amounts of UVB light are so striking that endocrinologist Michael Holick MD, and his colleagues at Boston University Medical Center in the US are studying the effects of providing artificial UVB light to older people. NASA has also contracted Holick to put this special light into spaceships for long missions to counteract the effects of weightlessness on bone.[63]

Early morning or late afternoon sun exposure is the safest. I personally take a forty-five-minute walk about four mornings per week during the warm months, wearing shorts and a tank top to ensure adequate sun exposure. When I can't get out in the morning, I try for late afternoon or early evening, when there is still some sunlight available but when the risk of overexposure is minimal. Other than these 'vitamin D-enhancing times' I wear sunscreen.

Avoid midday sun and sunburn. Almost all skin cancers are associated with the harmful effects of sun overexposure without adequate antioxidant protection. In fact, UV exposure beyond pre-erythema levels (reddening of the skin) doesn't enhance your vitamin D levels. In other words, vitamin D reaches maximum levels in light skin twenty minutes after exposure.

Other easy ways to get a little vitamin D enhancement are opening the window in your car as you drive, riding in an open-top vehicle, or even opening the windows in your house. Why not create a sunroom or sun corner – a place where you can easily open a window and expose yourself to warm sunlight without even having to go outside? This is a good option for city dwellers.

What to Do When You Can't Get Enough Sunlight

Vitamin D is an essential hormone. In the absence of sunlight, you must get it in your diet. While it is nearly impossible to get the high levels of vitamin D you need in your blood without adequate sun exposure, vitamin D supplementation has definitely been shown to help women build or maintain bone mass.[64]

People under sixty-five should take 400–800IU per day. People sixty-five and older should take 800–1,200IU per day unless they have a known sensitivity to it. (You may need more or less. The point is that sunlight is more reliable than any supplement.) Good food sources of vitamin D are liver, cod liver oil, and egg yolks.

Why Fortified Milk Isn't the Vitamin D Answer

Though all of us have been taught that it's possible to get all the vitamin D we need from fortified dairy foods, that's not always the case. When Dr Michael Holick studied the vitamin D content of fortified milk, he found that there's often not enough vitamin D present because of processing problems. In fact, up to 50 per cent of the milk tested had less vitamin D than noted on the label. Fifteen per cent of the milk had no vitamin D at all! And in skimmed milk there is a problem getting vitamin D into the solution because vitamin D is fat soluble and requires some fat to blend with the product. That's why skimmed milk products may have little or no vitamin D whatsoever.[65]

When in Doubt, Measure

If you have any evidence of osteoporosis from either bone density screening or a urine test, then I'd recommend getting a serum vitamin D level as well. This is a simple blood test. A blood level of vitamin D of 20–25nmol/l or lower indicates a severe deficiency. You want to aim for a level that is in the upper range of normal, about 75–250nmol/l. Levels greater than 100nmol/l have been shown to decrease hypertension.[66] Levels of 75nmol/l and above slow the progression of osteoarthritis. Studies of lifeguards and farmers – people who are out in the sun all the time – show that they have vitamin D levels of around 100nmol/l. You may also want to have your serum levels checked if you're healthy but you are in doubt about how much vitamin D you're getting or manufacturing from sun exposure. If your levels are low, get more sun exposure to prevent later problems, even if your bones seem healthy now.

I once did a consultation for a woman in her mid-forties who spent her summers in northern latitudes and ran regularly for exercise while covered in sunscreen and clothing. Though she lived most of the year in an area with abundant sunshine all year round, she avoided the sun at all costs because she was worried about skin cancer. When I ordered a serum vitamin D level, it came back at 25nmol/l, indicating severe deficiency. Since then, she has been taking daily fifteen-minute early morning sun baths in her garden. Within two months her serum vitamin D level had increased to a very healthy range, and both her mood and her immune system improved dramatically. Within six months her bone density had also improved. She discovered some other benefits as well: she completely recovered from a tendency to catch colds and have aches and pains.

Should You Use a Tanning Salon?

Though dermatologists cringe at tanning salons because of the danger of overexposure, I recommend them for those who are at high risk of osteoporosis, depression, or certain cancers and who have no other way of getting UVB radiation.

A short five- to ten-minute sun bath in a salon once or twice per week in the winter months can boost your brain serotonin levels, lift depression, help build bone, help calm arthritis, and maybe also help prevent some cancers. The key, as with natural sun exposure, is to be sure you never burn or get red skin, and also that your body is fortified with antioxidants.

Take Antioxidants

Increasing numbers of studies have shown that antioxidants such as vitamin E, vitamin C, proanthocyanidins, and beta-carotene help protect the skin from sun damage, and also help it heal more quickly. (See chapter 11 for further information.)

Beware Drug-induced Sun Sensitivity

Remember that many very common drugs actually increase sun sensitivity and will therefore increase your chances of getting sunburned if you stay out too long. These include the following: antibiotics such as azithromycin (Zithromax), minocycline (Minocin), tetracycline, and sulphonamides; diabetic medications of the sulphonylurea family; skin treatments such as Retin-A and Isotrex; and diuretics of the thiazide family. It's always best to check with your chemist.

Shore Up Your Earth Connection with Plant Medicine

Traditional herbalists teach that when we consume plants regularly, our bodies take in their energetic qualities as well as their vitamins and minerals – a perfect way to help us connect with nature and shore up our first emotional centres. Oats *(Avena sativa)* and oat straw (the grass, leaf, and flower of the oat), for example, thrive in chilly, wet climates characterised by harsh winds and sudden storms. These hardy plants are rich in calcium, iron, phosphorus, B complex, potassium, magnesium, and vitamins A and C.[67]

The noted herbalist Susan Weed has found that regular consumption of herbal infusions with their highly bioavailable nutrients help increase bone density as well as providing other benefits. One of my nutritionist colleagues also recommends them. I've started to use oat straw infusion regularly and highly recommend this or other infusions of your choice.

How to Make an Herbal Infusion

Infusions are stronger than herbal teas. Use 1oz (30g) of dried leaves (two handfuls of cut-up leaves, or three handfuls of whole leaves). Put in a litre jar. Fill jar with boiling water, put the lid on, and steep for four hours at room temperature. This can be kept in the refrigerator.[68] Use 2 cups daily.

When using oat straw or other plant medicines, open yourself to the wisdom of the earth and nature as they have manifested in the plant you are taking into your body. Be patient and persistent. Feel your bones becoming as strong and sturdy as the mountains and rocks that form the backbone of the planet.

THIRTEEN

Creating Breast Health

I remember the many evenings I sat in the labour and delivery wards of the hospital with one of my midwife colleagues. Though her own children were nearly grown up, this woman would sometimes clutch her chest when she heard a baby cry or saw a particularly adorable newborn. 'My breasts are tingling so much, I feel as though I could feed this child myself,' she would say at such moments.

Breasts are both literally and symbolically a source of nurturance. Their dual role is in part the result of a brain hormone known as prolactin. This chemical, which is activated after a woman gives birth, keeps the breasts full of milk and also enhances the process of bonding, so that when a mother breast-feeds, prolactin facilitates the flow of both milk and love to the child. The mother in turn is rewarded not only with pleasurable physical sensations, but with the emotional fulfilment that comes from providing for a being she deeply loves. Prolactin has such a powerful effect that many women experience the let-down reflex, which fills the breasts with milk, even when they're not actually nursing. Merely thinking about their child or hearing the child's cries can set the reflex in motion.

But prolactin secretion doesn't occur only during breast-feeding. Prolactin levels have been found to increase in both men and women when they are involved in pleasurable, mutually beneficial relationships. Not surprisingly, the emotions of love and compassion, which nourish our very souls, are often accompanied by the same tingling sensation in the breasts that nursing mothers feel – and that my midwife colleague described so eloquently.

I like to think of that tingling as proof that the 'milk of human kindness' is more than a mere metaphor. Love is wired into our biology. That's why nurturing and supporting others feels so good to most women, and why we so often find ourselves 'mothering' others. When the emotion of love can flow freely, our bodies are filled with the same hormone that sustains all human bonds, and our breasts are bathed in the energy of health.

Our Cultural Inheritance: Nurturing and Self-sacrifice

Love has a healing, life-enhancing effect if our relationships are truly reciprocal, allowing us to receive as much as we give. But this ideal is not so common. Most women have been brought up to nurture others in ways that often require us to put our own well-being at risk. Throughout history, we women have been revered for our ability to sacrifice ourselves for the good of those around us. It is no wonder that Tammy Wynette's song 'Stand by Your Man' is the best-selling country song of all time. But as it turns out, the man Tammy was standing by for much of her married life was beating her, which brings home very powerfully the degree to which our nurturing tendencies can tip the balance towards dangerous self-sacrifice.

Our breasts are the part of our anatomy most identified with nurturing. And they are also perhaps the most highly charged area of our bodies, flagrantly exploited by the culture we live in as our most potent weapon in the battle to win the love and approval of a man. Powerful symbols, these breasts. In the film *Erin Brockovich* the sassy legal-assistant heroine is asked by her astounded boss how she has managed, without any experience or training, to accumulate so much sensitive, damning information concerning a large utility company's environmental pollution practices. Looking resplendently voluptuous in her overflowing bustier, actress Julia Roberts replies, 'They're called boobs, Ed.'

No wonder one of my friends, when she heard I was getting divorced, asked if I was going to get breast implants. Our culture leads us to believe that without a stunning new set of breasts, it would be impossible for a woman at midlife to attract a new man. What more vivid proof could we find of our need for love – and the lengths to which we are willing to go to get it?

The Midlife Breast Challenge

Midlife is when we hear the wake-up call that demands that we start honouring our own needs. Our children are leaving home or long gone, the time for the kind of self-sacrifice demanded by bringing up a family is coming to an end, and we now have the opportunity to re-examine our lives. If we are involved in relationships that are getting in the way of self-realisation, we need to think about how we can change them. Perimenopause challenges us to be honest, to create relationships that are true partnerships with people who will love us for who we really are.

Breast Cancer Risk Factors

Midlife is also the time when, statistically speaking, your chances of getting breast cancer are on the rise. In fact, for women living in industrialised societies, age is first on the list of established risk factors for breast cancer.[1]

- Age (over fifty years old)

- Early onset of menstruation (before the age of twelve)

- Family history of breast cancer, in either a first-degree relative (mother, sister, daughter) or a second-degree relative (aunt, grandmother)

- Late menopause (after the age of fifty-five)

- Giving birth to a first child after the age of thirty

- Hormone replacement therapy

- Benign breast disease with biopsy showing atypical hyperplasia

- Regular alcohol consumption

Note: Early or surgically induced menopause decreases the risk of breast cancer.

Learning to form such mutually nurturing relationships, as part of a commitment to love and nurture ourselves on every level, will improve the health of every organ in the body. But the breasts are particularly likely to be affected, because the breasts are located in the fourth emotional centre, which is associated with the ability to express joy, love, grief, and forgiveness, as well as anger and hostility. If those emotions are blocked, then the health of all the organs in the fourth emotional centre, which include the lungs and heart as well as the breasts, may suffer.

Forming loving relationships that nurture us, and nurturing ourselves directly through the choices we make about how we live our lives, can help us to create breast health. Such nurturing is not selfish; in fact, it allows us to have within us something that is worth giving to others. Here again we can look to breast-feeding for the wisdom inherent in our bodies. Both the quality and quantity of a mother's milk are improved when the mother herself is well rested, well nourished, and happy. We need to remember this lesson at midlife, when the opportunity for transformation is boundless and the costs of turning our backs on it may be very high.

The Emotional Anatomy of Breast Cancer

Like all diseases, cancer has an emotional component as well as a physical one. Many women with breast cancer have a tendency to hide their emotions behind a stoic face and to stay in relationships where they give much more than they receive.

The refusal to honour and express our own emotions can sometimes reach pathological extremes. A woman once came to see me because she said she was having trouble breathing. She arrived alone and unsupported, and the tests I had done on her soon confirmed my fear that her breast cancer, which had been diagnosed a year before, had spread to her lungs. She had never sought treatment for her condition because she had not wanted to 'inconvenience' her husband or her children. In fact, she had not even let them know about her condition. I told her as gently as possible that her choices, though made in the spirit of generosity and self-sacrifice, were not really helping anyone, least of all herself. She needed support and nurturance, and her family needed to be included in what was happening to her.

In my experience, many women have been denying their needs for so long that they do not even know they have them. One of my friends recalled growing up with a mother whose automatic response to any desire she ever expressed was 'Don't ask, don't even think about it.' Imagine what that does to a person's ability to ask for what she needs, to express her feelings honestly. No wonder so many women will do almost anything to avoid appearing self-centred – to the point of putting themselves at risk of dying of terminal illness.

There are now many scientific studies confirming the idea that our emotional style may influence both the incidence of breast cancer and our ability to recover from it. One study, for example, involving 119 women between the ages of twenty and seventy who were referred for breast biopsy because of suspicious breast lumps, looked into the impact of adverse life events on the likelihood of the breast lump being cancerous. Severe crises such as divorce, death of a loved one, or loss of a job in the five years preceding the breast lump did indeed increase the chance of its being cancerous. But interestingly, the way in which a woman dealt with adversity was also a significant factor in whether she developed cancer. Those who had allowed themselves to experience their grief fully when they confronted devastating losses were three times less likely to suffer from breast cancer than those who hid their emotions behind a brave face or submerged their grief in various forms of activity.[2]

Not allowing ourselves to grieve uses up vital energy, depriving us of the resources we need to heal. At times of loss we must go through the painful and difficult process that I refer to as radical surrender: we must surrender to a power and order that is bigger than we are. Call it what you will – God, the universe, whatever – we must allow this power to heal our lives, and this can happen only through the full experiencing of our grief.

Another study showed that a woman's feelings about the communication between her and her family, and about the availability of help from her family, affected the function of her immune system and therefore her ability to recover. Women with breast cancer who perceived a lack of social support were found to have immune system depression and a poorer prognosis.[3] On the other hand, social support doesn't have to be from your family to have a positive impact on survival. Studies have shown that breast cancer or other support groups characterised by open and honest sharing of experience are associated with increased longevity and decreased rate of tumour recurrence.[4]

MARY: THE TEN-YEAR PLAN

Mary was forty-one when she called my research partner Dr Mona
Lisa Schulz for an intuitive reading. Married to a fiercely competitive
businessman who spent more time on the road than he did at home,
Mary longed for the day when her husband's business would finally
be self-sustaining enough to allow him to stop travelling so much. She
herself had once been a high-powered executive in the computer
industry but was now a stay-at-home mum with two children, aged
six and nine. As part of the ten-year plan for work, finances, and
family that she and her husband had developed, she had left her career
in order to devote herself full time to bringing up the two children
they had and the two they were planning to have in the time
remaining on that plan.

The problem was, only five years into the plan, Mary was
exhausted. As she told Dr Schulz, she was putting off having a third
child until she could get a handle on why she felt so terrible all the
time. She wanted to know what her body was trying to tell her
through her fatigue. That was why she had scheduled a reading with
Mona Lisa.

The reading Dr Schulz did on Mary revealed an energy pattern that
was like that of 'a widow pacing back and forth on a widow's walk,
forever looking out to sea, waiting and pining for her husband to
return'. On the basis of what she had read energetically, she told Mary
that she, like other women with this pattern of behaviour, could have a
tendency to form hormonally sensitive densities in her breasts.
(Since Dr Schulz does not make diagnoses during readings, she would
never use the term 'breast cancer' or even 'benign breast lump', both of
which are diagnostic terms.)

At this point, Mary revealed that she had, in fact, been diagnosed
with breast cancer four years earlier. The surgery, chemotherapy, and
radiation seemed to have successfully eradicated the cancer, but she
still felt completely drained by the experience.

Dr Schulz asked Mary what she thought was going on in her life.
Mary knew that something was painfully out of balance, but she
didn't know exactly what. She missed her old job and was aware that
staying at home didn't suit her temperament, but she felt that she
should just learn to make the best of it in the interests of the plan she
had agreed to. She was also aware of how much she longed for her
husband to share in the bringing up of their children, but felt she

couldn't voice this longing because it would interfere with his ability to complete his part of the ten-year plan.

Dr Schulz explained to Mary that all illness is a hologram that contains genetic, environmental, physical, nutritional, emotional, spiritual, and behavioural aspects simultaneously. For Mary, the understanding of that hologram would require her to question the validity of the plan that had locked her and her husband into a way of life that was in fact unsatisfactory to both of them. Her breast cancer had been a signal to her, and the fatigue that had enveloped her ever since then was another signal. Her task was to awaken to the message that her body was trying to give her. She needed to accept the fact that she was not temperamentally suited to be a stay-at-home mother. Some women would, of course, thrive in such circumstances if, like Mary, they had the economic wherewithal to support that lifestyle. Mary just didn't happen to be one of them.

But Mary hadn't allowed herself to own her dissatisfaction consciously because she and her husband were both wedded not just to their plan, but to an outdated view of gender roles: the woman is to be the full-time nurturer, the man the good provider. Mary's unhappiness seemed to her to be her own fault, a sign that she was not a good mother – so it was something she thought she needed to fight against, not act on.

Programme for Creating Breast Health Through Full Emotional Expression

The following is the programme Dr Schulz and I put together for Mary and other midlife women who are ready to create breast health more fully.

• *Be honest about what you're feeling.* Dr Schulz noted that Mary was too sweet and nice, despite being in a very difficult situation. She'd say things like 'It's not that bad. It's OK, I can handle it.' And then two seconds later she'd tell Dr Schulz how frustrated she actually was with her situation. Her response reminded me of an episode of the old TV sitcom *Golden Girls,* in which Blanche was trying to come to grips with her son's decision to marry a much older woman who was pregnant with his child. When a friend of hers asked her what she planned to do, she replied, 'Do what mothers always do. Tell my son I love him and that anything he does is fine with me, then complain like hell to anyone else who will listen.' This pattern, though funny in a sitcom, is exactly what creates disruption in the energy of our fourth emotional centre.

Creating health instead of havoc in your emotional centres requires you to extinguish those 'I'm fine' phrases from your vocabulary when they are covering up real and painful emotions that need to be expressed. You may need to work with a therapist to help you learn how to be honest first with yourself, and then with your mate or other family members.

You also need the courage to be honest with yourself about any aspect of your life that you aren't ready to change. Given our cultural inheritance about our breasts, it is little wonder that women's fear of breast cancer far overshadows our risk of those things that are more likely to kill us either directly or indirectly, such as heart disease or being battered by a husband or boyfriend. I've come to believe that the fear of breast cancer serves to numb us to what we're really afraid of – being abandoned and left alone while continuing to pine for true love and the improvement of the relationship we're in. One of my patients, a woman with breast cancer who was also supporting her husband financially and had the means to change her life, finally admitted to me that she continued to stay in her loveless marriage because it felt so much easier for her to die than to risk being the one to be abandoned or left alone first.

• *Create a life plan.* Draw up a one- or two-year life plan just for yourself (not for your mate or family members). Spend at least thirty minutes dreaming about how you'd like to fill your time, where you'd like to go, whom you'd like to be with, and so on. When we went over the life plan concept with Mary, she admitted that even the thought of having a third child exhausted her. Gradually she began to come to terms with the fact that the two additional children called for in their infamous ten-year plan might not be right for her. Clearly Mary's body in general, and her breasts in particular, had been trying to tell her this for a long time.

• *Create an energy budget.* Draw up a balance sheet with one column listing the activities that rejuvenate you and the other listing the activities that drain you. Then make a daily expenditure plan that tips the balance in favour of rejuvenation. (If you have young children, for example, I'd suggest that you share child care with other mothers or grandmothers locally.) Commit yourself to engaging in at least one activity per week that is pleasurable to you – regardless of what your family members think of it. Understand that this is a process, not a destination. It took me four years to tell my husband that I was having massages. Until then, even though I had made them part of my regular schedule, I didn't have the courage to admit to him that I was actually spending time and money on something so nurturing and pleasurable.

• *Maintain a relationship with your own creativity.* Keep your mind engaged. Mary felt hers was rotting away. She was clearly someone who needed the stimulation of a job. Don't allow your mind and your creativity to wither or permit your true self to get lost in the daily grind of living. If you're not working regularly, consider taking a class or engaging in some other stimulating activity on a regular basis. I've found time and again that the very act of having a routine tends to help us conserve and direct our energies. (I always practised my harp with much greater focus when I knew I had a performance coming up.) There is no substitute for having some order, discipline, and structure in your daily life. Just be sure that you are creating the structure, not the other way around.

• *Periodically re-evaluate your goals and plans.* I do this each year around my birthday, and also during the solstices and equinoxes of the year – times when the creative energies of the earth are maximally available to us. Let go of anything that is clearly obsolete and incompatible with your emerging inner wisdom. Mary told us later that when she asked her husband how *his* body was responding to their ten-year plan, he told her that his old ulcer had been acting up lately. But he hadn't wanted to share that with her, because he felt that he needed to show his love and support for his family by remaining a 'good provider'. This is a good example of how a basically good marriage can change and grow when people are honest with each other – and themselves – about their needs.

Lifestyle and Breast Health

Though I'm convinced that the most important part of creating daily breast health is achieved through the energetic influence of self-nurturance and mutually reinforcing relationships, the health of our breasts, like that of every other bodily organ, is also affected by what we eat and by other lifestyle choices.

The Fat Connection

A substantial body of research has linked the consumption of dietary fat with various breast symptoms and breast cancer. For years I advised my patients, particularly those at high risk of breast cancer, to follow a low-fat, high-fibre diet – the one that I felt was the most likely to keep breast tissue healthy. Because this type of diet was so often nutritionally superior to the ones my patients had been on previously, they often experienced improvement in symptoms such as breast pain and the lumpiness of fibrocystic breasts. (Though often termed a 'disease', this is simply an anatomical variation in which the glandular areas are more prominently palpable to the touch.) A low-fat, high-fibre diet also increases the excretion of excess oestrogen, thus lowering potential overstimulation of oestrogen-sensitive breast tissue.

However, some recent research suggests that the breast cancer–fat connection is not as straightforward as previously thought. It comes from an analysis of the diets of 88,795 women, aged thirty to fifty-five, from the famous Nurses' Health Study of nurses in the US, who had completed detailed questionnaires about their eating habits every four years from 1980 to 1994. This phase of the study focused on fat because it was known that Asian women, who eat a diet much lower in fat than ours, also have a much lower rate of breast cancer. However, breast cancer was found to be no more common among the women in the Nurses' Study who ate a lot of fat than among those who consumed less than 20 per cent of their calories in the form of fat. Furthermore, there appeared to be no difference in breast cancer incidence among those who ate saturated fats, or even the infamous trans fats, versus those whose fats were derived mainly from vegetable sources or from fish!

In response to these surprising results, the study's leading author, Dr Michelle Homes, an instructor of medicine at Harvard, said, 'Our research indicates it's highly unlikely that women who consume a low-fat diet are protected against breast cancer. Equally, it appears that a high-fat diet also poses no increased risk for the disease.'[5]

Though I would have been surprised by this study back in the 1980s, I'm not surprised now. Breast cancer is multifactorial, with nutritional, emotional, and genetic aspects. Nutritionally, I'm convinced that sugar and refined carbohydrates are a far bigger risk factor for breast cancer than dietary fat content, but unfortunately they weren't taken into account in this study. Nor were other factors that may help account for the low rate of breast cancer in Asian women. The different micronutrient intake, the high intake of plant hormones such as the isoflavones found in soya, and a lower amount of refined carbohydrates in their diet may all turn out to be factors that lower breast cancer risk.[6]

The Sugar–Insulin Connection

One thing we do know from recent research is that breast cancer is associated with a substance known as insulin-like growth factor (IGF-1). This substance affects the growth of breast cells in utero, during puberty, and during adult life. Abnormal IGF-1 activity is caused by insulin levels that are too high – a direct result of a diet too high in refined carbohydrates. (See chapter 7.) High insulin levels also suppress sex hormone-binding globulin (SHBG), which ordinarily circulates through the body binding oestrogen and lowering its activity. With less SHBG in the bloodstream, more biologically active oestradiol reaches the breast tissue. Over the course of many years, this relative excess of oestrogen may increase the risk of breast cancer.[7]

Alcohol Consumption

Many studies have linked the consumption of alcohol with increased risk of breast cancer. The risk increases with the amount of alcohol consumed. In the Nurses' Health Study, for example, researchers found that the risk of breast cancer in women who had one or more drinks per day was 60 per cent higher than the risk in women who did not drink.[8] Part of this is due to alcohol's effect on the liver's ability to process oestrogen effectively.

For women who are taking oral oestrogen replacement therapy, the risk of drinking alcohol may be even higher. In one study, women on oral oestrogen and synthetic progestogen replacement who drank the equivalent of half a glass of wine experienced increases in oestradiol levels in their blood of 327 per cent, a rise that didn't happen in women not on oral hormone replacement. Significant rises in oestradiol were noted within ten minutes of drinking the alcohol.[9] In the Nurses' Health Study participants this was prevented in those women whose average intake of folic acid was at least 600mcg per day. Alcohol is a known inhibitor of folic acid, and folic acid is required for DNA repair mechanisms. High folic acid intake may therefore prevent some of the gene mutations that lead to cancer.[10]

Another part of the alcohol–breast cancer link is that women too often use alcohol as a way to stay out of touch with the painful feelings

of sorrow, anger, and pining for love and relationship that may be associated with increased risk of disease emanating from the fourth chakra.

Smoking

A study published in the *Journal of the American Medical Association*
in 1996 noted that a flawed enzyme present in millions of Americans
(in half of all white women and in an even larger number of those of
Middle Eastern descent) may raise the risk of breast cancer in women
who smoke. Of those with the flawed enzyme, heavy smokers who
had reached menopause had about four times the risk of breast cancer
as non-smokers. Postmenopausal women who had the flaw and who
had smoked any amount at or before the age of sixteen also ran a
similar risk, which supports the theory that exposure to certain toxic
substances may be harmful during the stages of life when breast tissue
is developing.[11]

Smoking, like alcohol consumption, tends to shut down the energy
of the fourth emotional centre, rendering us numb to the situations
we're in and less capable of doing anything to change them for the
better.

Exercise

Regular exercise decreases the risk of breast cancer considerably,
along with all its other well-documented benefits. That's because
regular exercise normalises insulin and blood sugar levels and also
tends to decrease excess body fat, all of which keep oestrogen levels
normal. Women who exercise for about one hour four times per week
reduce their breast cancer risk by at least 30 per cent.[12] You don't need
to do strenuous exercise to get this benefit. Walking, gardening, and
dancing would all be fine.

Eating for Breast Health

Based on current evidence, I'd suggest that you follow the insulin-
balancing diet I've already outlined in chapter 7. Above all, I urge you
to nurture yourself fully every day by eating food that is delicious as
well as healthy. Eat well, because doing so is a way of reaching your
full potential.[13]

I have a fundamental problem with any approach, dietary or
otherwise, that promises to 'prevent' anything. Although there is an

extensive body of evidence supporting the hormone-balancing and health-enhancing effects of the nutrient-dense, insulin-balancing diet I've suggested, there's a problem. Even women who eat perfectly sometimes get breast cancer. If you make food choices only out of the desire to 'prevent' something, then by the law of attraction, you'll actually be carrying the energy of the disease you're afraid of right into your body along with the healthy food!

In the study mentioned above, for example, the nurses who ate the lowest amount of fat (less than 20 per cent of their daily calories) actually had the highest rate of breast cancer in the group. Though surprising at first glance, these data support a link between breast cancer and self-sacrifice, an association that has been scientifically documented. If you are afraid of breast cancer, it will not be helpful for you to become a dietary martyr, always depriving yourself of the foods you love and find nurturing. Imagine eating a small green salad, all the while craving something more substantial, and thinking, 'Well, I'll deprive myself because I'm preventing breast cancer.' Does this feel nurturing or healthy to you? It doesn't to me.

That said, let me review the basics.

• *Eat lots of fruits, vegetables, and linseed.* Research has shown that women who excrete the highest amount of lignans – which are formed in the intestinal tract from plant materials – have the lowest risk of getting breast cancer.[14] The food source with the highest known concentration of health-promoting lignans is flaxseed (linseed). I suggest that you consume 1/4 cup of freshly ground linseed daily. Diets high in plant materials also tend to be higher in fibre, which has been shown to help the body excrete excess oestrogen in the stool.[15]

Numerous studies have also demonstrated that fruits, vegetables, and seasonings such as broccoli, kale, cabbage (the cruciferous vegetables), tomatoes, turmeric, garlic, and onions contain antioxidants and other phytochemicals that protect against cell damage and mutation caused by free radicals. They may also block carcinogens from reaching or reacting with critical target sites throughout the body.[16]

• *Keep refined carbohydrates to a minimum.* Breast tissue is sensitive to excess androgens as well as excess oestrogen, both of which are normalised with a diet that keeps insulin and blood sugar normal. Over time this will become your favourite way of eating.

• *Eat soya.* Whole soya foods often help women with breast tenderness and pain, and they may even offer protection for women with breast cancer, or with high risk for it, thanks to soya isoflavones, which protect oestrogen-sensitive tissue against overstimulation by oestrogen.[17] It is best to get your isoflavones from whole foods, rather than from the purified extracts of soya found in isoflavone tablets or capsules. The more soya you eat, the greater your protection.

Some women have expressed concern about the phyto-oestrogens in soya and in some herbs recommended in menopause. None of the breast cancer risks associated with oestrogen replacement apply to the consumption of these plant hormones. The plant hormones found in whole soya food, dong quai, chaste berry, and black cohosh have never been associated with the promotion of breast cancer in any study. In fact, many studies have shown that they are protective because of their adaptogenic qualities, meaning their ability to modulate the activity of oestrogen in our bodies in a healthy, balanced way.

• *Eat omega-3 fats.* Studies have shown that women whose diet is high in omega-3 fats have a lower risk of developing breast cancer. Research has also shown that supplementing the diet with omega-3 fats can create a healthier ratio of omega-3 to omega-6 fats in breast tissue within three months.[18] I've had several patients who have had significant softening of firm scar tissue around their breast implants when they've supplemented their diets with omega-3 fats daily. A diet that contains adequate amounts of omega-3 fats also results in balanced eicosanoids, which will help prevent inflammation and tumour growth throughout the body. You can get enough omega-3 fats by eating salmon, sardines, or swordfish two or three times per week. Or you can take 100–400mg per day of DHA. Another convenient source of omega-3 fats is ground linseed. As mentioned above, I consider linseed a true perimenopausal superfood and recommend 1/4 cup per day to all women.

• *Get enough vitamin D.* Moderate doses of sunlight increase bone density and also decrease the risk of breast cancer. Oral vitamin D supplementation can also help in the absence of sunlight. (See chapter 12.)

• *Take coenzyme Q₁₀.* Coenzyme Q_{10} (also known as ubiquinone) is present naturally in the body and in organ meats (eg liver and kidneys). It has been shown to improve immune system functioning. Hundreds of studies have also demonstrated its ability to help those with congestive heart disease. Several studies have demonstrated that women with breast cancer have deficiencies in coenzyme Q_{10}. Taking coenzyme Q_{10} in relatively high doses, 90–350mg per day, has been associated with partial or complete remission of breast cancer.[19] In chapter 7 I recommended that all perimenopausal women take 10–100mg per day. If you are at high risk of breast cancer, I'd increase the dose to 70–100mg per day. Since statin drugs (prescribed to lower cholesterol) decrease levels of coenzyme Q_{10}, all women on these drugs should take this supplement.

Breast Cancer Screening

Most women have been taught that regular mammograms and breast self-examinations are the key to breast health. And there is indeed heartening evidence that the mortality rate for breast cancer is decreasing as a result. Recently ultrasounds have also been found helpful in the early diagnosis of breast cancer.

Though screening is an important part of early detection, keep in mind that it cannot actually *prevent* breast cancer. At best, it diagnoses it at an earlier and therefore more treatable stage. My fear, however, is that the massive national campaigns aimed at getting women to have regular mammograms have taught an entire generation that breast cancer screening is synonymous with creating breast health. Participating in disease screening is no substitute for learning the self-care techniques that could transform us.

Depending on individual circumstances, I recommend mammograms, breast self-examinations, and all the other screening technologies. But every perimenopausal woman needs to know about the limitations of screening and take responsibility for creating healthy breast cells daily by nurturing herself with healthy food, avoiding excessive alcohol, stopping smoking, and engaging in mutually satisfying relationships.

The Pros and Cons of Early Detection

The idea that breast cancer can be cured by early detection and prompt treatment rests on the belief that all breast cancers grow at the same rate. They don't. Some cancers grow rapidly and others slowly, which is one of the reasons why just about every one of us has heard about or knows a woman whose regular mammogram screening was normal but who was diagnosed with breast cancer several months later. One possible explanation for this is that mammography screening may be more likely to detect slow-growing, non-aggressive tumours than the kinds of cancers those women had. A study conducted at Yale–New Haven Hospital in the US of all the women who received their first treatment for breast cancer in 1988, for example, showed that those women whose cancers were detected via mammography screening alone had an excellent prognosis, not just because of early detection, but because the cancers so detected were relatively slow-growing or even dormant, thus requiring minimal therapy. Many of the women, for example, had a condition known as ductal carcinoma in situ (DCIS), a type of breast pathology that very often remains completely dormant for a woman's entire life.

In fact, autopsy studies of women who died of other causes, such as accidents, have shown that 40 per cent have some degree of DCIS in their breasts.[20] Other studies have confirmed that the incidence of DCIS has increased more than fourfold since 1980; this type of cancer now accounts for nearly half of all cancers detected by mammogram. The main reason for this dramatic increase is the widespread use of mammographic screening. Dr Gilbert Welch, a researcher at the US Dartmouth–Hitchcock Medical Center, puts the dilemma well when he writes, 'Our ability to detect subtle forms of breast cancer is a two-edged sword. On the one hand, it offers the hope of preventing some cases of advanced breast cancer through early detection and treatment. On the other hand, it fosters increased worry and labels more women as having disease, many of whom would never develop invasive cancer.'[21]

The DCIS Dilemma

DCIS presents a real dilemma for women and doctors alike. Although our increasingly sensitive technology keeps improving our ability to detect early forms of breast cancer, our understanding of what to do with this knowledge is lagging behind. What is clear is that in the majority of women DCIS does not go on to become invasive cancer, which means that only minimal treatment is necessary. Yet many women with DCIS are subjected to very aggressive treatment: surgery, sometimes followed by radiation or tamoxifen or both. The Yale investigators noted, for example, that of the thirty-one women with DCIS in their study, all of whom survived without recurrence, fully 48 per cent underwent mastectomies. The authors noted, 'Since none of these patients had cancer death or recurrence, regardless of the extensiveness of treatment, the need for aggressive forms of therapy might be reconsidered.'[22] That's one of the understatements of the decade. The high rate of DCIS that is picked up on mammograms may also be a factor in the much-celebrated reduction in breast cancer mortality that we've seen over the past twenty years; the women so diagnosed would not have died in any case.

Breast-screening Concerns

Several years ago I gave a lecture to a group that included doctors, allied health care professionals, and others interested in a more holistic approach to health. I presented the data on mammograms and DCIS and suggested that women may want this information when making decisions about if, when, and how often to have mammograms. I was dismayed by the reaction.

In the ladies' room during a break, women from the audience were confused and upset. They deeply believed in mammograms and felt safe when they had them. I had introduced doubt. I couldn't help wondering if, by telling the truth about the diagnosis and treatment questions raised by our improved technology, I had inadvertently broken my Hippocratic oath: 'First, do no harm.' But I decided that confusion is often the first step on the road to clarity and personal power. If a period of uncertainty and questioning was required for these women to rely more on their inner wisdom, then I decided that in the long run I'd done more good than harm. After all, there is nothing benign about surgery, radiation, and drug therapy, with all their well-known side effects, when they aren't absolutely necessary.

When I came back from the ladies' room I was met by an infuriated radiologist who ran a breast-screening centre. 'You're dangerous. Do you know that?' he spat at me. 'I cannot believe that you're telling women this stuff. I am so disappointed in you. You're putting women's lives at risk.' He wasn't interested in the scientific reasons for my statements, and it was clear to me that we weren't going to have a balanced discussion about the mammogram issue. His mind was made up. Then and there I learned directly and painfully that when it comes to breasts and mammograms, emotions run very high, and this has nothing to do with science.

In 1996 the US National Institutes of Health appointed a panel of prestigious experts who spent six weeks reviewing more than a hundred scientific papers and hearing thirty-two oral presentations on this issue. They concluded that there wasn't enough evidence to recommend routine mammography screening for all women aged forty to fifty. Women in the UK are recommended to have three-yearly screening after the age of fifty.

My Breast-screening Suggestions

• *Have a yearly breast exam from a health care professional.* The next time you have a medical check-up or go for your smear test, ask the doctor or nurse to go over your breast anatomy with you so that you can know exactly what normal feels like. (Far too many women think that their breasts are lumpy when they're simply feeling normal glandular tissue.) Once you know what normal feels like, get to know your breasts at different times during your menstrual cycle, because they feel different depending upon hormone levels. Breasts are usually easiest to examine during the first half of the menstrual cycle, when hormonal stimulation is at a minimum. During perimenopause, however, when menstrual periods are erratic and irregular, there's no way to tell for sure what part of the cycle you are in. Breasts may feel swollen and 'premenstrual' for weeks at a time. This is generally because progesterone levels are low, not because something is wrong. It's important to appreciate this variation.

• *Do regular breast self-examinations.* Every woman should know how her breasts feel and be familiar with their anatomy. Remember, without any coaching whatsoever, women find the great majority of breast cancers themselves. However, it is good to learn to do this in a non-mechanical way. As Dr Francis Moore of the US Harvard Medical School wrote, 'What man would enjoy lowering his trousers in front of a mirror once a month and examining both testicles carefully, by rigorous palpation, looking for testicular tumors?'[23]

What I recommend instead is a monthly breast self-massage. (Do not do this if you have been diagnosed with breast cancer, because it may increase tumour spread.) Many women never touch their breasts with love or tenderness, having been led to believe that their breasts are the property of their mates and not really part of their own bodies. Invite your breasts into your life by getting to know them and touching them regularly. Then your regular breast self-examination becomes an opportunity for healing. Breast massage activates lymph drainage, increases blood flow, and oxygenates tissue – all good ways to help create breast health. After all, for millions of years of human evolution, women nursed babies for most of their reproductive years, a process that provides a great deal of breast stimulation. This massage can also be done by your partner in a non-sexual, supportive way.

Here's a technique developed by Dana Wyrick, who practises lymphedema therapy at Mesa Physical Therapy/San Diego Virtual Lymphedema Clinic in San Diego, California in the US.[24]

SELF-MASSAGE OF CHEST AND BREAST

Do each side of your chest independently. Instructions below are for the left side; simply reverse 'hand' instruction to do your right side. Use a light touch. Your object is to *move the skin,* not to massage the muscles. The following routine, when done properly, will assist the lymphatic capillaries in removing toxins and impurities from the body tissue. The stroking will also accelerate transport of impurities to the lymph nodes, where they will be processed and rendered harmless. Finally, cleansed lymph will be returned to the bloodstream, where the now harmless impurities may be carried to the lungs, kidneys, and colon for elimination.

1. With the first three fingers of your right hand, locate the hollow above your left collarbone. Stroking from your shoulders towards your neck, lightly stretch the skin in the hollow. Repeat this movement five to ten times.

2. Now cover the hairy part of your left armpit with the fingers of your right hand held very flat. Stretch the skin of your armpit upwards five to ten times.

3. Next, again using a flat right hand, lightly stroke ('pet') the skin from the breastbone to the armpit. Do this above the breast, over the breast, and below the breast, repeating each path five to ten times.

4. Finally, using a flat right hand, lightly stroke from your waist up to your armpit on your left side, repeating five to ten times.

Now change hands and massage the right side of your chest.

FIGURE 19: THE LYMPH SYSTEM

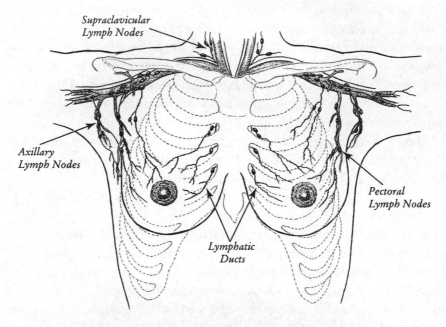

Supraclavicular
Lymph Nodes

Axillary
Lymph Nodes

Pectoral
Lymph Nodes

Lymphatic
Ducts

Every cell in the breasts and other organs is bathed in lymph.
Lymph carries nutrients and immune cells thoughout the body and filters
waste products through the lymph nodes, where they can be detoxified.
Stimulating lymph circulation through regular massage of the breast and
chest wall area can help maintain healthy breast tissue.
© 2001 by Northrup and Schulz

• *Mammograms for women ages thirty-five to fifty.* Consider having
a biennial mammogram and/or ultrasound or other screening if you
have a positive family history of breast cancer or if you find that
getting this screening puts your mind at ease. (Peace of mind produces
very positive biochemical changes in the body.) If you have a close
relative who got breast cancer before the menopause, consider annual
screening mammograms starting five years before the age your
relative was diagnosed. You may need to pay for this privately if your
doctor does not agree that it is indicated on the NHS. Contact your
local private hospital who will usually arrange this, either as part of a
women's health screening, or as simply an ultrasound or mammogram.

Note: The breasts of women under the age of fifty (and some who
are fifty and older) can be extremely dense because of normal ductal
connective tissue. This makes mammograms difficult to read and

interpret, since the X-rays can't penetrate the dense tissue. In older women this dense tissue is often replaced with fat, making mammograms more accurate. In women with dense breasts, about fifty out of a thousand will require further diagnostic procedures, such as additional mammograms, ultrasounds, and even biopsies, to determine whether or not they have breast cancer. Of these, it is estimated that only two will have breast cancer.[25] The others will often go through a great deal of anxiety, which I wish could be avoided!

• *Mammograms for women aged fifty and over.* All major medical associations agree that after the age of fifty, mammograms result in early detection and decreased mortality from breast cancer. Ideally, you may like to have a yearly or two-yearly mammogram. The NHS provides them three-yearly and you would need to arrange the additional tests privately yourself.

If You Find a Breast Lump

• *If you find a lump, get a diagnosis.* It's important to see your doctor who can help you through the process of finding out whether your breast lump is benign or cancerous. You will usually be referred to a specialist breast clinic.

• *Always take someone with you.* Many women who have found a breast lump are too frightened and overwhelmed to ask questions and explore all their options with their consultant. Having a companion can help you focus; if he or she takes notes, you can review them together later.

• *Don't let anyone rush your decision.* Many options are available for the diagnosis and treatment of breast lumps, ranging from breast cyst aspiration to needle biopsy to open biopsy. Most breast lumps or thickenings actually turn out to be benign. Many are simply fluid-filled cysts, which can be aspirated on an outpatient basis. If the fluid is clear, you have both your diagnosis and treatment at the same time. Nothing further needs to be done. Often breast lumps or thickenings are the result of hormonal stimulation and will go away after you get your period. This is particularly true during perimenopause, when oestrogen overstimulation of breasts is so common. One of my patients developed large, painful lumps in both of her breasts throughout her perimenopause. This really scared her and also made it difficult to tell what was really going on in her breasts. After she finally had her last period, however, her breasts returned to their normal consistency, and her lumps went away for good.

• *Get a second opinion if you're not completely comfortable with the first.* Even if you do have cancer, in the vast majority of cases your treatment will not be compromised if you take a couple of weeks or even months to find a doctor you trust and feel comfortable with.

• *If you're diagnosed with breast cancer, ask about sentinel node biopsy instead of removal of all your lymph nodes.* Removal of the lymph nodes in the armpit of the affected side, a procedure known as lymphadenectomy or lymph node dissection, is often done routinely to assess the extent of a tumour. This is called tumour staging and is done to determine treatment options. The problem with removal of the nodes, however, is that the procedure often results in painful and disabling swelling of the arm (known as lymphoedema) for years to come – a pretty high price to pay for staging of small breast tumours in which the lymph nodes are nearly always free of tumour.

An increasingly popular alternative to lymph node dissection is known as the sentinel node biopsy, in which the surgeon removes a single axillary lymph node, the sentinel node, which is the first to receive malignant cells from a breast tumour. The procedure is done in partnership with a radiologist, who injects a dye into the lymph system that guides the surgeon to the right location and also provides information about the status of the lymph nodes. In the vast majority of women with breast cancer who don't have obviously enlarged lymph nodes in the armpit, the sentinel node biopsy will be negative. This spares them from a complete lymph node dissection.[26] If your breast surgeon doesn't do this procedure, seek a second opinion.

Putting Breast Cancer Risk in Perspective

Most women grossly overestimate their risk of breast cancer. Recent surveys of women between the ages of forty-five and sixty-four show that 61 per cent feared cancer (predominantly breast cancer) more than any other disease. Only 9 per cent feared heart disease the most,

If You Have Been Diagnosed with Breast Cancer

Join a breast cancer or other support group in your area. Studies have shown that support groups characterised by open and honest sharing are associated with increased longevity and decreased rate of recurrence of tumour. Besides, a support group is a very safe place to learn how to ask for what you need – or even discover those needs in the first place.

The following books are personal accounts by women who have had breast cancer or who have helped others find their way through the experience. They provide powerful support for your inner wisdom during this time, as well as a wealth of practical information.

Sacred Choices: The Gentle Art of Disarming a Disease and Reclaiming Your Joy, by Judie Chiappone (Holistic Reflections, 2000).

My Healing from Breast Cancer, by Dr Barbara Joseph (Keats Publishing, 1996).

Fighting Spirit: The Stories of Women in the Bristol Breast Cancer Survey, edited by Heather Goodare (Scarlet Press, 1996).

A Cancer Battle Plan, by Anne E. Frähm with David J. Frähm (Tarcher–Putnam, 1997).

despite the fact that it is the leading cause of death in women, claiming more women's lives each year than the next fourteen causes combined.[27] Breast cancer isn't even the leading cause of death from cancer in women. That distinction goes to lung cancer.

Though every one of us probably knows a woman with breast cancer, and though breast cancer is the most common cancer among British women, the lifetime risk of breast cancer – the widely touted one-in-twelve-women figure – applies only if you live beyond the age of eighty-five.[28] The one woman in twelve who does develop breast cancer has a 50 per cent chance of receiving the diagnosis after the age of sixty-five and a 60 per cent chance of dying from another cause.

Kelly-Anne Phillips and her colleagues at Princess Margaret Hospital in Toronto, Ontario, Canada, have constructed a very helpful chart based on the 1995 incidence and mortality rates in the Ontario Cancer Registry. Here's what it shows.

Out of 1,000 females born healthy and alive:

- Aged 35–39: 986 will be alive. Of these, 1 will get breast cancer, 0 will die from it, and 2 will die of other causes.

- Aged 40–44: 983 will be alive. Of these, 5 will get breast cancer, 1 will die from it, and 4 will die of other causes.

- Aged 45–49: 977 will be alive. Of these, 8 will get breast cancer, 2 will die from it, and 6 will die of other causes.

- Aged 50–54: 968 will be alive. Of these, 11 will get breast cancer, 3 will die from it, and 11 will die of other causes.[29]

The irrational fear of breast cancer creates a great deal of suffering for women and prevents many from enjoying the benefits of peri-menopausal treatments – such as high-dose soya, bioidentical progesterone, low-dose bioidentical oestrogen – that can relieve symptoms and help prevent diseases that are far more likely to be a threat to longevity or quality of life.

The Breast Cancer Gene: Should You Be Tested?

Approximately 5 to 7 per cent of all breast cancer is attributable to inherited mutations in two different genes: BRCA1 and BRCA2. Women who inherit a BRCA1 mutation have a higher risk than those with a BRCA2 mutation. They have a 56 per cent lifetime risk of breast cancer and also an estimated 15 per cent risk of developing ovarian cancer by the age of seventy. Though less is known about the BRCA2 mutation, it is estimated that it will account for an additional 40 per cent of hereditary breast cancers.[30]

The true frequency and implications of breast cancer gene mutations are still uncertain, in part because the BRCA1 gene is very large and many different mutations have been found within it. One particular BRCA1 mutation has now been detected in approximately 1 per cent of Jews of Eastern European descent. Different mutations have been found in other populations. In addition, there are other gene pathways besides those governed by BRCA1 and BRCA2 mutations that may lead to breast cancer. When you add to this the technical problems of sequencing an entire gene, it is clear that genetic testing for breast cancer risk is an incomplete science. A negative test for the gene may have little meaning in a setting of a strong family history of breast and ovarian cancer.[31] On the other hand, if there is only one individual in the family with breast or ovarian cancer, the chances of this cancer occurring due to a mutation in either BRCA1 or BRCA2 are quite small.

Dr Francis Collins of the National Center for Human Genome Research in Bethesda, Maryland, in the US, summarised the current dilemma associated with testing positive for the breast cancer gene:

We are still profoundly uncertain about the appropriate medical care of women with these mutations. Despite the general usefulness of mammograms for the early detection of breast cancer in women over the age of 50, there are no data to instill confidence that regular mammography at a younger age, in concert with self-examination and examination by doctors or nurses, will reduce the risk of death from metastatic breast cancer among very-high-risk women with BRCA1 mutations. We do not yet know the appropriate use of more drastic measures, such as prophylactic mastectomy, especially given the anecdotal evidence that cancer can still occasionally arise in the small amount of epithelial tissues remaining after surgery .... Clinical research is urgently needed to address all these uncertainties.[32]

Testing also raises the potential for health insurance discrimination, life and disability insurance discrimination, and discrimination in employment.[33]

Here's the bottom line: though a negative test for the breast cancer gene can be a great relief for an individual with a positive family history for breast cancer, it's not a guarantee against getting breast cancer. I do not recommend being tested unless you have at least two or more close family members who've had breast or ovarian cancer. You should also undergo thorough genetic counselling from a professional with extensive knowledge and training in the field, both before and after getting your test results. If your test is positive, seek medical advice from a professional who is actively engaged in research protocols to further our knowledge of these troubling disorders. For further information contact Cancerlink or Bacup (see Resources).

The Effect of HRT on Breast Health

Despite the fact that most women, with or without supplemental hormones, will not get breast cancer, the link between hormones and breast cancer is worrying for everyone concerned. Nearly every woman asks, 'What is the effect of hormones on my risk of breast cancer?' The answer depends on which hormones she is taking, what her dosage is, and what her inherent risk factors are to begin with. These issues were raised by a letter I received from a man concerned about his wife's hormone supplementation programme.

> My wife has recently switched from taking Premarin, which she originally took to quell hot flushes, to taking natural proges-terone in the form of a skin cream. As a result, her breast pain and tenderness have gone away and so have her headaches. What's more, my wife has had almost complete relief from her hot flushes, too. But, as a result of some things I have read about the possible connection between progesterone and breast cancer, I want to be reassured that my wife is on the right track – and that no unscheduled trains will be coming down that track which could cause her harm in the future.

The experience of the woman described in this letter beautifully illustrates the side effects that often result from taking Premarin, the most commonly prescribed drug for perimenopausal symptoms. Breast pain is one of the most common adverse reactions to oestrogen replacement of all kinds, with anywhere from 20 to 35 per cent of women complaining of it when given standard, non-individualised doses.[34] This is especially frightening for women who have a personal or family history of benign breast disease (also known as fibrocystic breast disease), which, in the past, was felt to be associated with an increased risk of breast cancer. Newer research, however, has failed to show any consistent association between benign breast disease and increased risk of breast cancer. Nor does hormone replacement therapy seem to add to the risk for women in this group.[35]

Headaches are also a common side effect, since oestrogen can be metabolised into a substance that is similar to adrenaline and can result in pounding temporal headaches. Bioidentical progesterone, on the other hand, has been shown to stop hot flushes and has none of these side effects.

Many people, however, are uncertain about potential long-term health problems resulting from progesterone, because of a recent study from the US National Cancer Institute (NCI), which documented an increased breast cancer risk for those women on long-term oestrogen/progestogen hormone replacement. What most people (including doctors) do not understand is the difference between the synthetic hormones used in the NCI study and bioidentical oestrogen and progesterone.

Here are the facts. The National Cancer Institute study was a large epidemiological study involving 48,355 women who were on both oestrogen and progestogen for varying periods of time between the years 1980 and 1995. Women of normal weight who took the hormone combination for five years had a 40 per cent increased risk of breast cancer compared to those who were not on hormone replacement. (Intriguingly, women who were overweight did not have this increased risk.) They also had a greater risk of developing breast cancer than those on oestrogen alone.[36]

Though the 40 per cent increased-risk figure sounds very scary, here's what it really means: if you take 100,000 normal-weight women, aged between sixty and sixty-four, who are not on hormone replacement, you could expect 350 cases of breast cancer to develop over a five-year period. If all these women took a combination hormone replacement consisting of conventional oestrogen with progestogen, then the number of cases would increase to 560. As you can quickly see, the vast majority of women would not get breast cancer, with or without hormones.

Here's another way of saying this: statistically speaking, out of 1,000 women who have never taken conventionally prescribed hormones, 77 will get breast cancer by the age of seventy-five. For women who have taken hormones for five years, that figure climbs to 79; after ten years, it is 83; and after fifteen years, it is 89. Again, the vast majority of women who take hormone replacement therapy of any kind do not get breast cancer.

The other key point to keep in mind is that virtually all the women in this study – and in most of the other studies that link hormone replacement with breast cancer – were using non-individualised doses of conjugated oestrogens (usually Premarin) in combination with the synthetic progestogen Provera. Premarin has been the most-prescribed oestrogen either alone for women without a uterus, or in combination with norgestrel as Prempac-C. Each of these non-bioidentical hormones has its own risks.

Studies have shown that when Prempac-C is metabolised in the body, its breakdown products are biologically stronger, and therefore potentially more apt to promote cancer, than the breakdown products of bioidentical oestrogens.[37] It has also been demonstrated that there can be a greater than tenfold variance in blood levels of oestrogen among women on the *same* standard dose of Prempac-C – usually 0.625mg.[38] What is even more disturbing is that many of the women in these studies are on even higher doses, 1.25mg per day.

Synthetic progestogens present their own set of problems. They can bind to both oestrogen and androgen receptors in cells and thus stimulate unhealthy tissue growth. They can also *increase* the biological activity of oestrogen. This may explain why women in the National Cancer Institute study who were on both oestrogen and synthetic progestogen had an even greater risk of developing breast cancer than those women who were on oestrogen only.[39] If you are on hormone replacement therapy, you may want to check to see whether or not you are taking anything containing the following synthetic progestogens: medroxyprogesterone acetate – MPA (brand names Provera, Depo-Provera); norethisterone; or norgestrel (see pages 155–6). If you are, you might consider a change to bioidentical hormones.

What it boils down to is this: if you use hormones that are not identical to those produced by a woman's body, at doses that may be too high, you may be incurring a higher than necessary risk of breast cancer, as well as the adverse and additive effects of the metabolites of these hormones.

Bioidentical Hormones and Cancer Risk

There is good reason to believe that the long-term use of bioidentical low-dose oestrogen, balanced with bioidentical progesterone, would result in a very limited increase in breast cancer risk, if any.[40] Here's what every woman should know.

Oestrogen

The breasts are glandular organs that are exquisitely sensitive to cyclical hormonal changes in the body. In the first half of the menstrual cycle oestrogen tends to increase breast tissue growth; in the second half progesterone stabilises and refines this growth. During our menstrual periods our breasts are at their smallest, with both hormones at their lowest levels. During perimenopause, which is characterised by oestrogen dominance and a relative lack of progesterone, a woman's breasts may become larger and more tender with no cyclical waxing and waning to keep breast tissue more stable.

For decades numerous studies have demonstrated that, with the exception of phyto-oestrogens in whole foods, oestrogen of all kinds, even that produced by our own bodies, can promote breast tissue growth. In susceptible individuals, this may be associated with an increased risk of breast cancer.[41] It is this sensitivity to long-term, uninterrupted oestrogen exposure that explains breast cancer risk factors such as early menarche, late menopause, no children, and obesity. Therefore, to preserve breast health, use the least amount of bioidentical oestrogen that gives you the results you seek. And get your salivary hormone levels tested regularly to make sure you're not getting overdosed.

If you have a family history of breast cancer (grandmother, mother, sister, or maternal aunt) or have the gene for breast cancer, you will probably want to avoid oestrogen replacement despite its known benefits, and despite the fact that some very good studies have found that oestrogen replacement doesn't promote breast tumour growth even in those who have had breast cancer. *There are currently no clinical studies showing that oestrogen increases the rate of relapse among women who have had breast cancer.*[42]

Opting not to use oestrogen doesn't mean you have to suffer in silence. Many alternatives can relieve your symptoms, improve your health, and also protect your breasts: exercise, dietary improvement, whole soya, herbs, and natural progesterone. These alternatives can offer good results even if you have a strong family history of osteoporosis or Alzheimer's disease, and are concerned about not being able to get the benefits of oestrogen.

OESTRIOL: Preliminary studies have shown that women who excrete the highest levels of oestriol in their urine appear to have a lower risk of breast cancer. For that reason, many doctors, including me, have sometimes used oestriol, a non-patentable bioidentical oestrogen, in their patients' hormone replacement regimens. Oestriol is biologically weaker than oestradiol and oestrone, the two other oestrogens produced naturally in the body; as already discussed in chapter 9, it works very well when applied locally to oestrogen-sensitive tissue such as the vagina. Since oestriol, which is widely used in Europe, has been found to stimulate endometrial cells in the uterus, it may stimulate breast tissue as well. Nevertheless, in individualised doses, oestriol is a perfectly reasonable oestrogen to use for replacement.

Progesterone

Though the widely publicised study from the National Cancer Institute mentioned previously suggested that synthetic progestogen is not protective against breast cancer, its conclusions cannot be applied to the natural, bioidentical progesterone found in such preparations as ProGest or ProJuven creams. In fact, it makes biological sense that adding bioidentical progesterone (which has no androgenic or oestrogenic activity) to oestrogen replacement regimens could actually help protect the breasts against overstimulation from oestrogen and thus further decrease the risk of breast cancer. Bioidentical progesterone has been shown to reduce oestrogen-receptor production on breast cells and also to decrease the production of oestrogen within breast cells. Some women experience transient breast tenderness in the first week or so of bioidentical progesterone use, since it initially increases oestrogen receptors in the breasts. However, this effect is very short-lived and goes away after several days. There is no convincing evidence that bioidentical progesterone causes continued growth of breast tissue. In fact, it appears to do just the opposite.

At this time we simply do not have enough data on women using bioidentical oestrogens and progesterone. Most of the studies on hormone replacement therapy – including the huge, ongoing, US government-funded Women's Health Initiative – have been done using non-bioidentical hormones. We urgently need long-term epidemiological studies of bioidentical, individualised hormone replacement therapy, in order to provide adequate guidance to women and their doctors. But given the politics of medicine and research (including the fact that bioidentical hormones cannot be patented), we're not likely to have these studies for a long time to come.

Genes, Hormones, and Breast Cancer: The Cell Growth–Cell Death Cycle

If we were to do a very large, long-term study on natural proges-terone, we would probably find that it offers protection to the breast, especially if used without oestrogen during perimenopause, when oestrogen dominance is so common. The reasons for this have to do with the fact that progesterone plays a role in cell death. Let me explain why this turns out to be a good thing.

Nature in all her wisdom has created a balance between breast tissue cell growth and breast tissue cell death. Breast cancer is one of the health problems that arises when there's an imbalance between these two processes. Breast cancer – like all cancers, actually – is characterised by two processes: (1) excessive and uncontrolled cell division, and (2) a lack of normal, healthy programmed cell death.[43] The signals that direct cell growth, cell development, and programmed cell death (called apoptosis) are directed by the interac-tion between our genes and our environment. Though this process is extraordinarily complex, we are beginning to understand it, thanks to advances in molecular biology. For instance, we now understand that a gene known as the BCL2 gene blocks cell death. This function is appropriate for the times when breast cell tissue needs to grow (such as at puberty and at the ovulatory stage of the menstrual cycle).[44] However, when the BCL2 function is not modulated by other factors, it can cause inappropriate cell longevity and possible uncontrolled growth, which can lead to an increased risk of breast cancer. BCL2 is known as a proto-oncogene, which means that it promotes cancer if its expression goes unchecked.

Another gene that influences breast tissue is p53. The p53 gene, in contrast to BCL2, is a tumour suppression gene; it halts uncontrolled cell division by increasing apoptosis (cell death). Activation of this gene helps to prevent cell overgrowth and subsequent cancer.

As it turns out, the p53 and BCL2 genes are influenced by sex hormones in ways that either favour cancer or protect against it. Oestrogen increases the expression of the BCL2 gene and thus promotes breast cell growth. As I already mentioned, this isn't necessarily a bad thing. But unabated expression of the BCL2 gene due to excessive amounts of oestrogen can result in increased growth of oestrogen-sensitive tissue in the breasts, uterus, and ovaries. It is well known that the risk of cancers in these organs is associated with excessive oestrogen stimulation.[45]

In contrast, progesterone decreases the expression of the BCL2 gene while increasing the expression of the p53 gene, leading to an increase in programmed cell death at an appropriate time and thus to a decreased risk of cancer in oestrogen-sensitive tissues.[46]

Oestrogen and progesterone also differ in the *kinds* of breast tissue they stimulate. Oestrogen causes breast cells known as ductal tissue to divide and grow. Unopposed oestrogen has the capacity to create uncontrolled growth of breast tissue – including cancerous growth. Progesterone, on the other hand, causes the breast cells to differentiate into lobular cells – nature's preparation for milk production if pregnancy were to happen. If a woman does not get pregnant, these lobular cells simply undergo programmed cell death, dying off naturally at the end of their life cycle. In other words, a well-differentiated lobular cell is not capable of growing into a cancer.

A very helpful analogy was given to me by Dr David Zava, a researcher with years of experience studying the effects of hormones on breast tissue.[47] Dr Zava likens the different parts of breast tissue to the different parts of a tree. The ductal tissue, whose growth is promoted by oestrogen, is like the trunk and branches of the tree. The lobular cells, whose growth is promoted by progesterone, is comparable to the leaves that grow from the ends of the branches. Once a tree cell becomes a leaf, it can never go back to being a trunk or a branch. It simply grows up, matures, and eventually dies at the end of its programmed life cycle. This is not true with the trunk or branches, however. Their cells can grow at any time and make an infinite number of branches or growths on the branches or trunk itself – just like the infinite cell proliferation of a breast cancer.

Given the processes I've just outlined, it makes sense that women subject to excessive oestrogen stimulation – whether the oestrogen is produced in their own bodies (eg, during periods of oestrogen dominance, so common during perimenopause, or from excessive production of oestrogen in body fat cells) or is taken in from the outside (through oestrogen replacement or through environmental agents with oestrogen-like activity) – would be at increased risk of getting breast cancer. But if they take enough progesterone to balance this oestrogen, the risk would diminish. And that is precisely what the scientific literature suggests.[48]

For example, a study of women with progesterone *deficiency* from anovulation, who were being followed at an infertility clinic, has shown those women to have a risk of premenopausal breast cancer 5.4 times greater than those in a control group. And in a 1995 study in which transdermal bioidentical progesterone was placed directly on the skin of the breast, researchers found that the progesterone was able to inhibit breast cell proliferation. The dosages used were approximately the same as when a woman is using a transdermal cream such as ProGest or ProJuven – in other words, a 1.5–3 per cent progesterone cream twice per day at recommended dosages. These levels are about equal to those found at ovulation in most women.[49]

Another study showed that those women who had physiologically adequate levels of progesterone at the time of breast cancer surgery had a decreased risk of recurrence, compared to women whose progesterone levels were low.[50] This study has been repeated with the same results, which has led some breast cancer surgeons to suggest that women use 1.5–3 per cent progesterone cream on their skin for a week or so before breast biopsy or surgery. It appears that bioidentical progesterone can enhance immune response. It also seems to make any tumour cells that may be released during surgery less apt to attach to other sites and grow. This may be why women with breast cancer who are operated on during the luteal phase of their menstrual cycles – when progesterone levels are the highest – have a significantly decreased rate of recurrence.[51]

A 1996 review of the evidence on progesterone and breast health concluded that bioidentical progesterone not only reduced the rate of spread of breast cancer, but may even be responsible for reducing the incidence of new cases.[52]

Though no one has done a definitive long-term clinical trial of bioidentical progesterone, my clinical experience and that of many of my colleagues, including Dr John Lee, a pioneer in bioidentical hormone research, has led me to believe that bioidentical progesterone can benefit many women, especially if used during perimenopause, and will very likely be found to decrease the risk of breast and other oestrogen-responsive cancers that may well get their start during this time of life.

Progesterone Preparations and Progesterone Receptor-positive Breast Cancer

One of the questions I'm frequently asked is whether a woman whose breast cancer has tested positive for progesterone receptors can safely take progesterone. There is a great deal of confusion about what it means to have a breast biopsy that shows that the tumour is positive for progesterone receptors, especially in those women who have been using bioidentical progesterone at the time of their diagnosis.

Here are the facts. All breast cancers that are positive for progesterone receptors are also oestrogen receptor–positive. Because oestrogen is known to stimulate growth of these types of cancer cells, many people automatically assume that progesterone must do the same. Just the opposite is true. Positive progesterone receptors indicate that a cancer is receptive to the balancing and anti-cancer effects of progesterone.

To understand this apparent paradox, remember that hormones in the bloodstream and the fluid surrounding cells work by uniting with receptors on the surface of the cell. The hormone fits the receptor like a key in a lock. If the right receptor is there, the hormone message makes its way to the chromosomes and turns on the appropriate gene to produce a specific cellular effect. Progesterone signals the cell to stop multiplying, while oestrogen signals the opposite. For that reason, bioidentical progesterone is probably beneficial for women with progesterone receptor–positive breast cancer.

In general, women with oestrogen- and progesterone-positive breast tumours have a good prognosis, since the presence of these receptors means that the tumour is very well differentiated and slower growing than more poorly differentiated tumours.

Though I'm convinced that bioidentical progesterone is safe and even beneficial for women with oestrogen- and progesterone-positive breast cancers, this is a controversial area. Use your inner guidance and consult with your doctor.

My Advice About Progesterone

• If you are currently perimenopausal and using a progesterone cream or another form of bioidentical progesterone such as Crinone, you are helping your body create hormonal balance that may well protect your breasts from overstimulation by oestrogen and androgen. I recommend that you continue to use it, unless your inner guidance tells you otherwise.

• If you are at risk of oestrogen or androgen dominance, consider adding bioidentical progesterone. Conditions associated with oestrogen dominance are the following: irregular periods, body fat percentage greater than 28 per cent, sedentary lifestyle, polycystic ovary syndrome, fibroid tumours of the uterus, breast tenderness, a low-fibre diet high in refined carbohydrates, heavy menstrual periods, and hormone replacement with oestrogen only. Androgen dominance is associated with acne, polycystic ovarian disease, and male pattern baldness.

• Though not all women's health experts agree on the progesterone question, I personally would recommend that every woman who is concerned about her breast health avail herself of the substantial benefits of bioidentical progesterone, especially during the perimenopausal period, when it is well known that she is likely to start skipping ovulations and therefore to have low progesterone levels. Substantial doses of soya protein would be a reasonable alternative to progesterone.

What About Testosterone?

Androgens such as testosterone and even DHEA can be converted into oestrogen in the body, which means that taking testosterone could theoretically increase your risk of breast cancer. Use the lowest dose that gives you the results you need, or try alternatives first.

Here's the bottom line. It is in our best interest to make the wisest choices we can if we opt for hormone replacement – which means using bioidentical, individualised hormone replacement therapy at the lowest doses that give us the results we want. Once we've done that, we simply have to let go of our illusion of control and realise that there are no perfect solutions. We all do the best we can with the information we have at the time. But that information, like us, keeps evolving and changing. This year's best solution may differ from next year's. Nevertheless, most of the time our bodies and our cells maintain their health – which is why the vast majority of women, either on or off hormone replacement, do not get breast cancer.

The Tamoxifen Dilemma

Tamoxifen (trade name Nolvadex) is commonly prescribed to women with breast cancer and also sometimes to prevent breast cancer in high-risk women. It is one of a class of drugs called selective oestrogen receptor modulators (SERMs). Other SERMs include raloxifene (Evista), which is used to prevent and treat osteoporosis. Tamoxifen's anti-oestrogenic effect has been shown to prolong the disease-free interval and overall survival in women with both hormone-receptor-positive and hormone-receptor-negative tumours, as well as in those with positive and negative lymph nodes. It has also been shown to reduce the incidence of breast cancer in high-risk women. Tamoxifen is currently being taken by almost a million women in the US and is the most commonly used cancer drug in the UK.

Although tamoxifen *blocks* oestrogen in some organs, it acts *like* oestrogen in others, including the bones and the cardiovascular system. Thus it has been found to lower cholesterol and reduce the rate of fatal heart attack if taken for five years. It also helps maintain bone density.

Tamoxifen is not without significant risks, however, sometimes due to its oestrogenic properties, other times due to its anti-oestrogenic effects. Some researchers are concerned that its anti-oestrogenic effects on brain tissue may put women at increased risk of dementia or depression.[53] It has been my experience that many women who are taking tamoxifen suffer from depression but don't tell their doctors because they don't want to bother them. In its oestrogenic mode, tamoxifen results in changes in the endometrial lining of the uterus, ranging from atypical hyperplasia (abnormal thickening) and polyps to invasive cancer. The longer you're on it, the greater the risk.[54] This means that any woman on tamoxifen needs to have regular uterine screenings by ultrasound or other means to make sure she doesn't develop uterine cancer.

Another problem with tamoxifen is that if a woman continues to take it for longer than five years, it may stop acting like an anti-oestrogen in her breasts and start to act like an oestrogen.[55] In other words, a woman may develop resistance to it, and, if she does get breast cancer again, it may even increase the chance of the cancer being resistant to treatment.[56]

FIGURE 20: THE BENEFITS AND RISKS OF OESTROGEN-BLOCKING DRUGS

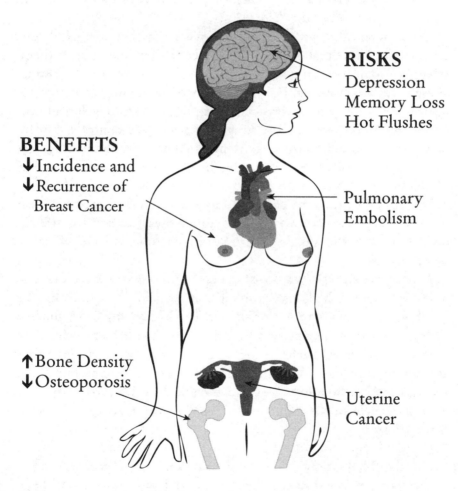

RISKS
Depression
Memory Loss
Hot Flushes

BENEFITS
↓Incidence and
↓Recurrence of
Breast Cancer

Pulmonary
Embolism

↑Bone Density
↓Osteoporosis

Uterine
Cancer

© 2001 by Northrup and Schulz

Tamoxifen for Breast Cancer Prevention

Tamoxifen is currently approved for and marketed to healthy women at risk of breast cancer in the US, but not in the UK. According to a study done by the US National Cancer Institute, the drug reduced the rate of expected breast cancers in a group of 13,000 women in the US and Canada from 1 in 130 women to 1 in 236 women. This represents a 50 per cent reduction in the risk of breast cancer in those women who took it prophylactically. Though two other studies, done in Europe, did not show any breast-cancer-decreasing benefits, the drug was recently approved in the US for prevention of breast cancer in women at high risk of the disease.[57]

Given women's own anxiety and overestimation of their breast cancer risk, I fear that many will take tamoxifen and subject themselves to its unnecessary and significant side effects when healthier alternatives are available. For example, women taking tamoxifen for prevention were two to three times more likely to develop uterine cancer or blood clots in the lung and legs than controls. Stroke, cataracts, and cataract surgery were more common with the drug, too. Most women also experienced some level of hot flushes and vaginal discharge.

So here's the problem. The encouragement to take tamoxifen feeds on women's sense of powerlessness about breast cancer by offering only one solution: taking a drug with significant side effects – including cancer!

Many women who get breast cancer don't have risk factors, and many who are at high risk won't get it. In addition, you can't do anything about many of your risk factors – like having had your first child late in life or having had a mother who had breast cancer. This risk factor approach keeps us focused on our breasts as though they are two premalignant, potentially deadly organs sitting on our chests like ticking time bombs – which is a terrible distortion of reality.

In an article in the *New York Times*, breast specialist Dr Susan Love wrote:

[In the NCI study] tamoxifen was shown to decrease the incidence of breast cancer by 49 per cent in high-risk healthy women. But the number of women in the study who got cancer was relatively small: 4.3 per cent of women developed breast cancer in the placebo group, while 2.2 per cent developed it in the tamoxifen group. This means that 95.7 per cent took tamoxifen with no immediate or short-term benefits and risked side effects including a small but real increase in deaths from lung clots.

More important, perhaps, the women in this study who had had biopsies showing atypical hyperplasia [precancerous changes in the cells lining the milk ducts – a diagnosis that often overlaps with DCIS] and who took tamoxifen reduced their risk of developing breast cancer by 86 per cent. If it were easy to identify which women will develop these changes, we could select which women are most likely to benefit from tamoxifen. But as of now there is no equivalent of a Pap [cervical] smear for breast cancer.

Or if we had a way to monitor women on tamoxifen, we might be able to detect when the cells are beginning to become resistant before they have a chance to do damage …. Thus the real message for women is not that tamoxifen is bad or good, but that it is an interesting drug that we do not fully understand.[58]

My Advice on Tamoxifen and the Other Selective Oestrogen Receptor Modulators

• If you are already on tamoxifen, feel good about it, and are having no side effects, then I'd recommend that you stick with it for up to five years.

• If you've had breast cancer, discuss with your doctor whether your type of cancer has shown a response to tamoxifen, and, if so, how long you should take it.

• If you are at increased risk of breast cancer, decrease that risk by following the suggestions I've given earlier in this chapter.

• If you opt to take tamoxifen or another SERM, get regular medical care, including screening for endometrial abnormalities and cataracts.

• You can decrease some of the side effects of tamoxifen by taking soya, using supplements, and following the dietary guidelines given on pages 420–3.

• Don't take tamoxifen for longer than five years unless you and your doctor feel strongly that your individual situation warrants it.

Remember, the problem of breast cancer can't be solved only at the physical level. Don't be fooled into believing that you must always take a drug to help your body stay well. To create healthy breast tissue, each of us needs to be willing to participate in creating a life that is healthy in mind and spirit as well as body. Sometimes we may need drugs or surgery; at other times we need only the natural strategies I've emphasised in this chapter and throughout this book – eating healthily, taking exercise, stopping smoking, cutting down on or eliminating alcohol, expressing your feelings, loving, and being loved.

FOURTEEN

Living with Heart, Passion, and Joy: How to Listen to and Love Your Midlife Heart

The years around menopause are the time when women's risk of heart disease, hypertension, and stroke rise significantly as our hearts and the network of blood vessels that carries nourishment to every cell in our bodies call out to us more loudly than ever, demanding that we listen well and allow ourselves to feel the exquisite joy of life more fully than ever. Because heart disease in all its guises claims more lives than any other illness, midlife is a time when a change of heart may save your life.

Despite the fact that eleven times more women die of heart disease than breast cancer, failure to diagnose heart disease in a timely manner is rarely the subject of complaints, whereas complaints for failure to diagnose breast cancer are more common. Many women never realise that they have a heart problem until the disease is well established. Breast cancer, on the other hand, is seen as an invader from outside ourselves, so we tend to take a fighting stance towards it, for better or for worse.

When it comes to your heart, however, you can't fight it – you must instead follow its dictates if you are to achieve the vibrant cardiovascular health that will nourish and rejuvenate every organ in your body for the rest of your life. The heart teaches us directly and persistently. And it is quite forgiving if we will simply heed its messages.

The Heart Has Its Say at Menopause:
My Personal Story

In chapter 3 I wrote about my first experience of the 'empty nest':
how I had picked up my younger daughter from her holiday course,
taken her for a college tour, driven the three long hours home with
her sound asleep in the car – and then found myself face to face with
the realisation that her physical presence wouldn't heal my emptiness.
There is a sequel to that story. The next morning I went for a walk.
About halfway through I began to experience an ache in my throat
that radiated up into my jaw. No matter what I did, I couldn't make
the pain go away. It felt as though a lump of food were stuck in my
oesophagus refusing to go down. I kept walking, wondering what this
symptom was all about. When I got home the pain was still there and
impossible to ignore. So I called my friend Mona Lisa Schulz and
asked her to come over and help me through the situation.

The throat is in the fifth emotional centre, which has to do with
communication, so I wondered if there was something I needed to
say. Mona Lisa reminded me, however, that I've never had any trouble
expressing myself. Instead, my family legacy of stoicism and heart
disease pointed to challenges in the fourth emotional centre.

Together we sat down and took out the Motherpeace tarot cards to
try to get some clarity. My intuition, which was reflected in the cards,
suggested that my throat and jaw pain had in fact originated in my
heart. I was also reminded that the classic symptoms of heart attack in
women are often located in the neck, jaw, and upper chest. As I
reviewed the events of the previous twenty-four hours, I came to see
that my literal 'heartache' stemmed from my disappointment and grief
over my reunion with my daughter – a reunion in which my own
needs for partnership and companionship had not materialised at all.

Setting Myself Up for Heartache

Looking back, I see now how I had set myself up for heartache. For
several days before going to pick up my daughter, I had fantasised
about how loving and warm our reunion would be. I anticipated her
every emotional and physical need as I prepared for the trip. I thought
that her return would help me heal from the heartache of my divorce.
In retrospect, I see that by trying to be truly there for her, I was
actually treating her the way I wished someone would treat me. In

addition to the drive together, I had hoped that she'd want to spend some time shopping and having a meal with me. I didn't ask for this outright. I've never wanted to be the kind of mother who manipulates her children into taking care of her needs by staging after-all-I've-done-for-you-at-least-you-could-have-dinner-with-me kinds of scenes. Knowing that this approach confuses love with guilt and obligation, I went to the opposite extreme. It never occurred to me, for instance, that it was OK to ask my daughters to spend an evening or a day with me now and then. Instead, I had led my daughters – and myself – to believe that I didn't have any needs that I couldn't fulfil on my own.

The Stoic Heart: My Legacy

By asking for so little, I was unconsciously carrying on a legacy I had inherited from my stoic maternal line, a legacy that is a set-up for heart disease: if you don't ask for much, you won't be disappointed. Instead, you can earn love by providing service. And if you become strong enough and capable enough to meet your needs for yourself, you'll never have to feel vulnerable, never have to face possible rejection.

My frenzied redecorating in the three weeks prior to my younger daughter's return was not motivated purely by the desire to create a living space that was pleasing to me, though that was part of it. It was also meant to please and delight my daughters. I had envisioned the newly decorated family room as a space in which they could stay up late and watch films with friends with no fear of keeping me awake. I wanted their approval.

After my daughter and I arrived home, I eagerly showed her the new rooms, anticipating oohs, ahhs, and praise. She looked around briefly, said she liked it, wondered why I had chosen those particular cushions, and then settled into phoning the six friends who had left messages for her.

As I unpacked the car to the background of her enthusiastic conversations, I felt as though I had just provided a very nurturing taxi service. When my children were little, providing a warm, safe place for them to grow up was enough. Now I wanted more. But I didn't know that yet. I was simply aware of vague discontent within me. After all, my daughter's behaviour was completely normal for a healthy sixteen-year-old with a burgeoning social life.

Why was I so heartsick? Why did I get chest pain the next morning?

My daughter certainly wasn't responsible for that. What was my heart trying to tell me? Over the next few days I began to unearth and to let go of a big heartache-inducing legacy that was now obsolete.

Keeping the Peace at Any Price Is a Big Pain in the Heart

Like my mother before me, I had been brought up to believe that it was my job to keep the peace in the family and make a comfortable home for my husband and children. I did this – mostly single-handedly – for most of my marriage. After my husband and I separated, I characteristically ploughed ahead, believing that my good-natured efforts would make it OK for the children. The truth is that I was heartsick about putting them through the pain of my divorce and also about stepping down from my position as cheerful emotional buffer for the family. In all this I had neglected the fact that I, too, had emotional needs and that I, too, was hurting and grieving over the loss of my marriage.

In trying to protect my children from their own inevitable pain, I had been doing everything in my power to maintain the illusion that our lives hadn't changed. I shielded them from the reality of bills to be paid and a household to be maintained, and never asked for their help. But my heart was giving me the painful message that this coping style wasn't working.

Intellectually I knew that staying healthy on all levels was by far the biggest help and support I could provide for my daughters during this difficult time. My chest pain was a sign that I needed to tend to the needs and desires of my own heart if I was going to accomplish this. As soon as I began this process my upper chest and neck pain went away completely and have not returned.

At midlife I came face to face with an unconscious, deeply buried sense of unworthiness that had, for as long as I could remember, motivated me to prove myself to others through service. In the case of my family, this giving was laced with unconscious guilt for having and loving my career while simultaneously thinking that maybe I really should be spending more time as a stay-at-home mum. I made up for the time I spent on the job – or at least I told myself I did – by becoming as efficient and cheerful as possible, my nurturing providing steady background music in the lives of those closest to me. It was simply expected.

Part of my legacy of stoicism and unworthiness was that I had almost no 'receptor sites' in my own body and psyche for the experience of someone actually anticipating and making space for my personal emotional needs. In other words, even if someone had wanted to be there for me in the way I was there for my children and husband, I would not have been open to attracting or even recognising it. The music may have been playing, but my personal radio dial was always set on another station.

My divorce awakened me to the presence of those friends who had always been there for me – and who always would be. But I first had to open my heart and feel vulnerable and needy enough to allow myself to ask for help and then accept it when it was offered. This didn't come naturally or easily. But it was preferable to the old pattern.

Over the years I've observed that many women use pleasing behaviours to make themselves acceptable to others. One of my friends told me that whenever she feels that she doesn't belong or fit in, she does what she did in her family of origin to relieve the tension: she cooks, she cleans, she buys food, and she makes meals for others.

When we first recognise the patterns within us that shut down the energy of our hearts, our tendency is to beat ourselves up about them – which simply closes our hearts further. The first step we each must take is to acknowledge that the patterns that are causing us heartache in adulthood began as successful adaptations to difficult childhood circumstances. They worked for us then, and they have allowed us to become who we are. So the first thing we want to do when we recognise these patterns is to congratulate ourselves.

Yearning for Connection: Needing to Be Free

I'm not suggesting that at midlife we need to give up serving others. Participating in true service – where you're not in it for love and approval – is good for the heart. Most women, however, don't get to true service until we learn to balance our need for connection with our need to be free. Like the parasympathetic and sympathetic aspects of our autonomic nervous system, which so exquisitely control the minute-to-minute calibre of our blood vessels, we need both freedom and connection. Nanna Aida Svendsen, a writer and teacher originally from Denmark, eloquently articulates this balance:

> The heart, it seems, yearns for connection. A great grief arises when connection to others seems to come at the cost of connection to ourselves. I notice how dead I become inside, even if only subtly, when I try to conform to other people's idea of who and how I should be and forgo my own feelings – my connection to

myself. When the natural generosity, compassion, and caring of the heart becomes distorted or usurped, then all sense of aliveness, generosity, creativity, and true self-expression seems to go and I am left feeling empty and drained. It takes a great deal of energy to shape oneself to fit someone else's needs and expectations, to conform to their demands, to be co-dependent. And no matter how tempting it is in the hope of gaining love, or of being kept safe, it always costs. Just as it always costs to demand conformity to our needs by others – to be in a hierarchy when the heart is yearning for partnership. You can see that cost in the faces of so many couples. You can see the suppressed anger or the deadness that resides there. Though the heart may long for connection and love, it also, it appears, longs to be free.[1]

Cardiovascular Disease: When the Flow of Life Is Blocked

Cardiovascular disease results, in part, from an accumulation of oxidised fat in blood vessels that calcifies and eventually causes blood vessel and heart damage. Strokes, which kill ninety thousand women in the US and sixty thousand women in the UK per year, can be likened to a heart attack in the head. Both heart attacks and strokes are caused by clogged vessels; what differs is their location. In addition to arteriosclerotic plaque deposits, emotions such as depression, anxiety, panic, and grief have been shown to cause constriction in blood vessels, thereby impeding the free flow of blood.[2]

Your heart beats a hundred thousand times per day and thirty-six million times per year. Anything that causes constriction in your blood vessels makes your heart and your vessels work harder to do their job. Clearly both emotional and physical factors are involved in creating or maintaining heart health. Over my years in practice I've seen happy, joyful women with high cholesterol counts live healthy lives into their eighties and even nineties, while much younger women whose lives were characterised by depression, anxiety, or hostility might have their first heart disease symptoms in their early fifties despite normal cholesterol levels.

Heart Disease Facts

- Heart disease is rare in premenopausal women.

- Heart disease (including hypertension and stroke) is the most frequent cause of death in women over the age of fifty.[3]

- Heart attack, though usually occurring later in life, is twice as deadly in women as in men.[4]

- One in two women will eventually die of coronary artery disease or stroke.

- Only one woman in twenty-five will die of breast cancer.[5]

Cardiovascular disease in any one area means that it is also present throughout your entire body. Though most of us wait until midlife to take steps to prevent or treat it, heart disease actually begins in childhood – the minute we learn to start shutting down our hearts to avoid feeling disappointment and loss.

At midlife our hearts ask us to wake up and live our personal truth so that there is a seamless connection between what we say we believe and how we actually live our day-to-day lives. As astrologer Barbara Hand Clow writes: 'The heart does not open if one is lying to oneself or others, is manipulating or controlling others, or is separated from other people.' She goes on to explain, 'The heart chakra is experienced very physically, and it is possible to actually feel the heart opening at midlife as the kundalini energy flows in: many of my clients, for example, report a burning in their heart areas.' If we don't follow our body's lead and fuel our hearts and lives with the energy of full emotional expression and full partnership, then heart attack, hypertension, stroke, and dementia are more likely to result.

When we have the courage to open our hearts at midlife, however, we are opening ourselves up to the possibility of living more fully and joyfully than we have since we were young children – only now we have the skills and power of an adult with which to direct our open-hearted energy. Clow writes, 'The heart chakra opening is the signal of "radical embodiment" – the soul totally in the body – which is the most exquisite experience available on Earth. The integrity of a person with an open heart is always astounding.'⁶

Palpitations: Your Heart's Wake-up Call

There's no question that heart palpitations at menopause are related to changing hormones. However, my experience has been that in many midlife women heart palpitations are primarily from increasing heart energy trying to get in and be embodied in a woman's life. At midlife our hearts and bodies often become increasingly sensitive to those things that don't serve us, like caffeine, aspartame, or monosodium glutamate, all of which may overstimulate our hearts. You also might need to avoid scary or violent news, films, books, or individuals.

The following letter from Terri, one of my newsletter subscribers, is typical of how midlife heart palpitations often present.

I am a forty-eight-year-old female with no major health problems. I do not take any prescription medicine. I walk five times a week and go to the gym about twice a week to do some light weight lifting. My periods are still fairly regular. I have a fairly healthy diet, although it could be better. I drink about a cup of coffee a day but usually don't drink soft drinks. About a month ago, after a fatty fast-food meal and a large cup of coffee in the early evening, I started experiencing heart irregularities. I felt like my heart was skipping a beat and was going to beat out of my chest! This went on for a couple of days and I went to see my doctor. She did an ECG, which was slightly abnormal, and scheduled me for a stress echocardiogram and Holter monitor. Of course, by the time I had these tests, the palpitations had stopped and they were normal. Then about a week later, they started again. I have cut out drinking coffee and started doing more yoga. I have also started taking more magnesium in addition to my multivitamins. I have monitored what is going on with my life and I can't seem to find any pattern to when these occur. Most nights when I lie down in bed they usually start up, especially when I lie on my left side. My doctor wants to start me on a low dose of a beta-blocker. I told her I would like to start using natural progesterone cream routinely for a couple of months because I feel these palpitations may be related to hormonal changes. I would really like to avoid taking heart medications. However, these palpitations can interrupt my sleep and are very uncomfortable. Are these palpitations hormonally related?

My suggestion to Terri was that she go through the programme for creating heart health I outline in this chapter. Her midlife heart is obviously becoming very sensitive, alerting her to the need to balance freedom and connection and also to nourish her heart fully. I concur with her intuitive desire to start on some natural progesterone as a way to balance potential oestrogen dominance. Besides, progesterone is known to be very calming to the nervous system. It may well help her with sleeping. In addition, her heart is telling her to stop caffeine. The caffeine in one cup of coffee can take up to ten hours to be metabolised in women, so it exerts a stimulatory effect on the central nervous system and the nerves of the heart for quite some time.

For many women, heart palpitations stop as soon as they begin to take progesterone cream or oestrogen and stop caffeine. But it's also important to find out what your heart is yearning for. One of my patients with heart palpitations found that they stopped soon after she asked for a promotion at work, something she hadn't had the courage to do before. She got the promotion and finds her work more fulfilling than ever. Her heart no longer has to speak so loudly.

The Brain–Heart Connection

Remember that the emotional and psychological changes of the perimenopausal years are to the entire life cycle as the week before one's period is to the monthly cycle. All the issues that have been occurring premenstrually and which perhaps had been avoided until now – 'Should I quit my job?' 'Should I stay in this relationship?' – now come up and hit us between the eyes rather relentlessly, demanding that they be dealt with at this time. Though women with palpitations often tell me that they have examined their lives and there don't appear to be any personal issues bothering them, my experience has been that our bodies speak to us only when we can't seem to 'hear' them any other way. When issues of love, issues of the soul, or issues of a woman's unmet passions cry out for attention, they often take the form of heart palpitations. If we are willing to be open to their meaning, we will be giving our hearts a chance to be heard. If we act on what we hear, the symptom often goes away.

FIGURE 21: THE HEART–EMOTION CONNECTION

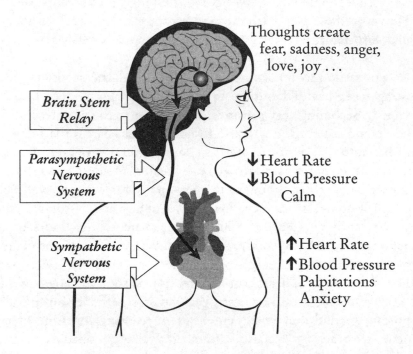

Thoughts create fear, sadness, anger, love, joy . . .

Brain Stem Relay

Parasympathetic Nervous System

↓ Heart Rate
↓ Blood Pressure
Calm

Sympathetic Nervous System

↑ Heart Rate
↑ Blood Pressure
Palpitations
Anxiety

Emotions have direct physical effects on the heart and cardiovascular system, via the sympathetic and parasympathetic nervous systems.
© 2001 by Northrup and Schulz

In his foreword to the book *The HeartMath Solution,* Dr Stephan Rechtschaffen writes that 'the heart is a physical object, a rhythmic organ, and love itself'.[7] We need to think of our hearts as all of these things simultaneously and care for them with this perspective in mind. Because of the intricate connections between our brains and our hearts, our thoughts and emotions can and do have a powerful effect on the heart's rhythm.

Let's take the dramatic example of sudden, unexpected cardiac death. This condition claims more than 450,000 lives per year in the US, and research, which focuses on the physical condition of the heart itself, has made relatively little headway in decreasing these numbers. Sudden cardiac death is caused by a fatal arrhythmia known as ventricular fibrillation (VF), a disorganised, self-perpetuating electrical instability of the heart muscle that results in a failure of the heart to pump blood.

VF can occur spontaneously in a completely normal heart and is usually seen when there is some pathological hindrance to the flow of blood in the heart vessels, a condition that often happens in humans in association with some psychosocial stress, such as bereavement, job insecurity, or marital strife. Whether or not a stressor affects the heart physically is dependent on the meaning that stress has for a given individual.[8]

Gender Bias and Heart Disease: Our Cultural Inheritance

For thousands of years our culture has valued male hearts more than female hearts. The heart-strengthening dreams and aspirations of women, as well as the vulnerable and tender hearts of men, have all suffered as a result. Here are the facts:

• The vast majority of research on both heart disease and its treatment has been done on men, even though the female's cardiovascular system is different from the male's.

• Women's brain connections to the heart are different from men's. Men's brains are more lateralised than women's, which means that in general most men use only one hemisphere at a time, usually the left, which is associated with linear, logical thinking. Women, on the other hand, use both hemispheres simultaneously, and they have more frequent access to their right hemispheres. The right hemisphere is associated with music, emotions, intuition, and a deep experience of oneself. Here's where things get interesting. There are more neuronal connections between the heart and the right hemisphere of the brain than between the heart and the left hemisphere. So in any given moment a woman has a greater neurological and emotional connection to her heart than do most men.

• Given the difference in their brain–heart connections, women with heart problems have different symptoms from men.[9] Men who are having a heart attack typically present with chest pain that begins under the breastbone and spreads to the jaw and the left arm. Women with heart attacks may not have chest pain at all. Instead, they may experience primarily jaw pain and indigestion. Or the first sign of a heart attack in women may be congestive heart failure, with no evidence of the heart attack preceding it except for telltale changes on an electrocardiogram. They may die from this 'silent' heart attack.[10] Women who do have chest pain often experience more functional limitation than men, but fewer women are referred to cardiologists for a complete check-up.

• Until very recently, most doctors have not appreciated this difference. Consequently, serious heart problems go underdiagnosed and undertreated in women. In fact, women are only half as likely as men to undergo acute catheterisation, angioplasty, thrombolysis, or coronary bypass surgery. The risk of dying of heart disease in a hospital is twice as great for a woman as it is for a man.

• When a woman with chest pain or a racing heart turns up at a doctor's surgery or casualty department, she may appear anxious and depressed, and an affective disorder rather than heart disease may be the first diagnosis considered. While it is true that affective disorders, including depression, phobias, and panic and anxiety, are twice as common in women as in men, they aren't 'just in women's heads' – they affect the body as well. One of my most vivid memories of my maternal grandmother is how she often wrung her hands at night. Though she always maintained a wonderfully friendly and cheery demeanour, her hands belied her outward peacefulness. She died of a sudden heart attack at the age of sixty-eight.

• If a man turns up who appears to be under stress, his symptoms are more apt to be correctly associated with heart attack – even if he behaves in a hostile way.

• Women's blood vessels are smaller and have a different organisation from men's. This is one of the reasons why coronary bypass surgeries and angioplasties don't work as well in women as they do in men and also why more women die after these procedures. More women than men with so-called normal coronary arteries also have heart attacks, angina, and myocardial ischemia. As a result, a normal angiogram (blood vessel study) in a woman with symptoms doesn't necessarily mean that she doesn't have heart disease.

• The rate of early death after heart attack is higher for women than men, even if the women receive treatment. Researchers don't know if this difference is caused by older average age at diagnosis, narrower vessels, greater frequency of co-existing illnesses, or inadequate or delayed medical care.

• The thought patterns and behaviours that are associated with heart disease in women are different from the patterns associated with heart disease in men. In research on men, sudden death from heart attack is related to hostility – so-called type A behaviour. This hasn't yet been demonstrated in women. This doesn't mean that men are inherently more hostile than women. In women, hostility just gets expressed differently. Recent studies have shown a correlation between hostility and hardening of the arteries in both men and women starting as young as the age of eighteen.[11] But men tend to act out their anger and frustration physically in the outer world, whereas women are taught that this is unacceptable and unladylike. Therefore women learn to hold these feelings inside, where they can ultimately set the stage for a great deal of heart trouble.[12]

Let's use the analogy of two pans of water on a cooker. The pan on the right – the woman – is on simmer, with a lid on top. The pan on the left – the male – has no lid, and the heat is on high. The heat of the male's anger will cause the water in the pan to boil vigorously, with a lot of steam and noise. In a typical male heart attack, the pan boils over. The woman's pan will never boil over, but the heat is there nonetheless, and the next thing you know, the water has evaporated and the pan has cracked. But because there was no noise and steam, no one was alerted to the problem. The same thing happens with a woman's cardiovascular system.

In the past few years, doctors have been warned about these differences and have been advised to do a cardiac evaluation of women with symptoms such as anxiety and chest pain. As we move towards a partnership society, our awareness of gender bias in heart disease treatment is becoming stronger. It is encouraging to know that the National Institutes of Health and the FDA in the US have called for the inclusion of women in cardiac-related clinical trials.

Arteriosclerosis: Reducing Your Risk

Arteriosclerosis is a thickening or hardening of the arterial wall. It underlies all coronary artery disease and is responsible for the majority of deaths in the Western world. I'll use a case from Dr Mona Lisa Schulz's intuitive practice to show how emotional factors become entwined with family history and other risk factors.

KAREN: A HEART AT RISK

When Karen rang Mona Lisa, she provided nothing more than her age, fifty-three, with a request for a reading. Mona Lisa quickly became aware that she was burned out from meeting the demands of her family. She also saw that Karen hid her emotions behind a brave and stoic face, especially her feelings of frustration, exhaustion, and weariness. She never complained.

When Mona Lisa proceeded to a physical reading on Karen's head, she saw decreased flexibility in her blood vessels. These stiff blood vessels were also present in her heart. Mona Lisa perceived that she had symptoms of dizziness and an odd imbalanced feeling. She also sensed blurred vision and a change in her heart rhythm. In addition, she saw that Karen was profoundly fatigued.

After this initial reading, Karen told Mona Lisa that she had become the mother of a combined family when she remarried. She cared not only for her three children, but also for her husband's children from his first marriage. One of Karen's children suffered from multiple disabilities and cerebral palsy. His medical problems made his care very complicated. But Karen told Dr Schulz that God had always been good to her and that although her family burden was great, she didn't feel she should complain. It seemed to Karen that others had it worse than she did. After all, she was a nurse and had seen this first hand. She finally admitted that she allowed herself to be used by her children but didn't feel that she had the verbal skills to do anything about it. She had recently picked up her stethoscope and heard a blockage in the carotid artery in her neck. Frightened, she went to her doctor and was sent to a cardiologist, who told her the carotid artery was 75 per cent blocked and that there were some blockages in her coronary (heart) arteries as well.

Illness has many different aspects. It is in part genetic, partly due to diet, and partly due to environmental toxins. The area that medical intuition focuses on is the emotional and behavioural aspects of health. Karen's history combined all of these factors. Her mother had died of a stroke and her father of a heart attack. Her father had always been very careful about his diet but had still had high cholesterol and hypertension despite good medical care. Her mother had always been overweight, no matter how hard she tried to lose the extra pounds. Both parents were stoics who brought up their kids on very little money and with little support from the extended family. Karen had never heard either of them complain, get angry, or even have a disagreement. Clearly Karen took after her parents, both genetically and emotionally. And her risk of blood vessel disease was the same as theirs.

Even if your family history looks like Karen's, you can break this chain of inheritance and lower your risk. The first step is a review of exactly what hardening of the arteries is, why it happens, and what to do about it.

The Anatomy of an Artery

Arteries carry blood away from the heart to all the organs and tissues of our body. They are lined with endothelial cells, which actually secrete anticoagulants (molecules that prevent blood clots, coronary occlusion, heart attacks, and embolic strokes) as well as pro-clotting proteins (which prevent bleeding or haemorrhagic strokes). If this endothelial lining is damaged or overproduces the pro-clotting factors associated with stress and subsequent imbalanced eicosanoids, the risk of heart attack or stroke rises.

Blood vessels undergo changes beginning in childhood, depending upon diet, genetic tendencies, and how we learn to handle emotional expression. In the famous Bogalusa Heart Study, for example, the beginnings of heart disease were discovered in children as young as nine.[13]

The following describes the three stages of development of arteriosclerosis:

1. Deposition of fatty streaks. These can be found in children. Immune cells called macrophages, which lie on the surface of the blood vessel endothelial cells, swallow LDL cholesterol as it floats by. The fat droplets accumulate, causing fatty streaks to develop in the coronary arteries and the aorta. LDL cholesterol and other components of arterial plaques won't stick to the endothelial lining of vessel walls unless there is some kind of damage to these walls in the first place – usually the result of free-radical damage to cells from environmental toxins (such as cigarette smoke), chemicals caused by stress, a nutrient-poor diet, or a combination of all of these.

2. Formation of fibrous plaques. Over time the fatty streaks enlarge, causing scarring in the underlying endothelial lining, and these scars can eventually grow into plaques, which are elevated areas of scarred or fibrous fatty tissue in the aorta, the coronary arteries, and the carotid arteries in the neck that bring blood to the brain and are often involved in strokes. (This is where Karen heard the disrupted flow of blood.) These domelike bulges have a central core of cholesterol crystals.

3. Complicated lesion. The dome of the lipid plaque eventually grows large enough to narrow blood vessels significantly, which eventually results in decreased blood flow and thus decreased flow of nutrients and oxygen to tissue – in the same way that mineral build-up clogs plumbing. The calcified plaque may begin to ulcerate. When this happens, there is a much greater risk of blood vessel rupture and bleeding, resulting in a stroke or haemorrhage. Bits of calcified artery can also break off and be propelled by the flow of blood into distant areas where they lodge in a vessel and further cut off blood flow, thus resulting in stroke (dead brain tissue), heart attack (dead heart tissue), or dead tissue in other areas of the body.

Disorders that are characterised by arteriosclerosis include diabetes, insulin resistance, hypertension, a diet too high in refined carbohydrates and too low in antioxidants, decreased thyroid hormone, and a genetic tendency towards producing too much homocysteine.

How Do You Know if Your Vessels Are Healthy?

Only rarely will a doctor be able to diagnose arteriosclerosis from hearing an odd sound (known as a bruit) in the carotid artery, or from hearing a click or abnormal rhythm in the heart. If you have diabetes or high blood pressure, are significantly overweight, never exercise, follow a poor diet, or are a smoker, the chances are good that you already have at least the beginnings of arteriosclerosis.

Most of the time, arteriosclerosis is not diagnosed until an individual has a cardiac event of some kind, such as a stroke or heart attack. Individuals with chest pain or difficulty walking because of

Factors Associated with an Increased Risk of Cardiovascular Disease

- You are/were a habitual smoker.

- You have high LDL ('bad') cholesterol (greater than 4.0m.mol/L).

- Your HDL cholesterol ('good' cholesterol) is low (less than 0.9m.mol/L).

- You have high triglycerides (greater than 4.5m.mol/L).

- You have high blood pressure (greater than 130/85).

- You have high levels of the amino acid homocysteine in your bloodstream.

- You are too fat (body mass index greater than 25) with an apple-shaped figure (a preponderance of body fat above the level of the hips).

- You have periodontal disease.

- You have diabetes.

- You are sedentary and don't exercise.

- You have a history of significant clinical depression.

vascular insufficiency often undergo an X-ray test known as an angiogram, which visualises blood vessels that are injected with dye. Sometimes an ultrasound technology known as a Doppler device will be used to diagnose vessels that are blocked.

The good news is that arteriosclerosis can be largely prevented or reversed by diet and lifestyle factors. In fact, the famous Nurses' Health Study, which has followed more than eighty-four thousand women for over fourteen years, has demonstrated that the risk of arteriosclerosis is very low in those women who exercise regularly, abstain from smoking, and follow the kind of diet I recommend in chapter 7.[14] I'll discuss selected risk factors in more detail below. If you are perimenopausal you may like to get a complete check-up from a doctor who is qualified to evaluate your cardiovascular status. This evaluation should include, as a minimum, a thorough history and physical examination, ECG, blood pressure check, and lipid profile. You will probably need to go privately for this. Many private hospitals (such as BUPA) do these screenings.

Cholesterol

A lipid profile is a measure of your total cholesterol, LDL cholesterol, HDL cholesterol, and triglyceride levels. Here are the numbers to aim for on the lipid profile.

TOTAL CHOLESTEROL: Below 5.2m.mol/L.

HDL (HIGH-DENSITY LIPOPROTEIN): HDL – the 'good' cholesterol – should be 0.9m.mol/L or higher. Low HDL cholesterol has been shown to be a more potent risk factor in women than it is in men. Women with low levels of this cholesterol subtype (a reading of 0.7m.mol/L or less) have a sevenfold increase in heart disease risk compared to those whose HDL levels are normal.[15]

LDL (LOW-DENSITY LIPOPROTEIN): LDL – the 'bad' cholesterol – should be 3.5m.mol/L or below if you have other risk factors or 4.0m.mol/L or below if you do not. LDL cholesterol rises after menopause in many women, a fact that has been used to promote oestrogen replacement, which decreases LDL levels. If your LDL is greater than 4.0m.mol/L, you're considered at high risk for coronary artery disease.

TRIGLYCERIDES: This number should be 2.3m.mol/L or lower. Triglycerides are an independent risk factor for women. A woman with a triglyceride level of greater than 4.5m.mol/L has a 14 per cent risk of developing coronary artery disease.

RELATIONSHIP OF TOTAL CHOLESTEROL TO HDL: Neither type of cholesterol is inherently bad or good. Both are necessary for good health. Like eicosanoids, they need to be balanced in the body. Divide your total cholesterol by your HDL cholesterol. If the resulting number is 4 or less you are at low risk. The ratio of total cholesterol to HDL is a much better predictor of risk than simply your total cholesterol number. Ask your doctor to give you a copy of your lipid profile so that you can get to know your numbers. It's very moti-vating to watch your lipid profile improve every year when you commit to becoming healthier than ever before at midlife.

Currently 40 per cent of women over fifty-five have elevated cholesterol levels.[16] Though interpretation of lipid profile results will vary from lab to lab, a total cholesterol level as high as 5.7 to 6.0m.mol/L does not necessarily indicate that a woman is at increased risk of heart disease if her HDL cholesterol is also high (0.9m.mol/L or above). Because most of the studies of heart disease and blood lipid levels have been done on men, we still don't know exactly what levels of blood lipids are optimal for women. What we do know is that women can have higher total cholesterol levels than men and not be at increased risk of heart disease.

Get the lipid profile repeated at least every five years if it's normal. If your blood sugar is high, get the test repeated more frequently.

If your cholesterol levels are high and you cannot institute lifestyle improvements, or if they haven't worked for you after an honest six-month trial, consider taking one of the 'statin' drugs, such as prava-statin (Lipostat) or simvastatin (Zocor). These drugs have been shown to result in a 24–38 per cent reduction in cardiac events, including stroke.[17] They can adversely affect liver function, so this must be monitored, and they also lower levels of the antioxidant coenzyme Q_{10} (see page 476).

High Blood Pressure

Blood pressure is also important; it should be 130/85 or less. (Some experts use 140/90 as the cut-off figure.) About 20 per cent or more of British women between the ages of forty-five and sixty-four have mild to severe high blood pressure, a condition that, in the famous Nurses' Health Study, has been found to increase the risk of coronary artery disease by 3.5 times.[18]

Blood pressure can be significantly lowered by any one of the following lifestyle changes: regular exercise (such as brisk walking), biofeedback, dietary improvement, or weight loss. Even in very over-weight women, losing only 10 to 20lb will often lower blood pressure significantly. If these measures fail, then it's advisable to use blood-pressure-lowering medication, even though these medications can have side effects such as dizziness, headaches, and fatigue.

Be sure to get your lipid profile and blood pressure checked again within three to six months.

Note: If you follow the insulin-normalising diet I recommend at perimenopause, you can expect substantial improvements in your lipid profile, your blood sugar, and your blood pressure within two to four weeks.

Homocysteine

Elevated blood levels of the amino acid homocysteine, which is found in high amounts in animal protein, constitutes a strong risk factor for cardiovascular disease. At least 10 per cent or more of the population has a genetic tendency for elevated levels of homocysteine. When high homocysteine levels are reduced, the incidence of heart attack is cut by 20 per cent, the risk of blood-clot-related strokes decreases by 40 per cent, and the risk of venous blood clots elsewhere in the body plunges by an impressive 60 per cent. Studies have shown that dietary intake of vitamins B_{12}, B_6, and folate can help combat an elevated homocysteine level, as can cutting back on the amount of animal-based protein in your diet. Blood tests to determine plasma homocysteine levels, B_6 (pyridoxine), B_{12} and red cell folate can be arranged by a doctor so you can make adjustments to your diet and supplement programme if indicated.

Periodontal Disease and Cardiac Risk

Periodontal disease (inflammation and infection of the gums) is present in a significant percentage of adults in the UK. In recent years, a number of compelling studies have shown that gum disease is a risk factor for coronary artery disease and stroke. Although no one can say that periodontal disease directly causes cardiovascular disease, research has clearly shown that periodontal disease is more prevalent in patients with acute and chronic heart disease. This association may be due, in part, to the fact that inflammation plays a central role both in gum disease and in hardening of the arteries. It has also been shown that the inflammation seen in periodontal disease is associated with narrowing of the carotid arteries, a risk factor for stroke.[19]

Periodontal disease is easily treatable through proper brushing, flossing, and regular visits to the dentist for professional evaluation and cleaning. Caring for your teeth and gums is a practical and easy way to decrease at least one risk factor for cardiovascular disease or stroke.

Smoking

Smoking is responsible for 55 per cent of the cardiovascular deaths in women under sixty-five years old. The Nurses' Health Study

---

How to Give Up

You have to want to give up to be successful. With each subsequent attempt, however, the chances for successfully staying off tobacco increase. The biggest problem women have with successfully giving up smoking is that they often have to change their friendships and behaviour patterns and begin to think of themselves as non-smokers.

Acupuncture can help people give up, because it's helpful for detoxing addictions. Some women also do well with Quit Smoking programmes or with one of the nicotine patches.

I recommend calling your local library as they may know what is available. Or discuss stopping smoking with your doctor.

---

followed more than 117,000 female nurses aged thirty to fifty-five. In that study the relative risk of total coronary artery disease among smokers was four times higher than that of women who never smoked. But in women who stopped smoking, the relative risk of coronary artery disease immediately decreased to 1.5. Two years after stopping smoking, the risk dropped to that of a woman who has never smoked. Smoking is also responsible for approximately 29 per cent of all cancers. Since 1987 lung cancer has been the leading cause of cancer deaths among women.[20]

At least thirteen studies have shown that smokers cease menstruation one to two years earlier than non-smokers. The effect is dose-dependent, and the difference persists after weight factors have been taken into consideration. Female smokers sixty years old and older also have significantly reduced bone mineral density of the hip compared with non-smokers.[21]

Age

The only reason that age is a risk factor for heart disease is that by the time you reach fifty or so, the processes that clog arteries are often well established. Coronary artery disease starts in many by the teenage years. It's the result of your day-to-day decisions on all levels: emotional, physical, and psychological. To treat it, reverse it, or prevent it, you need to change those day-to-day actions that led to it in the first place.

A large study of coronary risk factors in fifteen-year-olds and young adults, for example, showed that of 197 males and 197 females, 31 per cent of the males and 10 per cent of the females had calcifications of their coronary arteries by the age of fifteen. We know that these calcifications are closely associated with heart attack, stroke, and aneurysm in later life. To further figure out which individuals were more likely to have these lesions, the investigators found that the following factors were most predictive of coronary artery pathology: high body mass index and low HDL ('good') cholesterol.[22]

Powerful Versus Powerless

If you perceive that you are valuable and powerful in the world and have choices, then your heart will be more apt to work optimally. The opposite is also true. At least two studies have shown a relationship between a woman's job and her health. One study found that women who are employed and married have the best health, with or without children. If their husbands are supportive, so much the better. Good health is also associated with more complex and challenging jobs characterised by autonomy.

But if you feel that you have no autonomy, the risk for heart disease goes up. Clerical workers whose supervisors are demanding and whose job situations do not allow them to express anger are at increased risk of developing heart disease. Time pressure is also a risk factor that has been associated with poor health.[23]

If a woman's heart isn't in her work, she cannot express her anger about this, and she perceives that she can't leave, this conflict hits her right in the heart, an organ that is exquisitely sensitive to the effects of excessive catecholamines over time. A woman in a stressful job in which she feels she doesn't have a say is also more likely to smoke, which results in higher blood pressure and cholesterol – both additional risk factors for heart disease.

SHARON: DYING FOR HER BENEFITS

Sharon had been a patient of mine for years. Though she was about 1½ stone (9kg) overweight, she walked regularly and was in a very happy, supportive relationship. Her blood pressure and cholesterol were normal, and she was in good health. She was also on Premarin and Provera – two hormones that had been prescribed for her at the beginning of her menopause for hot flushes. She had done well with this approach and there was no reason to change the prescription. (At the time, we didn't have the data on alternatives that are now available.) At the age of fifty-four Sharon developed chest pain, and a cardiac check-up showed that she had narrowing of her coronary arteries. She underwent bypass surgery. When I asked Sharon if she was going through any unusual stresses around the time of her chest pain, she told me that she had been hoping she could take early retirement from her job as a university professor. She and her husband had bought a holiday home, where they spent as much time as possible. But she discovered that if she took early retirement, she wouldn't be eligible for her full pension benefits. So she halfheartedly decided that she had no choice but to stay another ten years. It was shortly after she made this decision that she developed her chest pain. As I did her annual pelvic and breast examination, I asked her if she really felt it was worth it to stay another ten years in a job that was literally shutting off the joy to her heart. And I was reminded that people who stay in jobs they hate strictly for their benefits rarely get to use them.

Studies suggest that low educational standing is consistently associated with higher risk of coronary artery disease in women. This isn't necessarily related to formal education, however; rather, it is tied more to the fact that those who are better educated tend to take better care of themselves and to know that they have choices. Also, body mass index and cigarette smoking are inversely related to educational attainment. Vigorous leisure-time activity is also related to educational attainment. Fitness levels assessed by treadmill have been directly related to educational attainment in women but not in men.[24] The good news is that you don't need to go back to college for an advanced degree to change your perception and take charge of your lifestyle.

The number and diversity of your friends and associates also contributes to heart health or lack of it. Women with greater numbers of children and too many demands on their time combined with a lack of emotional support have been shown to be at greater risk of heart disease. But women who perceive that their families are supportive are at lower risk.

Depression

Depression is consistently related to a high risk of heart disease in both men and women. In a recent survey of my newsletter subscribers, 46 per cent listed their biggest health concern as depression and anxiety. In contrast, only 18 per cent indicated that heart disease was their greatest concern. What these and most other women don't realise is that the emotions associated with sadness or grief, anger or depression, and fear or anxiety are very much connected to heart disease (as well as bone health).

Women's blood vessels are smaller than men's and are extremely sensitive to the biochemical changes that occur in response to the emotions of daily life. These biochemical changes result in either constricted or dilated blood vessels. When your blood vessels constrict in response to emotions such as anger, grief, and fear, they do so because of an outpouring of chemicals from the sympathetic nervous system; blood flow is reduced, and tissue damage and high blood pressure are the result.

Because at least 25 per cent of women suffer from depressive episodes at some point in their lives, and because women are more apt to suffer from depression than men, depression emerges as a very important and modifiable risk factor for women. Though it is well documented that both men and women often suffer from depression after a heart attack, newer data conclude that depression is an important independent risk factor for heart disease. A study from the Ohio State University College of Medicine and Public Health in the US recently showed just how profoundly depression affects coronary artery disease in women. Even after adjusting for other factors such as smoking, obesity, and lack of exercise, the risk of non-fatal coronary artery disease was 73 per cent higher in depressed women compared to a control group.[25] In their research, depressed women were also shown to be twice as likely to develop coronary artery disease as were normal, non-depressed women.

Carbohydrates, Sugar, and Heart Health: What Every Woman Should Know

By now you know that overconsumption of refined carbohydrates plays a role in developing type 2 or adult-onset diabetes, a disease whose incidence is rapidly increasing as our population grows fatter

and fatter. But what most women don't know is that the same carbohydrate consumption pattern that results in obesity, poor skin, and
hormone imbalance is also a potent risk factor for heart disease,
hypertension, and stroke. The diet most commonly prescribed for
treatment and prevention of heart disease in both men and women is a
high-carbohydrate, low-fat approach. Unfortunately, this diet may
have exactly the opposite effect. When compared to a higher-protein,
higher-fat diet with exactly the same number of calories, the high-
carbohydrate diet has been shown to increase risk factors for ischemic
heart disease, such as high triglycerides and insulin, in healthy postmenopausal women. It also lowers HDL cholesterol.[26] Eating a high-
carbohydrate meal has also been shown to trigger angina sooner and
reduce exercise tolerance in patients with known heart disease. This
is probably because high insulin levels can cause constriction of
arteriosclerotic coronary arteries.[27]

The experience of many women whose husbands go on high-
carbohydrate, low-fat diets following heart attacks is that the men
lose weight and lower their total cholesterol while their wives gain
weight and may lose some of their HDL ('good' cholesterol) on
exactly the same food plan. To prevent this, women need to be sure to
eat only those carbohydrates that don't raise insulin levels too high or
too quickly.[28] (See chapter 7.)

To understand how excessive carbohydrate intake can contribute
to heart disease, we have to return to the subject of insulin. When you
eat carbohydrates that are converted into sugar rapidly, your body
pours insulin into your blood from your pancreas. Insulin is necessary to move the sugar from your bloodstream into your cells, where
it is used for energy. But insulin doesn't simply regulate your blood
sugar; it also helps control the storage of fat in your body. And heart
disease is basically a disease associated with too much fat in our
arteries.

Here's how it happens. Insulin directs amino acids, fatty acids, and
carbohydrate breakdown products into our body tissues. It also regulates the body's production of cholesterol. Insulin tells the liver to
begin making LDL cholesterol ('bad' cholesterol), which at high
enough levels – and under the right circumstances – actually sticks to
the blood vessel walls and forms a plaque. And that is the essence of
coronary artery disease and also cerebrovascular disease – the kind
of arterial disease that affects brain function and enhances your risk of
stroke and also dementia.

If you eat a lot of sugar or a lot of high-glycaemic-index carbohy-drates such as pasta, bread, sweets, biscuits, and potatoes (and/or alcohol), and you are prone to high blood sugar or insulin resistance (as about 75 per cent of us are), your liver may well increase its synthesis of LDL, which tends to stick to your blood vessels, forming plaques and subsequently causing arteriosclerosis, or hardening of the arteries.

Insulin also drives your kidneys to retain fluid, in a way that is similar to the kind of fluid overload that is seen in coronary artery disease and congestive heart failure. Excess insulin therefore poses a significant risk for hypertension, coronary artery disease, obesity, and high cholesterol levels, not just diabetes. Fluid retention from insulin is the reason why susceptible individuals can easily put on 3 or 4lb after a single large carbohydrate-rich meal.

Insulin and Blood Vessel Wall Thickening

In addition to all its other important roles, insulin is also a growth factor in the body. Excess insulin promotes smooth muscle growth in your blood vessel walls, which contributes to the formation of plaque, causing your artery walls to thicken and become rigid. Excess blood sugar from chronic carbohydrate consumption irreversibly attaches to the LDL cholesterol molecules that are already stuck to the blood vessel walls. This disease process in blood vessels is a set-up for free-radical damage, a type of cellular damage that is akin to rust on a car.[29]

Here's the bottom line. If you think you're lowering your risk of heart disease by lowering your fat intake and increasing your intake of carbohydrates, you may be doing just the opposite, depending upon your genetic heritage. If you eat too many high-glycaemic-index carbohydrates and don't exercise, and if you have a tendency towards carbohydrate addiction, then your body will convert those carbohydrates into excess blood sugar, fat, and LDL cholesterol. In addition, the higher your intake of refined carbohydrates, the higher your cellular levels of series 2 eicosanoids. These have repeatedly been shown to favour cell overgrowth, such as cancer, and also tissue inflammation – which is a well-documented risk factor for heart disease.[30]

Follow a diet that keeps insulin levels low – the same diet that also prevents middle-age spread, balances your hormones, and improves your skin. Currently a major controversy is raging in the medical profession about which diet is healthiest – a low-fat, high-carbohydrate diet or one that includes moderate fat, adequate protein, and moderate carbohydrates. The truth is that neither diet is right for everyone. We are all different. The best choice for you will depend upon what risk factors you have for cardiovascular disease and insulin resistance.

Some women are able to keep their weight and cholesterol levels normal by eating a lot of complex carbohydrates, including whole-grain breads, and others – like me and millions of others – are not. You can't go wrong, however, if your diet consists mostly of lean meats, low-fat dairy produce, and lots of fruits and vegetables. Choose the most colourful ones, such as blueberries, strawberries, leafy greens, pumpkin, and kale. These are the highest in antioxidants. Hundreds of studies have confirmed that foods rich in flavonoids, carotenoids, and other antioxidants can reduce your risk of cardiovascular disease. Women who routinely eat four to five servings of fruits and vegetables per day (particularly the green, leafy, cruciferous, and citrus varieties) have a 28–35 per cent decreased risk of stroke – an estimated 7 per cent decrease in risk for each serving.[31]

The isoflavones and other substances in soya have definitely been shown to have a beneficial effect on blood lipids. An analysis of thirty-eight controlled clinical trials found that the consumption of soya protein rather than animal protein resulted in significantly decreased levels of total cholesterol, LDL cholesterol, and triglycerides.[32] Regular consumption of soya protein and ground flaxseed (linseed) is also associated with lowered cholesterol and a decreased risk of arteriosclerosis.[33]

Last but not least, avoid partially hydrogenated fats whenever possible.

Cardioprotective Supplements

The following is a list of the best-studied cardioprotective foods and supplements. You don't need to take all of them. Many will be present in a good comprehensive formulation for women. But others, like a higher dose of vitamin C, a cup of green tea daily, or a clove of garlic, are easy to add to your day.

Magnesium

Among its many roles in the body, magnesium helps stabilise electrical conduction in the cardiac muscle. It also helps relax the smooth muscle in blood vessels.[34]

Magnesium deficiency is relatively common; because commercial agriculture today relies heavily on inorganic fertilisers, our food supply tends to be poor in this mineral. Food processing results in decreased magnesium as well. Chronic emotional and mental stress is also associated with magnesium deficiency because the stress hormones cortisol and adrenaline release magnesium from the cells; eventually it is excreted in the urine. Diuretics result in the loss of magnesium in the urine, too, which is why the chronic use of diuretics has been associated with sudden cardiac death. If you're on diuretics for high blood pressure or any other reason, make sure that you take additional magnesium, potassium, and zinc. Excessive use of the stomach acid inhibitors cimetidine (Tagamet) and ranitidine (Zantac) can result in magnesium deficiency as well. Take 400–1,000mg per day in divided doses with meals.

Calcium

Calcium is needed by every cell in your body, including the electrical system of the heart. Adequate calcium intake helps keep blood pressure normal. This mineral works in tandem with magnesium, and therefore it's important to take both together. In general you want to be sure that your calcium is balanced with magnesium in either a 1:1 or 2:1 ratio. Take 400–1,200mg/day with meals, depending upon how much calcium is present in the diet.

Antioxidants

Thousands of studies have documented the ability of antioxidants to help your heart, blood vessels, and every other tissue in your body resist free-radical damage and thus stay healthy. Here's an overview of my favourites – though there are others.[35]

COENZYME Q$_{10}$: This nutrient is concentrated in organ foods such as liver, kidney, and heart. It helps produce ATP, the basic energy molecule in every cell of the body. It is also a powerful antioxidant. Numerous studies have documented its beneficial effects on the heart, both in maintaining health and in healing from disease. (High doses have even been found to reverse some types of cardiomyopathy.)[36]

Coenzyme Q_{10} improves the ability of the heart to pump effectively and has also been shown to help reduce high blood pressure and congestive heart failure in those who already have heart disease. Coenzyme Q_{10} is also very important for breast health. Coenzyme Q_{10} levels in heart muscles can be ten times greater than in other tissues because the heart functions continuously, without resting. That's why any condition that impairs the ability of the heart to do its work leaves this organ more susceptible to free-radical damage.

Coenzyme Q_{10} can be depleted in women who take statin drugs, including pravastatin (Lipostat) and atorvastatin (Lipitor), to lower their cholesterol.[37] These drugs interrupt many biochemical pathways, which may put the body at risk of other problems such as breast cancer.[38] Studies have shown that almost half of patients with hypertension have coenzyme Q_{10} deficiencies. Taking 50mg twice a day for ten weeks has been shown to lower blood pressure significantly.[39] For those individuals already on medication for elevated blood pressure, the need for antihypertensive medication declined gradually in about four and a half months in half of the patients who took coenzyme Q_{10} (225mg per day); some were able to stop taking blood pressure medication altogether.[40]

The minimum dose of coenzyme Q_{10} I recommend is 30mg/day. For anyone with any family history of heart disease, I'd recommend 60–90mg/day to help prevent the disease from developing. The dose can go up to 300–400mg per day for those with advanced heart disease.[41]

CAROTENOIDS: There are dozens of studies that show that individuals who consume high amounts of pigment-rich foods are at lower risk of heart disease. These foods are loaded with carotenoids such as beta-carotene, which has been shown to decrease risk of free-radical damage to the heart and blood vessels. In one study of individuals who had already had unstable angina and had undergone coronary artery bypass, the addition of beta-carotene to their diets decreased subsequent major cardiovascular events such as heart attack, stroke, need for additional bypass procedures, and cardiac death by 50 per cent.[42] Beta-carotene prevents the lipoprotein LDL ('bad' cholesterol) from becoming oxidised. The usual dose of beta-carotene is 25,000IU (15mg) per day in supplement form.

However, a mix of the carotenoids is better than taking just one. For example, lutein is present in HDL ('good') cholesterol and may help prevent LDL cholesterol from oxidising. The best way to get lutein is in fruits and vegetables, but it is also available in health food shops as a supplement; take 3–6mg per day. Lycopene is another good antioxidant; eating tomatoes a couple of times a week will give you all the lycopene you need.

VITAMIN E: This antioxidant has been shown to keep blood platelets 'slippery', thus decreasing the risk of blood clots. Vitamin E is an anti-inflammatory in the heart muscle. It may also inhibit arrhythmia and cardiomyopathy. In the Nurses' Health Study, participants taking 400–800IU of vitamin E per day exhibited a lower rate of heart attack. The Cambridge Heart Study, which looked at the effects of vitamin E on two thousand patients with documented heart disease, found that those who took between 400 and 800IU of vitamin E per day had a 77 per cent decrease in cardiovascular disease over a year's time.[43] Dosage is 200–800IU per day of d-alpha-tocopherol (natural vitamin E; check the label) or mixed tocopherols.

TOCOTRIENOLS: These newer vitamin E-related compounds have recently been found to have very powerful antioxidant activity. Sometimes they are included in a vitamin supplement and sometimes they are available separately. Fresh fruits, dark green leafy vegetables, almonds, peanuts, and wheatgerm also contain tocotrienols and the other types of vitamin E. The usual dose is 40–80mg/day.

SELENIUM: This antioxidant has been shown to decrease the risk of free-radical damage to blood vessel walls. Usual dose is 50–200 mcg per day.

OLIGOMERIC PROANTHOCYANIDINS (OPCS): The proanthocyanidins are in the class of foods known as the flavonoids. Cardiovascular disease risk is inversely proportional to flavonoid intake.[44] OPCs are derived from grape seeds or pine bark (one brand is Pycnogenol). This is a supplement I wouldn't live without because of its many benefits. OPCs are quickly absorbed into the bloodstream, help to regenerate the body's levels of vitamin E, and also prevent the oxidation of LDL cholesterol by free radicals. In addition, they improve blood vessel and skin elasticity by helping prevent free-radical damage to collagen, reduce or eliminate the discomfort of arthritis, help prevent circulation problems, and reduce excessive blood clotting. They also help prevent all the symptoms of allergy and hay fever. The usual dose is 40–120mg/day.

L-CARNITINE: This supplement helps to keep triglycerides low, raises HDL cholesterol, and helps prevent heart disease by enhancing the overall health of the heart muscle and helping to prevent cardiac arrhythmias.[45] It also helps the body utilise energy within the mitochondria of each cell and is therefore helpful for fat loss. The usual dose is 500–2,000mg/day.

ALPHA-LIPOIC ACID (ALA): Alpha-lipoic acid is a unique antioxidant in that it is both water- and fat-soluble. That means that it can stand guard against free-radical damage in every part of the cell. It has also been shown to help preserve intracellular levels of vitamins C and E and to help regenerate another antioxidant known as glutathione. Alpha-lipoic acid is also helpful for the metabolism of insulin, and in Germany it has been approved for the treatment of diabetic neuropathy (nerve damage). It has been shown to improve blood flow both to the nerves and to the skin. The usual dose is 50–200mg/day.

VITAMIN C: This powerful antioxidant helps protect the endothelial lining of your blood vessels and has also been found to aid the absorption of calcium and magnesium, two key minerals for heart health. A dose of 1,000mg per day has been shown to reduce systolic blood pressure significantly, though the mechanism is not clear. I recommend taking it in the form of plain old ascorbic acid. If you have a sensitive stomach, use the ascorbate form. The usual dose is 1,000–3,000mg/day.

B Vitamins and Folic Acid

Over half of all women don't get the folic acid they need. This not only puts their babies at risk of neural tube defects such as spina bifida, but also increases their risk of arteriosclerosis and heart disease. It has been found that the individuals with the highest homocysteine levels also have the lowest levels of folic acid, B_{12}, and B_6. A higher dose of folic acid than the RDA is associated with a lower risk of heart attack (it may inhibit platelet aggregation and prolong clotting time) and is also the antidote for high homocysteine.[46] Women with adequate B vitamin and folate levels have a definite decreased risk of heart disease.[47]

The usual doses are: vitamin B$_6$, 40–80mg per day; vitamin B$_{12}$, 20mcg per day; folic acid, 400–800mcg per day. It's always best to take these together with the entire B complex. (See chapter 7.)

Foods for Heart Health

FISH: Studies have shown that 3g per day of fish oil containing both EPA and DHA is cardioprotective because of its effects on eicosanoid balance.[48] Alternatively, you can eat three servings of cold-water fish per week, such as salmon, mackerel, swordfish, or sardines. One 4oz (113g) serving of salmon contains about 200mg of DHA.

If you don't eat fish regularly, supplement your diet with omega-3 supplements, from either fish oil or algae-derived DHA (good for vegans). The usual dose is 100–200mg per day.

GREEN TEA: The flavonoids in green tea are known as polyphenols. These substances have powerful antioxidant effects that may be greater than or equal to that of vitamins C and E. As little as one cup of green tea per day will provide protection.[49]

GARLIC: Garlic has a long history of use in the treatment of hypertension. One pilot study showed that high doses of garlic (2,400mg of deodorised garlic per day) significantly lowered both diastolic and systolic blood pressure. Like alpha-lipoic acid, garlic appears to increase the activity of the endothelial cells that produce nitric oxide, which is a blood vessel relaxant.

Numerous studies have also shown that regular consumption of garlic reduces cholesterol by 10 per cent or more and lowers triglyceride levels by up to 13 per cent. It may also inhibit platelet aggregation and blood clot formation.[50]

The German Commission E, which evaluates therapeutic claims for natural substances, recommends a dosage level equivalent to 1 to 4 cloves of fresh raw garlic a day. This is the amount estimated to provide 4,000mcg of allicin, one of garlic's most beneficial compounds. Many good garlic supplements are on the market. Look for one with the active ingredient alliin, because this substance is relatively odourless until it is converted into allicin in the body. Products containing this substance supply all the benefits of fresh garlic but are more socially acceptable. A daily dose should be 10mg of alliin, or a total allicin potential of 4,000mcg. (See Resources.)

HAWTHORN: In her inspiring book *Herbal Rituals*, master herbalist Judith Berger points out that hawthorn leaf, blossom, or berry (*Crataegus oxycantha*) extracted into water or spirit-based preparations is a 'fierce and protective ally for those seeking to prevent heart-related conditions which are passed on from generation to generation'.[51] Hawthorn berry extract can calm palpitations, help restore blood vessel elasticity, ease fluid build-up in the heart, halt fatty degeneration of the heart, help dilate coronary arteries, and also reduce blood pressure. It can be used by those already on cardiac medication and may help you decrease your dosage. I take my hawthorn as a tea. You just buy a bag of organically grown hawthorn berries at a health food shop and steep them in hot water to taste. There is nothing standardised about this method, but I see myself as creating a healthy heart by drinking a little tea, not treating heart disease. Hawthorn has not been shown to have any adverse side effects.

If you prefer to take your hawthorn as a pill, look for a standard-ised extract, and use a product that contains 10 per cent proantho-cyanidins or 1.8 per cent vitexin-4''-rhamnoside. The usual dose is 100–250mg three times per day.

Sodium–Potassium Balance

Decreasing sodium and increasing potassium in your diet can help control high blood pressure, which is an important risk factor for heart and circulatory problems.[52] For the 60 per cent of individuals whose hypertension is related to sodium intake, the effect of sodium on blood pressure can be relieved by increasing one's intake of potassium. Dietary potassium deficiency is caused by a diet that is low in fresh fruits and vegetables and high in sodium. This is your basic fast-food diet! A diet rich in fruits, vegetables, and whole grains can supply you with 4,000–6,000mg of potassium a day. Drugs such as diuretics, laxatives, aspirin, and others can also deplete your potassium. Prolonged exercise is associated with loss of potassium as well – up to 3,000mg of potassium can be lost in one day by sweating. A diet high in potassium and low in sodium protects against high blood pressure, stroke, and heart disease. Potassium supplements have been shown to lower both systolic and diastolic blood pressure significantly, but these have side effects, including nausea, vomiting, diarrhoea, and ulcers, when given in pill form at high dosage levels. This won't happen if you increase your levels through diet alone.

Many Westerners have a potassium-to-sodium ratio of 1:2, but researchers recommend a 5:1 ratio. One trip to a fried-chicken joint or pizza place will mess up this ratio. Because fruits and vegetables like potatoes, bananas, and apples are such rich sources of potassium, don't get too worried about their high glycaemic indexes. Because they are whole foods, they will not raise your insulin levels high enough to really cause damage unless they are highly processed into something like french fries. It is the simple carbohydrates in white flour products that really mess things up as far as both insulin and potassium-to-sodium ratios are concerned. This is yet another reason why you want to try for five servings of fruits and vegetables per day in your diet.

Because magnesium and potassium work together at the level of the cell, they are often low at the same time.

Foods to Improve Your Potassium–Sodium Ratio

Potatoes	110:1 ratio of potassium to sodium
Carrots	75:1
Apples	90:1
Bananas	440:1
Oranges	260:1

What About Aspirin?

The FDA in the US has suggested that death rates from heart attack could be cut by nearly a quarter if doctors would give one-half of a standard (300mg) aspirin tablet during a heart attack and continue administration of the tablet for thirty days.

In 1982 Dr John Vane won the Nobel prize by showing that aspirin can inhibit the clumping of platelets in blood vessels. The regular use of aspirin (75mg) may decrease the risk of heart attack by preventing clots from forming in arteries that have been narrowed by arteriosclerosis. It inhibits the formation of series 2 eicosanoids, the cellular hormones that are associated with inflammation, platelet clumping, and build-up of arterial plaques. Studies strongly suggest that those who have evidence of ischemia of the heart muscles (decreased oxygenation of the heart) can definitely benefit from taking aspirin.[53]

Most studies suggest that you should use one junior aspirin or one standard aspirin a day (75–300mg per day) in order to maximise the effects without inducing gastrointestinal (GI) bleeding or upset stomach, common side effects of aspirin. *Caution:* Do not take aspirin if you are on an SSRI antidepressant such as fluoxetine (Prozac), paroxetine (Seroxat), or sertraline (Lustral). This is because these drugs plus aspirin increase your chances for having upper GI bleeding or ulcers. The non-steroidal anti-inflammatory drugs (NSAIDs), such as naproxen sodium (Synflex) or ibuprofen (Brufen, Fenbid), can also increase your risk for GI bleeding and stomach upset. When you take aspirin along with these, your risk of gastrointestinal problems is even higher.

Here's what I'd recommend. If you have any family history of heart disease, or fear of it, and aren't taking any SSRIs or NSAIDs regularly, then you might want to consider taking a junior aspirin a day, starting at about the age of fifty, if it feels right. (This age is arbitrary. Most studies were done on people who are sixty or older.) If it doesn't, think about the issue yearly to decide if the time is right. An antioxidant programme may offer similar benefits without risk of GI bleeding. OPCs (see page 478) or ginger tea are particularly good.

Get Moving!

Exercise provides all the cardiovascular benefits attributed to oestrogen and has been shown repeatedly to significantly reduce the risk of heart disease, hypertension, and stroke.[54] Exercise training after diagnosed coronary artery disease has also been shown to improve blood flow to the heart by improving the ability of the blood vessel lining (endothelium) to keep vessels open and also by recruiting collateral vessels in the heart muscle that help bypass vessels that have been blocked.[55] The benefits of exercise to help your heart even after a heart attack are evidence of just how forgiving the heart and blood vessels are when we care for them.

Your goal should be to exercise five or six days per week for at least thirty minutes. Walking is fine. Exercise decreases insulin and blood sugar levels and will give you a much bigger 'grace factor' in terms of your diet. In other words, when you exercise, you'll have a bit more leeway with your diet. Don't overdo it, however; if you use exercise simply as a way to keep your weight down, you are more apt to injure yourself – and, sooner or later, you'll regain the weight.

The Role of Lymph

One of the main reasons why exercise has such healing power is that it vastly increases the lymph circulation in your body. Lymph is the clear fluid that drains from around your body's cells into the lymphatic system, a network of thin-walled vessels found throughout every organ and tissue in your body. Lymph vessels contain small valves to keep the lymph from flowing backwards. Bean-shaped structures known as lymph nodes are found at frequent intervals along lymph vessels, with major centres occurring in the groin, neck, and armpits and alongside the aorta and the inferior vena cava in the chest and the abdomen. The function of the lymph nodes is threefold: (1) to filter out and destroy foreign substances, such as bacteria and dust; (2) to produce some of the white cells called lymphocytes that help fight tumours and other invaders; and (3) to produce antibodies that help in the body's immune surveillance system. All lymph eventually gets emptied into a large central vessel in our chest cavities, known as the thoracic duct, which eventually empties into our hearts, so that the lymph and blood get mixed together once again after our lymph nodes have removed the waste, bacteria, and other flotsam and jetsam from it.

In addition to its role in helping keep bacteria and other invaders in check, the lymphatic system is essential to the mechanism by which fats are processed by the body. Lymph vessels that drain the small intestine collect the digested fat from the foods we eat and pass it directly into the main blood circulation, bypassing the liver. Once fats are in the blood, they may or may not get laid down in the blood vessels of the heart, forming fatty streaks that eventually lead to hardening of the arteries and the beginning of cardiovascular disease. Whether or not this happens depends upon our diet, our exercise habits, and our emotional and psychological state.

I interviewed Jerry Lemole, MD, a leading cardiovascular surgeon from Philadelphia in the US, many of whose patients suffer from end-stage heart disease. His research on the role of the lymph system is both intriguing and motivating.

The HDL-Lymph Connection

The lymphatic system in the heart is intimately involved with the process that leads to coronary artery disease. LDL, the so-called bad cholesterol, is a large, fluffy fat molecule that can get into blood vessel walls through breaks in the intimal tissue that forms the blood vessel lining. This is especially apt to happen when LDL cholesterol becomes oxidised. Once LDL gets stuck here, it tends to break down and leave cholesterol deposits behind.

HDL cholesterol, the 'good' cholesterol, is a smooth football-shaped molecule that is small enough to actually get into the tissue around the blood vessel wall and vacuum up the cholesterol deposits left behind by the LDL.

In order for HDL to do its job of vacuuming up cholesterol deposits, it needs to get to where the cholesterol is located. It does this through lymph circulation. Dr Lemole likens HDL molecules that pick up cholesterol in the artery walls to taxis in New York City. If you view Manhattan from a helicopter, you'll see a certain number of taxis. At any given time, because traffic in New York is so often backed up in the tunnels that lead to and from the city, you'll have many taxis unavailable to passengers in the street who need to be picked up. If you could speed up the passage of the taxis through the tunnels, there would be more of them available on the streets.

The same is true with the cholesterol-carrying capacity of HDL. When lymph flow is sluggish, HDL molecules simply are not available to pick up excess cholesterol deposits. If you speed up the circulation time of lymph, you'll also improve the efficiency of HDL to scavenge excess fat from your arteries.[56]

How to Speed Up Lymph Flow

1. Don't sit for long periods of time. Women who sit for long periods of time at sedentary jobs are more likely to get heart disease because the lymphatic flow through their thoracic cavity is limited.

2. Breathe deeply and regularly. Breathing fully in through your nose and inhaling air down into the lower lobes of your lungs followed by a brisk exhalation massages the thoracic duct and all the lymph vessels and nodes in your chest cavity, which helps HDL get to the places it needs to go to do its work.

3. Move. Lymph flow depends upon the muscles in the body to move it along. Every time you walk, do yoga, breathe deeply, run, or move your muscles briskly, you are helping move the lymph along. Dr Lemole reports that the average turnover time for proteins in lymph is once to twice per day. But when you exercise regularly, you can increase this figure to three to five times per day. So exercising gives your body three to five times more opportunity to get rid of excess cholesterol deposits in the blood vessels around your heart.

4. Avoid overexercise. When we exercise, we actually increase the oxidative stress in our bodies, which results in the production of free radicals in our bodies. Over time this can do more damage than good. That's why so many endurance athletes have impaired immune function, which makes them more susceptible to infections and illness. This needn't be the case if you always breathe in and out fully through your nose as you exercise and never exert yourself beyond what is comfortable with this way of breathing. (For further information about this, read *Body, Mind, and Sport,* John Douillard (Three Rivers Press, 2001).)

Dr Lemole recommends that you walk at a pace of about 3.6–4.0 miles per hour, which means that it should take you about thirty to forty minutes to cover two miles. Any faster than that and you will incur a lot of oxidative stress in your body that will require you to take additional antioxidant vitamins to cover the potential damage. Remember that if you exercise so that you're breathing comfortably in and out through your nose, your body will also be operating at a pace that decreases free-radical damage, because comfortable nose breathing results in a balance between your sympathetic and parasympathetic nervous systems.

Exercise lowers many cardiovascular risks, including high blood pressure. In one study, those who did not engage in vigorous exercise regularly had a 35 per cent greater risk of hypertension than those who did. Though it helps to have been active at school and in college, you will not be protected unless you continue regular vigorous exercise throughout your life.

Is Oestrogen Replacement Necessary to Prevent Heart Disease?

Because the incidence of heart disease in women rises at about the age of fifty, the same time that oestrogen levels start to decrease, scientists have long assumed that heart disease after menopause must be related to an oestrogen deficiency. And because studies have demonstrated that oestrogen lowers LDL cholesterol, raises HDL cholesterol, and helps support blood vessel walls, the medical profession has quite naturally assumed that giving everyone oestrogen would solve the problem of heart disease.

Here's a summary of the documented effects of oestrogen replacement on the heart:

- Oestrogen exerts a cardioprotective effect on blood vessels and helps coronary arteries dilate (not constrict inappropriately).[57] It directly modifies and normalises the function of the endothelium and vascular smooth muscle.

- It has a favourable impact on lipoproteins, cholesterol, and fibrinogen levels and reverses some adverse effects of lipid metabolism.

- It decreases endothelium retention of LDL by coronary arteries.[58]

- Unopposed oestrogen works better than oestrogen in combination with progestogens. As I discussed in chapter 5, synthetic progestogens cancel out some of the beneficial effects of oestrogens.

- Oestrogen has been used as an alternative to cholesterol-lowering drugs such as lovastatin and pravastatin. There may even be an additive effect on cholesterol and lipoproteins by combining HRT and pravastatin.[59]

The PEPI study and several others that showed similar improvements in blood lipids from taking oestrogen have led many doctors to prescribe oestrogen replacement therapy routinely to all their post-menopausal patients as a way to prevent heart disease.[60] But the recent results of the HERS and ERA studies show that oestrogen replacement does *not* decrease the incidence of heart attack in women who already have heart disease, and in fact may even increase the risk for a while. This certainly has decreased the unbridled enthusiasm for prescribing Premarin that has characterised the medical profession for the last decade.[61]

And now, preliminary data from the large US randomised clinical trial known as the Women's Health Initiative, which is studying the effect of hormone replacement therapy on healthy women, has actually shown a small increase in heart attacks, strokes, and blood clots in women on Premarin and Provera, and even in those who are taking only Premarin without Provera. Though it looks as though this risk disappears after the first two years of use and that after this time oestrogen may be beneficial, these results have been very confusing to many.[62]

It will take years of further study to sort out the conflicting evidence about oestrogen. Despite extensive observational studies supporting a role for oestrogen in preventing heart disease, the HERS and Women's Health Initiative data have made one thing clear: Premarin plus Provera, and even Premarin alone, don't seem to be as cardioprotective as we've been led to believe. Until we have large, long-term studies on the individualised bioidentical hormone regimens I recommend, we won't have the data necessary to truly evaluate the benefits of hormone replacement for heart disease prevention. More than ever, women are going to have to use their own intuition and body wisdom when making this choice.

Despite these recent studies, many researchers feel strongly that oestrogen still has a role in heart disease prevention and that women who are on it should stay on it. Let's go over all the factors involved in keeping your heart healthy so that you can decide for yourself whether or not you might benefit from oestrogen replacement as a way to prevent heart disease.

Fact number one: No researcher has ever demonstrated a cause-and-effect relationship between low oestrogen levels and subsequent heart disease. If they had, oestrogen replacement would be the number-one drug prescribed for men over the age of forty! Oestrogen is only one factor that improves the blood lipids associated with heart disease. Exercise also increases HDL cholesterol, as does a diet that normalises insulin levels.

Fact number two: Heart disease was very rare in the West before the 1930s. (It is still very rare in non-industrialised areas such as rural China.) This is not because everyone died before they were fifty! Quite the contrary – if you survived the threat of childhood infectious diseases, your chances of living to a healthy old age were as good or better than they are now. In the 1930s our society shifted increasingly towards industrialisation, with much of the population moving from tightly knit farm communities to the city. Lack of community has been associated with increased rates of heart disease. Refined foods also gradually replaced whole foods grown or produced at home. A diet rich in refined sugar and white flour, and devoid of minerals and other nutrients, has been demonstrated time and again to be associated with cancer, obesity, and heart disease. When people moved into the cities, physical activity decreased dramatically. Regular exercise is a very well-documented way to keep your heart healthy – the heart is a muscle that requires regular exercise for proper functioning. Yet less than 40 per cent of all women exercise regularly.[63]

Fact number three: In addition to these huge cultural changes, another dietary change that has major health implications occurred at about the same time. Partially hydrogenated fats, which have a long shelf life, began to be added to the food supply, and margarine gradually replaced butter and lard. Now it is difficult to find any prepared baked goods that do not contain partially hydrogenated fats. But these fats have been directly linked with the free-radical damage to blood vessel walls that eventually results in heart disease. And though an excess of saturated fat in your diet is also not ideal, a small amount of saturated fat daily is far healthier than partially hydrogenated fat, which doesn't occur anywhere in nature!

Fact number four: In the studies that show a benefit from oestrogen replacement, the women on the oestrogen may have been healthier to begin with than those not taking oestrogen. This may have been the reason why the famous Nurses' Health Study showed a decrease in risk of cardiovascular disease of up to 50 per cent in HRT users.[64] Other studies have suggested this as well.[65]

Fact number five: There is no reason to believe that a normal life stage such as menopause would be automatically associated with disease.

Nature doesn't work that way. Many postmenopausal women maintain adequate oestrogen levels for years. Your body fat, liver, adrenal glands, and ovaries continue to produce oestrogen throughout your life if you are well nourished and are taking in the right building blocks for hormones. Before starting oestrogen replacement therapy, ask your doctor to determine your total oestrogen level and see how much you have on your own. If your serum oestradiol levels are between 50pg/ml and 150pg/ml, you are making enough of your own oestrogen.[66]

Though there are no studies directly comparing the heart disease risk of a group of healthy, physically fit postmenopausal women with sedentary postmenopausal women on a low-nutrient diet who also take oestrogen, we do have a few clues about how powerful lifestyle factors are in preventing heart disease. The Nurses' Health Study showed that women who had none of the risk factors for heart disease (only 3 per cent of the total number of study participants) – specifically, smoking, overweight, lack of exercise, and poor diet – had an 83 per cent lower risk of coronary events than the rest of the women.[67]

Fact number six: The energies of love, enthusiasm, joy, and passion actually enliven your heart. To promote a healthy heart, you must have a goal, a passion, a reason for living.

Many women get heart disease when, for any number of reasons, their heart is no longer in their work or their life. A very healthy eighty-five-year-old patient without any signs of heart disease recently told me that she didn't think she'd be around much longer. Her ninety-year-old husband had been hospitalised with heart disease and wasn't back to his usual state of health. She said, 'We've been married for sixty years. I couldn't go on living without him.' It is well known that elderly spouses often die within weeks of each other. Even in the medical profession this is known as 'dying from a broken heart'.

Fact number seven: Smoking is the number-one risk factor for heart disease in both men and women. Smoking literally shuts down the energy of the heart. If you are a smoker, notice when you feel like smoking. You may find that your desire to smoke is directly linked with an emotion that you don't want to feel. If you smoke and want to give up, I'd recommend trying nicotine patches and joining a Quit Smoking course.

My Advice About Hormones and Your Heart

Use bioidentical hormones as part of your heart protection plan in the following circumstances:

- If you've read all the pros and cons of oestrogen replacement and feel that it is right for you. Right now both the medical profession and society in general tend to believe that the benefits of oestrogen outweigh any risks. This belief, in and of itself, can have a therapeutic effect.

- If you honestly cannot exercise or change your diet right now.

- If you have a very strong family history of heart disease, feel you 'take after' those family members who've had heart disease, and feel you can't change that.

- If you're already on oestrogen for other reasons and you like the way you feel on it.

- If you find yourself worrying about your heart regularly and would fret less about your health if you were following conventional medical guidelines for protecting yourself.

- If you are still undecided. In this case, there is no harm to be done by giving oestrogen a trial run. Get your doctor to check your lipid profile after three months to see if there have been any improvements. Start with the lowest possible dose of bioidentical hormones that you can and see how you feel. If it isn't right, you can either change the type of HRT you are on or go off it very slowly, tapering down over a two-month period of time.

Avoid synthetic progesterone. As already noted, this synthetic hormone eliminates many of the benefits of oestrogen and may even increase the risk of heart attack.

As in all matters of health, there is no one magic bullet that will be the right answer for everyone. In reducing the complex matter of

heart health to whether or not to take oestrogen daily, the medical–
pharmaceutical industry has unwittingly done women everywhere a
disservice. But with the right information, and by following the
wisdom of your heart, you will be able to make the right decision for
yourself.

How to Love and Respect Your Midlife Heart

Though it has been said that 'home is where the heart is', in my experience home is also where the heart most easily gets broken. One of
the greatest challenges of midlife is to come home to ourselves. We
can do this only when we allow ourselves to get to the heart of the
matter – and our emotions will always lead us there. Too many
women use addictions – to food, alcohol, smoking, too much or too
little exercise, or recreational drugs – as a way to avoid the feelings
that will lead them home. It is only through achieving emotional
balance that we will truly reach the feeling of being at home within
ourselves. And it is only through learning emotional balance that we
will be willing to stick with the healthy diet, exercise, and supplement
programmes that will help our hearts. Though I suggest that you
follow the dietary and exercise guidelines I've outlined, I believe that
it is even more important to learn what it is to love and accept yourself. This journey home is always poignant and often painful, but
inevitably always worth it, too.

One of my perimenopausal friends whose mother had been
mentally ill, and who knew that she had always used food as a way to
cope with the craziness of having to care for both her mother and her
younger siblings, told me that when she reached forty-three she
finally was able to allow herself to really feel the pain of all those
childhood years and let it go. She said, 'I remember the first time I sat
in my therapist's office and actually allowed myself to feel the
absolute panic and terror within that was the result of fear that I'd
become just like my mother. And in that moment I knew why people
with severe weight problems often don't lose weight – or why they
put it straight back on. They prefer overeating and obesity to allowing
themselves to feel the depth of despair and pain within them.' Luckily
my friend has a very strong faith, and with the help of God she finally
allowed herself to get all those old feelings out in the open, a process
that took several months and a lot of tears.

She credits this to the fact that she sailed through menopause without a symptom. She no longer uses food to quell her emotions and has kept her weight stable for over ten years. The only way out was through!

Whether or not you have midlife heart symptoms such as palpitations, hypertension, high cholesterol, chest pain, jaw pain, arm pain, or any other evidence of heart disease, or if you simply want to prevent heart disease in the future, you owe it to yourself to learn the language of your heart.

The Heart-opening Effect of Pets

One of the first things I did after my husband moved out was to go down to the animal shelter and get two cats, something I'd wanted to do for a long time – my husband had been allergic to them. Few things have done me and my health as much good as my two cats, Buddy and Francine. One of my midlife friends, a professional woman with a high-powered job, recently got a dog. She said to me, 'It's really true that happiness is a warm puppy. What a wonderful thing to wake up each morning to such unconditional love! Everyone in my block of flats loves him. And when I take him for a walk, I make all kinds of new friends!' Scientific literature on the health benefits of pets proves beyond the shadow of a doubt that our hearts are touched and healed, quite literally, by the unconditional love that animals can bring to our lives.

Though animals can't offer all the different types of support that we humans need, they still provide companionship, security, and a feeling of being needed. They also help connect us to the world around us and give us a focus outside ourselves – which is very helpful for those who suffer from depression. Larry Dossey, MD, has extensively researched the healing power of prayer, and refers to companion animals as 'four-legged prayer'.

The presence of a pet is associated with decreased cardiovascular reactivity – which means that the influence of a pet helps us stabilise our blood vessels and heart rhythm. People have been found to have lower heart rates and lower blood pressure when they are with their pets. This translates into thousands of fewer heartbeats over months and years, which can slow the development of arteriosclerosis. Research at Brooklyn College in the US has shown that pets slow heart rate even among highly stressed, high-intensity type A personalities.[68]

Pets of all kinds lower blood pressure. Petting a dog has been shown to decrease the blood pressure of healthy college students, hospitalised elderly people, and adults with high blood pressure. When bird owners talk to their birds, their blood pressure drops an average of ten points. And watching fish in an aquarium has been shown to bring blood pressure below resting levels. Research has also shown that when children are sitting quietly and reading, their blood pressure is lower when a dog is in the room.[69]

Support from animal companions has been linked to increased survival in those with coronary artery disease. This survival was independent of marital status and living situation. In the US, University of Pennsylvania researchers Aaron Katcher and Erika Friedmann found that people with pets lived longer after experiencing heart attacks than those without pets.[70] Subsequent research has shown that among people who have heart attacks, pet owners have one-fifth the death rate of those who do not have pets.[71] If you can't own a pet yourself, volunteer at an animal shelter or visit other people's pets. They're a cardiac tonic with no side effects.

Whether or not you get a new pet, a new job, or a new mate, midlife is a time of rebirth. The newly opening midlife heart is tender, green, and new. Don't allow it to be stepped on. Learn how to protect yourself; ask for help and allow yourself to receive it. Open your heart, care for your heart, and let it lead you home.

The Calm After the Storm

One day during the winter after my divorce, I awoke at 6am to go to my regular morning exercise class. Though the weather report said it was raining, I opened the door and walked out into a snowstorm that was dumping about two inches an hour all around me. Nevertheless, I set out. After all, I'm a veteran of snowy winters. As I headed south, however, I could scarcely see, and I briefly considered turning around. But in my characteristically stoic fashion I continued, certain that the weather would soon improve. Suddenly my car started spinning in a circle, wildly out of control and heading for the railings. I braced myself for the crash, wondering simultaneously whether I would survive being hit broadside by the oncoming traffic. After my car slammed to a halt against railings cushioned by snow, I braced for further collisions. Miraculously, the cars behind me were able to stop in time. Not sure what to do next, I hesitantly put my car into gear. I was able to pull out onto the road, and I slowly continued my drive. As I entered the city the weather did indeed clear, and I ended up going to my class. Though I was shaken, the damage to my car was mostly cosmetic – I had shattered my left rear bumper, nothing else. I felt very lucky. I knew that I could have been killed.

My accident seemed like a swift energetic re-enactment of my perimenopause, complete with the shattering of my marriage and of the parts of my personality that now needed to die if I was to stay healthy and grow. The accident happened almost one year to the day from the time when my husband and I had separated and started divorce proceedings. For the past year my old life and personality had, like my vehicle on that icy road, been seized by a force beyond my control. Despite my worst fears, I had ended up able to move forward under my own power. And though at the time the impact of the break-up had felt as though it might destroy some essential part of me, the damage, like the damage to my car, turned out to be largely cosmetic. My life no longer looked as picture-perfect as it once had. Yet I discovered that the only thing of true significance that had been shattered was the closely guarded and comforting illusion that something or someone outside of myself could and should save me from living the life that I was destined to live. After twenty-four years of marriage, I had managed to spend a year without a man. I had survived a great deal of grief and pain, found that I was able to support my children and myself, and, though shaken, had emerged more fearless than ever before.

The morning after my accident I awoke to a beautiful sunny day, my two cats asleep on the foot of the bed. Yes, I was alone in the house. Yes, my nest was empty. But my heart was more full of love, joy, and anticipation for the future than it had been in over a year. I was free, and for the first time in my life I could create the rest of my life on my own terms instead of trying to please someone else – whether parents, teachers, husband, or children.

I also knew, right down in my bone marrow, that I needed to cherish my newfound moments of solitude in my own home, because they might not last for ever. If I meet a man with whom I can be fully myself, sharing both my vulnerability and my competence and valuing the same mix of qualities in him, then I would love to have a life partner again. For now, though, I know that my primary relationship has to be the one with myself. I can no longer lose myself in a relationship with anyone else or put anyone else's welfare ahead of my own. So at this transitional time of my life I am savouring every sunset and every morning of awakening to new possibilities, new adventures.

Whether or not I ever find that life partner, I know I am not alone. And neither are you, whether or not you're married, have children, or live in a community. You and I are part of a massive group of capable, healthy, and self-assured women who are redefining what it means to be a woman at midlife: physically, emotionally, financially, and spiritually. All of the things we were passionate about in our adolescence are now coming up for us again. But this time we have the skills, connections, and know-how to act on our passion and make it real. Once we truly become partners with our own spirits at midlife, we not only restore our faith in ourselves, but also become part of a force to be reckoned with.

Every morning I look at myself in the mirror, and I like the woman I see. I like her physical and emotional strength and her compassionate heart, a heart that has been broken but has now become courageous enough to love again – if (and only if) I can find someone who can love me in return without asking me to compromise any part of myself.

We're waking up together, you and I. Don't let anyone tell you that the passions that are now shaking you to the core are simply a hormonal storm. Don't let anyone tell you that you're asking too much or that you should be more 'realistic'. Your passions are real, and they are calling out to you to be acted upon. But don't panic if you feel some pain. Whenever we give birth to anything important, like the new relationship with our souls that is possible at midlife, there are going to be labour pains. You don't have to make this transition overnight. You have months, even years.

Never forget that the big wisdom of life comes at menopause. There is enormous power here. Though the mainstream media has tried to make midlife women all but invisible, we're at a turning point. There is a critical mass of us, and we're beginning to know our own power. No one yet suspects how much we can accomplish when we go into our businesses, churches, clubs, and families and, quietly and peacefully, like the stealth missiles we are, set about changing everything for the better.

What happens when each of us, in her own unique way, starts refusing to say the lines that have been handed to us, refuses to play the roles that we've inherited from the women before us – women who did the best they could but whose roles are now as obsolete as the role I chose to play in my marriage back in the 1970s?

It is estimated that by the year 2008 women between the ages of fifty and sixty-five will be the largest demographic group in the UK. And for the first time in human history, the money we will be using will be money we have earned ourselves. What happens when we wake up to the power that has always been there but that our mothers and grandmothers were talked out of? What happens when, because of our sheer numbers and the circumstances of our formative years, we wake up and realise that the people we've been waiting for are us?

As we flex our economic, mental, and physical muscles and put our money and energy where our ideals are, the world will change in ways that reflect our inherent women's wisdom, wisdom that has the potential to benefit every woman, man, child, and living being on this planet.

Notes

Chapter 1: Menopause Puts Your Life Under a Microscope

1. Sams, J., & Carson, D. (1988). *Medicine Cards* (p. 150). Santa Fe: Bear & Co.

Chapter 2: The Brain Catches Fire at Menopause

1. Seymour, L. J. (ed.) (April, 1999). News from Redbook. *Redbook*, p. 16.
2. Larsson, C., & Hallman, J. (1997). Is severity of premenstrual symptoms related to illness in the climacteric? *J. Psychosomatic Obstetrics & Gynecology, 18,* 234–243; Novaes, C., & Almeida, O. P. (1999). Premenstrual syndrome and psychiatric morbidity at the menopause. *J. Psychosomatic Obstetrics & Gynecology, 20,* 56–57; Arpels, J. C. (1996). The female brain hypoestrogenic continuum from PMS to menopause: A hypothesis and review of supporting data. *J. Reproductive Medicine, 41* (9), 633–639.
3. Schmidt, P., et al. (1998). Differential behavioral effects of gonadal steroids in women with and in those without premenstrual syndrome. *NEJM, 338* (4), 209–216.
4. Larsson, C., & Hallman, J. (1997). Is severity of premenstrual symptoms related to illness in the climacteric? *J. Psychosomatic Obstetrics & Gynecology, 18,* 234–243; Novaes, C., & Almeida, O. P. (1999). Premenstrual syndrome and psychiatric morbidity at the menopause. *J. Psychosomatic Obstetrics & Gynecology, 20,* 56–57.
5. Benedek, T., & Rubenstein, B. (1939). Correlations between ovarian activity and psychodynamic processes: The ovulatory phase. *Psychosomatic Medicine, 1* (2), 245–270.
6. Weitoft, G. R., et al. (2000). Mortality among lone mothers in Sweden: A population study. *Lancet, 355,* 1215–1219.
7. Herzog, A. (1997). Neuroendocrinology of epilepsy. In S. C. Schacter & O. Devinsky (eds.), *Behavioral Neurology and the Legacy of Norman Geschwind,* 235–236. Philadelphia: Lippincott, Williams & Wilkins; Moyer, K. E. (1976). *The Psychology of Aggression.* New York: Harper & Row; Albert, I., et al. (1987). Inter-male social aggression in rats: Suppression by medical hypothalamic lesions independently of enhanced defensiveness of decreased testicular testosterone. *Physiology & Behavior, 39,* 693–698; Post, R. M. (1992). Transduction of psychosocial stress into

the neurobiology of recurrent affective disorder. *Am. J. Psychiatry, 149,* 999–1010.

8. Linehan, M. (1993). *Skills Training Manual for Treating Borderline Personality Disorder,* 143. New York: Guilford Press.

9. Herzog, A. G. (1989). Perimenopausal depression: Possible role of anomalous brain substrates. *Brain Dysfunction, 2,* 146–154.

10. Ledoux, J. E. (1986). Sensory systems and emotions: A model of affective processing. *Integrative Psychiatry, 4,* 237–243. For a complete scientific discussion of this area, see Schulz, M. L. (1998). *Awakening Intuition,* 113–135. New York: Harmony.

11. Musante, L., et al. (1989). Potential for hostility and dimensions of anger. *Health Psychology, 8,* 343; Mittleman, M. A., et al. (1995). Triggering of acute MI onset of episodes of anger. *Circulation, 92,* 1720–1725. For an exhaustive listing of the scientific studies documenting the emotional risk factors for heart attack, see Schulz, M. L., op. cit. (chapter 9, 216–250).

12. Porges, S., et al. (1996). Infant regulation of the vagal 'brake' predicts child behavior problems: A psychobiological model of social behavior. *Developmental Psychobiology, 29* (8), 697–712; Porges, S. (1992). Vagal tone: A physiological marker of stress vulnerability. *Pediatrics, 90,* 498–504; Donchin, Y., et al. (1992). Cardiac vagal tone predicts outcome in neurosurgical patients. *Critical Care Medicine, 20,* 941–949.

13. Heim, C., et al. (2000) Pituitary-adrenal and autonomic responses to stress in women after sexual and physical abuse in childhood, *JAMA 284* (5), 592–596.

14. Schulz, M. L., MD, PhD, behavioural neuroscientist and neuropsychiatrist (personal communication, March 20, 2000).

15. Van Der Kolk, B. A. (1996). The body keeps the score: Approaches to the psychobiology of posttraumatic stress disorder. In *Traumatic Stress: The Effects of Overwhelming Experience on Mind, Body, and Society.* New York: Guilford Press.

16. Clow, B. H. (1996). *The Liquid Light of Sex: Kundalini Rising at Midlife Crisis.* Berkeley, CA: Bear & Co. This book comes complete with charts that allow the reader to determine exactly when their key life passages will or have happened, thus allowing one to take full advantage of what might otherwise be considered a crisis without meaning.

Chapter 3: Coming Home to Yourself:
From Dependence to Healthy Autonomy

1. I originally learned to do this through a process known as Proprioceptive Writing,™ taught by Linda Metcalf and Tobin Simon. (See Resources)

2. Brody, E. M. (1989). *Family at Risk in Alzheimer's Disease,* 2–49. DHHS Publication no. 89–1569. Bethesda, MD: National Institute of Mental Health.

3. The research of Julie Brines, a sociologist at the University of Washing-

ton who studies so-called status-reversal couples, was covered in 'Excuse Me, I'm the Breadwinner.' *Money for Women Magazine* (May–June, 2000), 16–17.

Here is the data: Men whose wives earn all of the family cash spend four fewer hours a week on housework on average than do men who earn just as much as their partners. When the husband works and his wife stays at home, the husband spends three hours per week on housework versus his wife's twenty-five hours. When both husband and wife work and earn equal amounts, the husband does nine hours of housework per week and his wife does seventeen hours. But when the wife works and the husband stays at home, the husband spends only five hours per week on housework, while his wife spends sixteen hours per week.

Chapter 4: This Can't Be Menopause, Can It?
The Physical Foundation of the Change

1. Randolph, J., & Sowers, M. F. (1999). Research on perimenopausal changes in 500 Michigan women, reported in *Midlife Women's Health Sourcebook*. Atlanta, GA: American Health Consultants.
2. McKinlay, S. M., et al. (1992). The normal menopause transition. *Maturitas, 14,* 103; Treloar, A. E., et al. (1981). Menstrual cyclicity and the perimenopause. *Maturitas, 3,* 249.
3. Munster, K., et al. (1992). Length and variation in the menstrual cycle – a cross-sectional study from a Danish county. *British J. Obstetrics & Gynecology, 99* (5), 422; Collett, M. E., et al. (1954). The effect of age upon the pattern of the menstrual cycle. *Fertility & Sterility, 5,* 437.
4. Rannevik, G. (1995). A longitudinal study of the perimenopausal transition: Altered profiles of steroid and pituitary hormones, SHBG and bone mineral density. *Maturitas, 21,* 103.
5. Coulam, C. B., Adamson, S. C., & Annegers, J. F. (1986). Incidence of premature ovarian failure. *Am. J. Obstetrics & Gynecology, 67* (4), 604–606; Miyake, T., et al. (1988). Acute oocyte loss in experimental autoimmune oophoritis as a possible model of premature ovarian failure. *Am. J. Obstetrics & Gynecology, 158* (1), 186–192; Coulam, C. B. (1982). Premature gonadal failure. *Fertility & Sterility, 38,* 645; Gloor, H. J. (1984). Autoimmune oophoritis. *Am. J. Clinical Pathology, 81,* 105–109; Leer, M., Patel, B., Innes, M., et al. (1980). Secondary amenorrhea due to autoimmune ovarian failure. *Australian, New Zealand J. Obstetrics & Gynecology, 20,* 177–179; International Medical News Service. (1985, November). Evidence of autoimmune etiology in some premature menopause. *OB-GYN News, 20* (21), 1, 30.
6. Sumiala, S., et al. (1996). Salivary progesterone concentrations after tubal sterilization. *Obstetrics & Gynecology, 88,* 792–796.
7. Aksel, S., et al. (1976). Vasomotor symptoms, serum estrogens and gonadotropin levels in surgical menopause. *Am. J. Obstetrics & Gynecology, 126,* 165–169. Judd, H. L., & Meldrum, D. R. (1981). Physiology

and pathophysiology of menstruation and menopause. In S. L. Romney, M. J. Gray, & A. B. Little, et al. (eds.), *Gynecology and Obstetrics: The Health Care of Women.* (2nd edn, 885–907). New York: McGraw-Hill.

8. Riad-Fahmy, D., et al. (1982). Steroids in saliva for assessing endocrine function. *Endocrine Reviews, 3* (4), 367–395; Dabbs, M. J. (1990). Salivary testosterone measurements: Collecting, storing, and mailing salivary samples. *Physiology & Behavior, 49,* 815–887; Lipson, S., & Ellison, P. T. (1989). Development of protocols for the application of salivary steroid analysis to field conditions. *Am. J. Human Biology, 1,* 249–255; Ellison, P. T. (1992). Measurement of salivary progesterone. *Annals of the N.Y. Acad. Sci., 694,* 161–176; Kahn, J. P., et al. (1988). Salivary cortisol: A practical method for evaluation of adrenal function. *Biological Psychology 23,* 335–349. Laudat, M. H., et al. (1988). Salivary cortisol: A practical approach to assess pituitary-adrenal function. *J. Clinical Endocrinology & Metabolism, 66,* 343–348;

9. Massoudi, M. S., et al. (1995). Prevalence of thyroid antibodies among healthy middle-aged women. Findings from the thyroid study in healthy women. *Annals of Epidemiology, 5* (3), 229–233.

10. Jeffries, W. McK. (1996). *The Safe Uses of Cortisone.* Springfield, IL: Charles C. Thomas.

11. Golan, R. (1995). *Optimal Wellness,* 203. New York: Ballantine; Baschetti, R. (1995). Chronic fatigue syndrome and licorice (letter). *New Zealand Medical Journal, 108,* 156–157; Stormer, F. C., et al. (1993). Glycyrrhizic acid in licorice: Evaluation of health hazard. *Federal Chemistry & Toxicology, 31,* 303–312.

12. Guthrie, J., et al. (1996). Hot flushes, menstrual status, and hormone levels in a population-based sample of midlife women. *Obstetrics & Gynecology, 88,* 437–442.

13. Leonetti, H., et al. (1999). Transdermal progesterone cream for vasomotor symptoms and postmenopausal bone loss. *Obstetrics & Gynecology, 94,* 225–228.

14. Freedman, R. R., & Woodward, S. (1992). Behavioral treatment of menopausal hot flashes: Evaluation by ambulatory monitoring. *Am. J. Obstetrics & Gynecology, 167,* 436–439; Stevenson, D. W., & Delprato, D. J. (1983). Multiple component self-control program for menopausal hot flashes. *J. Behavioral Therapy & Experimental Psychology, 14* (2), 137–140; Domar, A. D., & Dreher, H. (1997). *Healing Mind, Healthy Woman,* 291–292. New York: Henry Holt & Co.

Chapter 5: Hormone Replacement Therapy: An Individual Choice

1. Mosca, L. (2000). The role of hormone replacement therapy in the prevention of postmenopausal heart disease. *Arch. Intern. Med., 160,* 2263–2272.

2. Shen, L., Qiu, S., Chen, Y., Zhang, F., van Breemen, R. B., Nikolic, D., &

Bolton, J. L. (1998). Alkylation of 2'-deoxynucleosides and DNA by the Premarin metabolite 4-hydroxyequilenin semiquinone radical. *Chemical Research in Toxicology, 11,* 94–101; Bhavnani, B. (1998). Pharmacokinetics and pharmacodynamics of conjugated equine estrogens: Chemistry and metabolism. *Proceedings of the Society for Biological Medicine, 217* (1), 6–16; Zhang, F., et al. (1999). The major metabolite of equilin, 4-hydroxyequilin, autoxidizes to an σ-quinone which isomerizes to the potent cytotoxin 4-hydroxyequilenin-σ-quinone. *Chemical Research in Toxicology, 12,* 204–213.

3. Cole, W., et al. (1995, June 26). The estrogen dilemma. *Time,* 46–53 (cover story).

4. Shaak, C. (in press). Restoration of early luteal phase hormone levels in menopausal women by transdermal application of progesterone, estradiol, and testosterone. Note: Dr Shaak's study used the following patented formulation of bioidentical hormones, known as TransproET: 150mg progesterone, 0.5mg oestradiol, and 0.5mg of testosterone per cc of cream. Patients were instructed to use some portion of a teaspoon of cream ($1/8$–$1/4$tsp), usually twice daily, depending upon their baseline endogenous hormone levels. For further information, write to Dr Shaak at WomanWell, 405 Great Plain Avenue, Needham, MA 02492, USA. Tel.: 781-453-0321; Hargrove, J., et al. (1998). Absorption of estradiol and progesterone delivered via Jergens lotion used as hormone replacement therapy. Poster session presented at the annual meeting of the North American Menopause Society, Philadelphia.

5. Follingstad, A. (1978). Estriol, the forgotten hormone. *JAMA, 239* (1), 29–39; Lemon, H. (1977). Clinical and experimental aspects of the anti-mammary carcinogenic activity of estriol. *Frontiers of Hormonal Research, 5* (1), 155–173; Lemon, H. (1975). Estriol prevention of mammary carcinoma induced by 7,12-dimethylbenzathracene and procarbazine. *Cancer Research, 35,* 1341–1353; Lemon, H. (1973). Oestriol and prevention of breast cancer. *Lancet, 1,* (802), 546–547; Lemon, H. (1980). Pathophysiologic considerations in the treatment of menopausal patients with oestrogens: The role of oestriol in the prevention of mammary cancer. *Acta Endocrinologica, 233, suppl.,* 17–27; Lemon, H., Wotiz, H., Parsons, L., et al. (1966). Reduced estriol excretion in patients with breast cancer prior to endocrine therapy. *JAMA, 196,* 1128–1136.

6. Heimer, G. M. & Englund, D. E. (1992). Effects of vaginally administered oestriol on postmenopausal urogenital disorders: A cytohormonal study. *Maturitas, 3,* 171–179; Iosif, C. S. (1992). Effects of protracted administration of estriol on the lower urinary tract in postmenopausal women. *Archives of Gynecology and Obstetrics, 3* (251), 115–120; Kirkengen, A. L., Andersen, P., Gjersoe, E., et al. (1992, June). Oestriol in the prophylactic treatment of recurrent urinary tract infections in postmenopausal women. *Scandinavian Journal of Primary Health Care,* 139–142; Raz, K. & Stamm, W. (1993). A controlled trial of intravaginal

estriol in postmenopausal women with recurrent urinary tract infections. *NEJM, 329,* 753–756.

 7. Speroff, L., et al. (1999). *Clinical Gynecologic Endocrinology and Infertility* (6th edn, 56–64). Philadelphia, PA: Lippincott, Williams & Wilkins.

 8. Speroff, L. (1999, September). Commentary: Postmenopausal therapy reduces the risk of colorectal cancer. *OB/GYN Alert,* 35.

 9. Love, R. R., Cameron, L., Connell, B. L., Leventhal, H. (1991). Symptoms associated with tamoxifen treatment in postmenopausal women. *Arch. Intern. Med., 151,* 1842–1847.

10. Zimniski, S. J., et al. (1993) Induction of tamoxifen-dependent rat mammary tumors. *Cancer Res., 53,* 2937–2939; Powell-Jones, W., et al. (1975). Influence of anti-oestrogens on the specific binding in vitro of (3H)oestradiol by cytosol of rat mammary tumors and human breast carcinomata. *Biochem. J., 150,* 71–75; Vancutsem, P. M., et al. (1994). Frequent and specific mutations of the rat p53 gene in eptocarcinomas induced by tamoxifen. *Cancer Res., 54,* 3864–3867; Shuibutani, S., et al. (1997). Miscoding potential of tamoxifen-derived DNA adducts: Alpha-(N2-deoxyguanosinyl) tamoxifen. *Biochem., 36,* 13010–13017; Simon, R. (1995). Discovering the truth about tamoxifen: Problems of multiplicity in statistical evaluation of biomedical data. *J. Natl. Cancer Inst., 87,* 627–629.

11. Koenig, H., et al. (1995). Progesterone synthesis and myelin formation by Schwann cells. *Science, 268,* 1500–1503.

12. When I was a houseman in obstetrics and gynaecology at St Margaret's Hospital in Boston, US, in the mid-1970s, I routinely saw women in their late thirties and forties who had a number of children and continued to get pregnant year after year, until they welcomed a hysterectomy as a way to avoid further pregnancies. Their lives, beliefs, and biology stand in sharp contrast to today's thirty-six-year-old professional woman who started worrying that she wouldn't be able to get pregnant as soon as she reached thirty-five. Our beliefs have subtle yet powerful effects on our biology – effects that are confirmed by research. Brant Secunda is an American-born shaman who was trained by the Huichol Indians, who live in a remote region of Mexico. Brant reports that Huichol women routinely get pregnant in their fifties and some even in their sixties. The work of Dr Alice Domar, of the Beth Israel Deaconess Center for Mind-body Medicine in the US, reports a 50 per cent increase in pregnancy rates in previously infertile women, most of whom are professionals in their thirties and forties, when they participate in programmes characterised by group support, deep relaxation, and attention to self-care. These pregnancies become possible because of the ability of the mind and beliefs to effect hormonal levels that better favour conception.

13. Hully, S., et al. (1998). Randomized trial of estrogen plus progestin for secondary prevention of coronary heart disease in postmenopausal women. *JAMA, 280,* 605–618; Sullivan, J. M., et al. (1995). Progestin enhances vasoconstrictor responses in postmenopausal women receiving estrogen replacement therapy. *Menopause, 4,* 193–197; Williame, J. K., et

al. (1994). Effects of hormone replacement therapy on reactivity of atherosclerotic coronary arteries in cynomologous monkeys, *J. Am. Coll. Cardiol., 24,* 1757–1761; Sarrel, P. (1999). The differential effects of œstrogens and progestins on vascular tone. *Human Reproduction Update, 5* (3), 205–209.

14. Tang, G. W. K. (1994). The climacteric of Chinese factory workers. *Maturitas, 19,* 177–182.

15. Hammond, C. B. (1994). Women's concerns with hormone replacement therapy – compliance issues. *Fertility & Sterility, 62* (suppl. 2), 157S–160S.

16. The Postmenopausal Estrogen/Progestin Intervention (PEPI) trial (1995). Effects of estrogen or estrogen/progestin regimens on heart disease risk factors in postmenopausal women. *JAMA, 273,* 199–206.

17. Daly, E., et al. (1996). Risk of venous thromboembolism in users of hormone replacement therapy. *Lancet, 348,* 977–980; Jick, H., et al. (1996). Risk of hospital admissions for idiopathic venous thromboembolism among users of postmenopausal estrogen. *Lancet, 348,* 981–982; Grodstein, F., et al. (1996). Prospective study of exogenous hormones and risk of pulmonary embolism in women. *Lancet, 348,* 983–986.

18. Yaffe, K., Lui, L.-Y., Grady, D., Cauley, J., Kramer, J., & Cummings, S. R. (2000). Cognitive decline in women in relation to non-protein-bound estradiol concentrations. *Lancet, 356* (9231), 708–712.

19. Grodstein, F., Newcomb, P. A., & Stampfer, M. J. (1999). Post-menopausal hormone therapy and the risk of colorectal cancer: A review and meta-analysis. *Am. J. Medicine, 106* (5), 574–582.

Chapter 6: Foods and Supplements to Support the Change

1. Hudson, T. (1994). A pilot study using botanical medicine in the treatment of menopausal symptoms. Portland, Oregon, National College of Naturopathic Medicine and the Bastyr University of Natural Health Sciences.

2. Tyler, V. E. (1993). *The Honest Herbal: A Sensible Guide to the Use of Herbs and Related Remedies* (3rd ed.). Binghamton, NY: Haworth Press.

3. Elghamry, M. I., & Shihata, I. M. (1965). Biological activity of phyto-estrogens. *Planta Medica, 13,* 352–357.

4. Knight, D., & Eden, J. (1996). A review of the clinical effects of phyto-estrogens. Part 2. *Obstetrics & Gynecology, 87* (5), 897–904; Kaldas, R. S., & Hughes, C. L. (1989). Reproductive and general metabolic effects of phytoestrogens in mammals. *Reproductive Toxicology, 3,* 81–89.

5. Rose, D. P. (1992). Dietary fiber, phytoestrogens, and breast cancer. *Nutrition, 8,* 47–51.

6. Tamaya, T., et al. (1986). Inhibition by plant herb extracts of steroid bindings in uterus, liver, and serum of the rabbit. *Acta Obstetrica Gynecologica Scandinavia, 65,* 839–842.

7. Yoshiro, K. (1985). The physiological actions of tan-kwei and cnidium. *Bull. Oriental Healing Arts Institute USA, 10,* 269–278; Harada, M., Suzuki, M., & Ozaki, Y. (1984). Effects of Japanese *Angelica* root and peony root on uterine contraction in the rabbit *in situ. J. Pharmacol. Dynam., 7,* 304–311; Zhu, D. P. O. (1987). Dong quai. *Am. J. Chinese Medicine, 15,* 117–125.

8. Bohnert, K.-J. (1997, spring). The use of *Vitex agnus-castus* for hyperprolactinemia. *Quarterly Review of Natural Medicine,* 19–20; American Botanical Council (1992). *Kommission E monograph: Agnus casti fructus (chaste tree fruits).* Fort Worth, TX: Author.

9. Duker, E. M., et al. (1991). Effects of extracts from *Cimicifuga racemosa* on gonadotropin release in menopausal women and ovariectomized rats. *Planta Medica, 57,* 420–424, 1991.

10. Cassidy, A., Bingham, S., & Setchell, K. (1994). Biological effects of a diet of soy protein rich in isoflavones on the menstrual cycle of premenopausal women. *Am J. Clin. Nutr., 60,* 333–340; Anderson, J. W., et al. (1998). Effects of soy protein on renal function and proteinuria in patients with Type 2 diabetes. *Am. J. Clin. Nutr. 68* (6 suppl.), 1347S–1353S.

11. Wong, W. W., Heird, W. C., & Smith, E. O. (2000, April). Potential health benefits of soy in postmenopausal women. Data presented at the Experimental Biology Meeting, San Diego, CA.

12. Foth, D., & Cline, J. M. (1998). Effects of mammalian and plant estrogens on mammary glands and uteri of macaques. *Am. J. Clin. Nutr., 68* (suppl.), 1413S–1471S.

13. Scheiber, M., & Setchell, K. (1999, June). Dietary soy isoflavones favorably influence lipids and bone turnover in healthy postmenopausal women. The Endocrine Society's 81st Annual Meeting Synopsis.

14. Food & Drug Administration, U.S. Department of Health and Human Services (1999). FDA talk paper: FDA approves new health claim for soy protein and coronary heart disease (T99–48).

15. William, K. (1997, November). Interactive effects of soy protein and estradiol on arterial pathobiology. American Heart Association annual scientific sessions, Orlando, FL.

16. Girman, A., & Poole, C. (2000). *Preventing Osteoporosis with Ipriflavone: Discover the Proven, Safe Alternative to Estrogen Replacement Therapy.* Rocklin, CA: Prima Publishing.

17. Bennink, M. R., Thiagarajan, L. D., et al. (1999, September). Dietary soy is associated with decreased cell proliferation rate and zone in the colon mucosa of subjects at risk for colon cancer. Presented at the American Institute for Cancer Research Meeting, as reported on Reuters Health News Service.

18. Rao, L., et al. (1997). Anti-thyroid isoflavones from soybean: Isolation, characterization, and mechanisms of action. *Biochemical Pharmacology, 54,* 1087–1096.

19. Albertazzi, P., et al. (1998). The effect of dietary soy supplementation on hot flashes. *Obstetrics & Gynecology, 91,* 6–11.

20. Ibid.
21. Aldercreutz, H., et al. (1986). Determination of urinary lignans and phytoestrogen metabolites, potential antiestrogens and anticarcinogens in urine of women on various habitual diets. *J. Steroid Biochemistry, 25* (5B), 791–797.
22. Aldercreutz, H. (1984). Does fiber-rich food containing animal lignan precursors protect against both colon and breast cancer? An extension of the 'fiber hypothesis.' *Gastroenterology, 86* (4), 761–764; Jenab, M., et al. (1996). The influence of flaxseed and lignans on colon carcinogenesis and beta-glucuronidase activity. *Carcinogenesis, 17* (6), 1343–1348; Johnstone, P. V. (1995). Flaxseed oil and cancer: Alpha-linolenic acid and carcinogenesis. In S. C. Cunnane & L. U. Thompson (eds.), *Flaxseed in Human Nutrition.* Champaign, IL: AOCS Press; Serraino, M., et al. (1991). The effect of flaxseed supplementation on early risk markers for mammary carcinogenesis. *Cancer Letter, 60,* 135–142; Serraino, M., et al. (1992). The effect of flaxseed supplementation on the initiation and promotional stages of mammary tumorigenesis. *Nutrition & Cancer, 17,* 153–159.
23. Lampe, J. W., et al. (1994). Urinary lignan and isoflavonoid excretion in premenopausal women consuming flaxseed powder. *Am. J. Clin. Nutr., 60,* 122–128; Mousavi, Y., et al. (1992). Enterolactone and estradiol inhibit each other's proliferative effect on MCF and breast cancer cells in culture. *J. Steroid Biochemistry & Molecular Biology, 41,* 615–619.
24. Bierenbaum, M. L., et al. (1993). Reducing atherogenic risk in hyperlipemic humans with flaxseed supplementation: A preliminary report. *J. Am. College Nutrition, 12* (5), 501–504.
25. Middleton, E., & Kandaswami, C. (1994, November). Potential health-promoting properties of citrus bioflavonoids. *Food Technology,* 115–119.
26. I am indebted to Maureen Manetti, M.Ac., and her mother, Fern Tsao, for their assistance in preparing this section on traditional Chinese medicine and menopause.
27. Vernejoul, P., et al. (1985). Étude des meridiens d'acupuncture par les traceurs radioactifs [The study of acupuncture meridians using radioactive tracers]. *Bulletin Académie Nationale Médicine, 169* (7), 1071–1075.

Chapter 7: The Menopause Food Plan:
A Programme to Balance Your Hormones and Prevent Middle-age Spread

1. Fine, J. T., Colditz, G. A., Coakley, E. H., Moseley, G., Manson, J. E., Willett, W. C., & Kawachi, I. (1999). A prospective study of weight change and health-related quality of life in women. *JAMA, 282,* 2136–2142.
2. Fukagawa, N. K., et al. (1990). Effect of age on body composition and resting metabolic rate. *Am. J. Physiology, 259,* E233.
3. Ganesan, R. (1995). Aversive and hypophagic effects of estradiol. *Physiological Behavior, 55* (2), 279–285.

4. As of this writing, *Dr. Atkins' New Diet Revolution* has sold over eight million copies and has remained the number-one best-selling diet book of the late 1990s. The research supporting the book is sound, though controversial.

5. A clinical study of the Atkins diet presented at the Southern Society of General Internal Medicine in New Orleans (1999) by lead researcher Dr Eric Westman, assistant professor of Medicine at North Carolina's Duke University, US, failed to show any adverse effects on kidney and liver function in the forty-one mildly obese study subjects who limited their carbohydrate intake to less than 20g per day. They also took a multivitamin-mineral and fish oil supplement and exercised three times a week. The Durham study lasted for four months and test subjects dropped an average of 21lb each. Cholesterol levels dropped 6.1 per cent and triglycerides dropped by 40 per cent, while protective HDL cholesterol levels increased by about 7 per cent. Blood pressure and body composition also underwent favourable changes. The results of the Durham study were supported in a second, larger study of 319 overweight or obese patients conducted over a period of one year at the Atkins Center for Complementary Medicine in New York City, US. Results were similar, laying to rest any safety concerns. Under many perimenopausal conditions, however, even the Atkins diet may not be as effective as it is during other life stages, nor as it is for men.

6. Huang, Z., Willett, W. C., Colditz, G. A., Hunter, D. J., Manson, J. E., Rosner, B., Speizer, F. E., & Hankinson, S. E. (1999). Waist circumference, waist:hip ratio, and risk of breast cancer in the Nurses' Health Study. *Am. J. Epidemiol.*, *150* (12), 1316–1324.
   Dr Zhi-ping Huang from the US Harvard School of Public Health and his colleagues examined the association between waist circumference and waist-to-hip ratio with subsequent risk of breast cancer. Those with a waist circumference between 32 and 35.9 inches had a breast cancer risk 1.5 times greater than normal, while those with a waist circumference between 36 and 55in had a risk that was almost twice that of women whose waists were between 15 and 27.9in. Abdominal adiposity is associated with an excess of androgen and increased conversion of androgen to oestrogen in fatty tissue. The research also concluded that 'all postmenopausal hormone users were at increased risk of breast cancer regardless of central obesity'.

7. Wild, R. D., et al. (1985). Lipoprotein lipid concentrations and cardiovascular risk in women with polycystic ovarian syndrome. *J. Clinical Endocrinology & Metabolism, 61,* 946; Rexrode, K., et al. (1998). Abdominal adiposity and coronary heart disease in women. *JAMA, 280,* 1843–1848; Gillespie, L. (1999). *The Menopause Diet: Lose Weight and Boost Your Energy,* 18. Beverly Hills, CA: Healthy Life Publications.

8. Huang, Z., et al. (1999). Op. cit.

9. Groff, J. L., & Gropper, S. (2000). *Advanced Nutrition and Human Metabolism,* 147, 252, 447. Belmont, CA: Wadsworth.

10. Reaven, G. M. (2000). *Syndrome X: Overcoming the Silent Killer That Can Give You a Heart Attack.* New York: Simon & Schuster.

11. Eriksson, J., et al. (1989). Early metabolic defects in persons at increased risk for non-insulin-dependent diabetes mellitus. *NEJM, 321,* 337–343; Lillioja, S., et al. (1993). Insulin resistance and insulin secretory dysfunction as precursors of non-insulin-dependent diabetes mellitus: Prospective studies of the Pima Indians. *NEJM, 329,* 1988–1992.

12. Reaven, G. M. (1988). Role of insulin resistance in human disease. *Diabetes, 37,* 1595–1607; Zavaroni, I., et al. (1989). Risk factors for coronary artery disease in healthy persons with hyperinsulinemia and normal glucose tolerance. *NEJM, 320,* 702–706.

13. Fuh, M. M., et al. (1987). Abnormalities of carbohydrate and lipid metabolism in patients with hypertension. *Arch. Intern. Med., 147,* 1035–1038; Zavaroni, I., et al. (1987). Evidence that multiple risk factors for coronary artery disease exist in persons with abnormal glucose tolerance. *Am. J. Medicine, 83,* 609–612.

14. Nestler, J., et al. (1999). Ovulatory and metabolic effects of D-chiro-inositol in the polycystic ovary syndrome, *NEJM, 340,* 1314–1320.

15. Kazer, R. (1995). Insulin resistance, insulin-like growth factor 1 and breast cancer: A hypothesis. *International J. Cancer, 62* (4), 403–406.

16. Bruning, P. F., Bonfrer, J. M., van Noord, P. A., Hart, A. A., de Jong-Bakker, M., & Nooijen, W. J. (1992). Insulin resistance and breast-cancer risk. *International J. Cancer, 52* (4), 511–516; Seely, S. (1983). Diet and breast cancer: The possible connection with sugar consumption. *Medical Hypotheses, 11,* 319–327.

17. Bruning, P. F., et al. (1992). Ibid.

18. Kazer, R. (1995). Op. cit.

19. Gillespie, L. (1999). *The Menopause Diet Mini Meal Cookbook,* 3. Beverly Hills, CA: Healthy Life Productions.

20. Michnobicz, J. (1987). Environmental modulation of estrogen metabolism in humans. *International Clinical Nutritional Review, 7,* 169–173; Anderson, K. E. (1984). The influence of dietary protein and carbohydrate on the principal oxidative biotranformations of estradiol in normal subjects. *J. Clinical Endocrinology & Metabolism, 59* (1) 103–107.

21. Opara, E. C., et al. (1996). L-glutamine supplementation of a high fat diet reduces body weight and attenuates hyperglycemia and hyperinsulinemia in C57BL/6J mice. *J. Nutrition, 126* (1), 273–279; Rogers, L. L., et al. (1955). Voluntary alcohol consumption by rats following administration of glutamine. *J. Biological Chemistry, 214,* 503–507.

22. Cutler, R. G. (1984). Carotenoids and retinol: Their possible importance in determining longevity of primate species. *Proceedings of the National Academy of Sciences, 81,* 7627–7631.

23. Murakoshi, M., et al. (1992). Potent preventive action of alpha-carotene against carcinogenesis. *Cancer Research, 52,* 6583–6587.

24. Franceschi, S., et al. (1994). Tomatoes and risk of digestive-tract cancers. *International J. Cancer, 59,* 181–184.

25. Hornstra, G. (2000). Essential fatty acids in mothers and their neonates. *Am. J. Clin. Nutr., 71* (suppl.), 1262S–1269S.

26. I was introduced to this concept by Drs Mary Dan Eades and Michael Eades, authors of *Protein Power* (New York: Bantam, 1996), and have found it to be true. Remember, however, that it is possible to produce too much insulin from overeating anything and also during times of stress – even when there aren't any carbohydrates around.

27. Dulloo, A. G., Duret, C., Rohrer, D., Girardier, L., Mensi, N., Fathi, M., Chantre, P., & Vandermander, J. (1999). Efficacy of a green tea extract rich in catechin polyphenols and caffeine in increasing 24-h energy expenditure and fat oxidation in humans. *Am. J. Clin. Nutr., 70* (6), 1040–1045; Sinatra, S. (1998). *The Coenzyme Q_{10} Phenomenon.* New Canaan, CT: Keats.

28. Ianoli, P., et al. (1998). Glucocorticoids upregulate intestinal nutrient transport in a time-dependent substrate-specific fashion. *Gastrointestinal Surgery, 2* (5), 449–457.

29. McGuigan, J. E. (1994). Peptic ulcer and gastritis. In K. Isselbacher et al. (eds.), *Harrison's Principles of Internal Medicine, vol. 2* (13th ed., 1369). New York: McGraw-Hill.

30. Murray, M., & Pizzorno, J., (1998). *Encyclopedia of Natural Medicine,* 134–137. Rocklin, CA: Prima Publishing; van Marle, J., et. al. (1981). Deglycyrrhizinised licorice (DGL) and renewal of the rat stomach epithelium. *European J. Pharmacology, 72,* 219–275.

Chapter 8: Creating Pelvic Health and Power

1. Helms, J. M. (1987). Acupuncture for the management of primary dysmenorrhea. *Obstetrics & Gynecology, 69* (1), 51–56.

2. Lepine, L. A., et al. (1997). Hysterectomy surveillance – United States, 1980–1993. *MMWR, 46,* 1–15.

3. Bradley, L., & Newman, J. (2000). Uterine artery embolization for treatment of fibroids: From scalpel to catheter. *The Female Patient, 25,* 71–78.

4. West, S. (1994). *The Hysterectomy Hoax.* New York: Doubleday.

5. Garcia, C.-R., & Cutler, W. B. (1984). Preservation of the ovary: A reevaluation. *Fertility & Sterility, 42* (4), 510–514.

6. Hasson, H. (1993). Cervical removal at hysterectomy for benign disease: Risks and benefits. *J. Reproductive Medicine, 58* (10), 781–789.

7. Carlson, K., Miller, B., & Fowler, F. (1994). The Maine Women's Health Study. I. Outcomes of hysterectomy. *Obstetrics & Gynecology, 83,* 556–565.

8. Rohner T. J., Jr., & Rohner. J. F. (1997). Urinary incontinence in America: The social significance. In P. D. O'Donnel (ed.), *Urinary Incontinence.* St. Louis, MO: Mosby-Yearbook, Inc.

9. Resnick, N. (1998). Improving treatment of urinary incontinence. *JAMA, 280* (23), 2034–2035.

10. Pandit, M., et al. (2000). Quantification of intramuscular nerves within the female striated urogenital sphincter muscles. *Obstetrics & Gynecology, 95,* 797–800.

11. Bhatia, N., Tchou, D. C. H., et al. (1988). Pelvic floor musculature exercises in treatment of anatomical urinary stress incontinence. *Physical Therapy, 68,* 652–655; Diokno, A. (1996). The benefits of conservative management in SUI. *Contemporary Urology, 8,* 36–48.

12. Singla, A. (2000). An update on the management of SUI. *Contemporary Ob/Gyn, 45* (1), 68–85.

13. Burgio, K., et al. (1998). Behavioral vs. drug treatment for urge incontinence in older women: A randomized trial. *JAMA, 280* (23), 1995–2000.

14. Galloway, N., et al. (1998, June–July). *Multicenter trial: Extracorporeal magnetic resonance therapy (EMRT) for the treatment of stress urinary incontinence.* First International Consultation on Incontinence, Monaco. (Abstract no. 31.)

15. Eckford, S. D., Jackson, S. R., Lewis, P. A., et al. (1996). The continence control pad – a new external occlusion device in the management of stress incontinence. *British J. Urology, 77,* 538–540.

16. Lose G., & Versi, E. (1996). Pad-weighing tests in the diagnosis and quantification of incontinence. *International J. Urogynecology, 3,* 324–328; Versi, E., et. al. (1996). Evaluation of the home pad test in the investigation of female urinary incontinence. *British J. Obstet. Gynaecol.,* 103, 162–167.

17. Bergman, A., & Elia, G. (1995). Three surgical procedures for genuine stress incontinence. Five-year follow-up of a prospective randomized study. *Am. J. Obstetrics & Gynecology, 173,* 66–71.

18. Singla, A. Op. cit., 77.

19. Santarosa, R. P., Blaivas, J. G. (1994). Periurethral injection of autologous fat for the treatment of sphincteric incontinence. *J. Urology, 151,* 607–611; Bard, C. R. (1990). PMAA submission to U.S. Food & Drug Administration for IDE #G850010.

20. Burgio, K., et al. Op. cit.

Chapter 9: Sex and Menopause: Myths and Reality

1. Sarrel, P. & Whitehead, M. I. (1985). Sex and menopause: defining the issues. *Maturitas, 7,* 217–24.

2. Bergmark, K., et al. (1999). Vaginal changes and sexuality in women with a history of cervical cancer. *NEJM, 340,* 1383–1389.

3. Savage, L. (1999). *Reclaiming Goddess Sexuality,* 23. Carlsbad, CA: Hay House.

4. Love, P., & Robinson, J. (1994). *Hot Monogamy: Essential Steps to More Passionate, Intimate Lovemaking* (p. 371). New York: Dutton.

5. Hurlburth, D. F. (1991). The role of assertiveness in female sexuality: a comparative study between sexually assertive and sexually non-assertive

women. *J. Sex. & Marital Ther., 12,* 183–190; Hoch, Z., et al. (1981). An evaluation of sexual performance comparison between sexually dysfunctional couples. *J. Sex. & Marital Ther., 17,* 90–102.

6. Zussman, et al. (1981). Sexual responses after hysterectomy-oophorectomy: recent studies and reconsideration of psychogenesis. *Am. J. Obstetrics & Gynecology, 40* (7), 725–729.

7. Bachman, G. A. (1985). Correlates of sexual desire in postmenopausal women. *Maturitas, 3,* 211.

8. Sarrel, P. (1990). Sexuality and menopause. *Obstetrics & Gynecology, 75* (4, suppl.), 26S–35S; Sarrel, P. (1982). Sex problems after menopause: A study of 50 married couples treated in a sex counseling programme. *Maturitas, 4* (4), 231–239.

9. Sarrel, P. (1990). Op. cit.

10. Sarrel, P., et al. (1998). Estrogen and estrogen-androgen replacement in postmenopausal women dissatisfied with estrogen-only therapy. *J. Reproductive Medicine, 43* (10), 847–856; Sherwin, B., et al. (1985). Differential symptom response to parenteral estrogen and/or androgen administration in the surgical menopause. *Am. J. Obstetrics & Gynecology, 151,* 153–160.

11. Love, P., & Robinson, J. (1994). Op. cit. (pp. 73–76), commenting on the study of Schreiner-Engel, P. (1981). Sexual arousability and the menstrual cycle. *Psychosomatic Medicine, 43,* 1999–2212.

12. Collins, G. (2000). Safe sex: Important at any age. *The Female Patient, 20,* 4–8.

13. Love, P., & Robinson, J. (1994). Op. cit., 234–235.

Chapter 10: Nurturing Your Brain: Sleep, Depression, and Memory

1. Bliwise, D. L., et al. (1992). Prevalence of self-reported poor sleep in a healthy population age 50–65. *Social Science Medicine, 34* (49), 49.

2. Walsh, J. K., et al. (1992). Insomnia. In S. Chokroverty (ed.), *Sleep Disorders Medicine: A Comprehensive Textbook* (p. 100). Stoneham, MA: Butterworth.

3. Rapkin, A., et al. (1997). Progesterone metabolite allopregnenolone in women with premenstrual syndrome, *Obstetrics/Gynecology, 90* (5), 709–714.

4. Leathwood, P. D., et al. (1985). Aqueous extract of valerian root (*Valeriana officinalis* L.) reduces latency to fall asleep in man. *Planta Medica, 54,* 144–148.

5. Murray, M. (1998). *5-HTP: The Natural Way to Overcome Depression, Obesity, and Insomnia.* New York: Bantam Books.

6. Holm, E., Staedt, U., Heep, J., Kortsik, C., Behne, F., Kaske, A., & Mennicke, I. (1991). Untersuchungen zum Wirkungsprofil von D, L-Kavain: Zerebrale Angriffsorte und Schlaf-Wach-Rhythmus im Tierexperiment. [The action profile of D, L-kavain: Cerebral sites and sleep-wakefulness rhythm in animals.] *Arzneimittelforschung, 41* (7), 673–683; ANPA Committee on Research (2000). The use of herbal

alternative medicines in neuropsychiatry: A report of the ANPA Committee on Research. *J. Neuropsychiatry & Clinical Neurosciences, 12,* 177–192.

7. McKinlay, J. B., et al. (1987). The relative contribution of endocrine changes and social circumstances to depression in mid-aged women. *J. Health & Social Behavior, 28,* 345–363; Woods, N. F., Mitchell, E. S. (1996). Patterns of depressed mood in midlife women: Observations from the Seattle Midlife Women's Health Study. *Research in Nursing & Health, 19* (2), 111–123; Martinsen, E. W. (1990). Benefits of exercise for the treatment of depression. *Sports Medicine, 9* (6), 380–389; Morgan, J., et al. (1970). Psychological effects of chronic physical activity. *Medical Science & Sports, 2* (4), 213–217; Kessler, R. C., et al. (1993). Sex and depression in the National Comorbidity Survey. I: Lifetime prevalence, chronicity and recurrence. *J. Affective Disorders, 29,* 85.

8. Pratt, L. (1996). Depression, psychotropic medication and risk of myocardial infarction. *Circulation, 94* (12), 3123–3129; Michelson, D., et al. (1996). Bone mineral density in women with depression. *NEJM, 335,* 1176–1181; Denollet, J., et al. (1996). Personality as independent predictor of long-term mortality in patients with coronary heart disease. *Lancet, 347,* 417–421; Frasure-Smith, N., Lesperance, F., & Talajic, M. (1995). Depression and 18-month prognosis after myocardial infarction. *Circulation, 91* (4), 999–1005.

9. Sarno, J. (1991). *Healing Back Pain: The Mind-Body Connection,* 26–27. New York: Warner Books; Shealy, N. (1995). *Miracles Do Happen,* 250. Rockport, MA: Element Books.

10. Woods, N. F., Mitchell, E. S., & Adams, C. (2000). Memory functioning among midlife women: Observations from the Seattle Midlife Women's Health Study. *Menopause, 7* (4), 257–265.

11. Aleem, F. A. (1985). Menopausal syndrome: Plasma levels of beta-endorphin in postmenopausal women measured by a specific radio-immunoassay. *Maturitas, 7,* 329–334; Genazzani, A. R., et al. (1988). Steroid replacement treatment increases beta-endorphin and beta-lipotropin plasma levels in postmenopausal women. *Gynecology & Obstetrical Investigation, 26,* 153–159.

12. Roca, C. A., et al. (1999). Gonadal steroids and affective illness. *Neuroscientist, 5* (4), 227–237; Halbreich, U. (1997). Role of estrogen in post-menopausal depression. *Neurology, 48* (5, suppl. 7), S16–S20.

13. Garcia-Segura, L. M., et al. (1996, November). Effect of sex steroids on brain cells. In B. G. Wren (ed.), *Progress in the Management of the Menopause. The Proceedings of the 9th International Congress on the Menopause, Sydney, Australia,* 278–285. New York: Parthenon Publishing.

14. Young, R. J. (1979). Effect of regular exercise on cognitive functioning and personality. *British J. Sports Medicine, 13* (3), 110–117; Gutin, B., (1966). Effect of increase in physical fitness on mental ability following physical and mental stress. *Research Quarterly, 37* (2), 211–220.

15. Doogan, D. P., & Caillard, V. (1992). Sertraline in the prevention of depression. *British J. Psychiatry, 160,* 217–222; Eric, L. (1991). A prospective, double-blind, comparative, multicenter study of paroxitine and placebo preventing recurrent major depressive episodes. *Biological Psychiatry, 29* (suppl. 1), 254S–255S.
16. Pert, C. B. (1997, October 20). Letter to the editor. *Time, 150* (16).
17. Coppen, A. (1967). The biochemistry of affective disorders. *British J. Psychiatry, 113,* 1237–1264; Stewart, J. W., et al. (1984). Low B$_6$ levels in depressed outpatients. *Biol. Psychiatry, 19* (4), 613–616; Hall, R. C. W., & Joffe, J. R. (1973). Hypomagnesemia: Physical and psychiatric symptoms. *JAMA, 224* (13), 1749–1751; Lieb, J., Karmali, R., & Horrobin, D. (1983). Elevated levels of prostaglandin E2 and thromboxane B2 in depression. *Prostaglandins Leukot. Med. 10* (4), 361–367.
18. Fux, M., Levine, J., Aviv, A., & Belmaker, R. H. (1996). Inositol treatment of obsessive-compulsive disorder. *Am. J. Psychiatry, 153* (9), 1219–1221; Levine, J., et al. (1995). Double-blind, controlled trial of inositol treatment of depression. *Am. J. Psychiatry, 152,* 792–794.
19. Jorm, A. F., et al. (1987). The prevalence of dementia: A quantitative integration of the literature. *Acta Psychiatrica Scandinavia, 76,* 465–479; Aronson, M. S., et al. (1990). Women, myocardial infarction, and dementia in the very old. *Neurology, 40,* 1102–1106.
20. Nash, J. M. (2000, July 24). The new science of Alzheimer's. *Time, 156* (4), 51.
21. Snowdon, D., et al. (1996). Linguistic ability in early life and cognitive function and Alzheimer's disease in late life: Findings from the Nun Study. *JAMA, 275* (7), 528–532; Snowdon, D. et al. (1997). Brain infarction and the clinical expression of Alzheimer's disease. The Nun Study. *JAMA, 277* (10), 813–817.
22. Baldereschi, M., et al. (1998). Estrogen replacement therapy and Alzheimer's disease in the Italian Longitudinal Study on Aging. *Neurology, 50,* 996–1002; Kawas, C., et al. (1997). A prospective study of estrogen replacement therapy and the risk of developing Alzheimer's disease: The Baltimore Longitudinal Study of Aging. *Neurology, 48,* 1517–1521; Paganini-Hill, A., & Henderson, V. W. (1996). Estrogen replacement therapy and risk of Alzheimer's disease. *Arch. Intern. Med., 156* (19), 2213–2217; Tang, M. X., et al. (1996). Effect of œstrogen during menopause on risk and age at onset of Alzheimer's disease. *Lancet, 358,* 429–432; Ohkura, V., et al. (1994). Evaluation of estrogen treatment in female patients with dementia of Alzheimer's type. *Endocrinology J., 41,* 361–371; Henderson, V., et al. (1994). Estrogen replacement therapy in older women: Comparisons between Alzheimer's disease cases and nondemented control subjects. *Archives of Neurology, 51,* 896–900; Paganini-Hill, A., et al. (1994). Estrogen deficiency and risk of Alzheimer's disease in women. *Am. J. Epidemiol., 140,* 256–261; Brenner, D. E., et al. (1994). Postmenopausal estrogen replacement therapy on the risk of Alzheimer's disease: A population-based case control study. *Am. J. Epi-*

demiol., 140, 262–267; Honjo, H., et al. (1993). An effect of conjugated estrogen to cognitive impairment in women with senile dementia, Alzheimer's type: A placebo-controlled double-blind study. *J. Japanese Menopause Society, 1,* 167–171; Kantor, H., et al. (1973). Estrogen for older women. *Am. J. Obstetrics & Gynecology, 116,* 115–118; Caldwell, B. M. (1954). An evaluation of psychological effects of sex hormone administration in aged women. *J. Gerontology, 9,* 168–174.

23. McEwen, B. S., et al. (1999). Inhibition of dendritic spine induction on hippocampal ca-1 pyramidal neurons by nonsteroidal estrogen antagonists in female rats. *Endocrinology, 140,* 1044–1047.

24. Lerner, A. J., et al. (1996, October). Interactions of smoking history with estrogen replacement therapy as protective factors for Alzheimer's disease. Presentation at 26th annual meeting of the Society of Neuroscience, Washington, D.C.; Wilson, P. W. F., et al. (1995). Postmenopausal estrogen use, cigarette smoking, and cardiovascular morbidity in women over 50: The Framingham Study. *NEJM, 313,* 1038–1043; Falkeborn, N., et al. (1993). Hormone replacement therapy and the risk of stroke. Follow-up of a population-based cohort in Sweden. *Arch. Intern. Med., 153,* 1201–1209; Finucane, F. F., et al. (1993). Decreased risk of stroke among postmenopausal hormone users: Results of a national cohort. *Arch. Intern. Med., 153,* 73–79; Paganini-Hill, A., et al. (1988). Postmenopausal estrogen treatment and stroke: A prospective study. *British Medical J., 297* (6647), 519–522.

25. Manly, J. J., et al. (2000). Endogenous estrogen levels and Alzheimer's disease among postmenopausal women. *Neurology, 54,* 833–837.

26. Honjo, H., et al. (1993). Op. cit.; Ohkura, V., et al. (1994). Evaluation of estrogen treatment in female patients with dementia of Alzheimer's type. *Endocrinology J., 41,* 361–371; Henderson, V., et al. (1994). Estrogen replacement therapy in older women: Comparisons between Alzheimer's disease cases and non-demented control subjects. *Archives of Neurology, 51,* 896–900; Henderson, V. W. (1999, spring). Estrogen and Alzheimer's disease: A current status. *Menopausal Medicine: A Quarterly Newsletter of the Am. Soc. Reproductive Medicine, 7* (1), 1–4; Schmidt, R., et al. (1996). ERT in older women: A neuropsychological and brain MRI study. *J. Am. Geriatric Society, 51,* 896–900; Jacobs, D. M. (1998). Cognitive function in nondemented older women who took estrogen after menopause. *Neurology, 50,* 386–373; Marder, T., et al. (1998). Postmenopausal estrogen use and Parkinson's disease with and without dementia. *Neurology, 50,* 1141–1143; Shaywitz, S. E., et al. (1999). Effect of estrogen on brain activation patterns in postmenopausal women during working memory tasks. *JAMA, 281* (13), 1197–1202; Erikson, P. S., et al. (1998). Neurogenesis in the adult human hippocampus. *Nature Medicine, 4* (11), 1313–1317; Sarrel, P. M., et al. (1994). Estrogen actions in artery, bone, and brain. *Scientific American* (1994, July–August), 44–53.

27. Evans, P. H. (1991). Cephaloconiosis: A free radical perspective on the

proposed particulate-induced etiopathogenesis of Alzheimer's dementia and related disorders. *Medical Hypotheses, 34* (3), 209–219.

28. Freedman, M., et. al. (1984). Computerized axial tomography in aging. In M. L. L. Albert (ed.), *Clinical Neurology of Aging.* New York: Oxford University Press; Lehr, J., & Schmitz-Scherzer, R. (1976). Survivors and non-survivors: Two fundamental patterns of aging. In H. Thomas (ed.), *Patterns of Aging. Findings from the Bonn Longitudinal Study of Aging.* Basel: S. Karger; Benton, M. L., et al. (1981). Normative observations on neuropsychological test performance in old age. *J. Clinical Neuropsychiatry, 3,* 33–42.

29. Baldereschi, M., et al. (1998). Op. cit.; Schneider, L. S., et al. (1996). Effects of estrogen replacement therapy on response to tacrine in patients with Alzheimer's disease. *Neurology, 46,* 1580–1584; Brinton, R. D., et al. (1997). 17-beta-estradiol increases the growth and survival of cultured cortical neurons. *Neurochemical Research, 22,* 1339–1351; Brinton, R. D., et al. (1997). Equilin, a principal component of the estrogen replacement therapy Premarin, increases the growth of cortical neurons via an NMDA receptor-dependent mechanism. *Experimental Neurology, 147,* 211–220; Matsumoto, A., et al. (1985). Estrogen stimulates neuronal plasticity in the deafferented hypothalamic arculate nucleus in aged female rats. *Neuroscience Research, 2,* 412–418; Okhura, T., et al. (1995). Estrogen increases cerebral and cerebellar blood flow in postmenopausal women. *Menopause, 2,* 13–18; Singh, M., et al. (1994). Ovarian steroid deprivation results in a reversible learning impairment and compromised cholinergic function in female Sprague-Dawley rats. *Brain Research, 644,* 305–312; Singh, M., et al. (1996). The effect of ovariectomy and estradiol replacement on brain derived neurotrophic factor messenger hippocampal brain expression in cortical and hippocampal brain regions of female Sprague-Dawley rats. *Endocrinology, 136,* 2320–2324.

30. Sherwin, B. (1997). Estrogen effects of cognition in menopausal women. *Neurology, 48* (suppl. 7), S21–S26.

31. McEwen, B. S., & Wooley, C. S. (1994). Estradiol and progesterone regulate neuronal structure and synaptic connectivity in adult as well as developing brain. *Experimental Gerontology, 29,* 431–436; Wooley, C. S., & McEwen, B. S. (1993). Roles of estradiol and progesterone in regulation of hippocampal dendritic spine density during the estrous cycle in the rat. *J. Comparative Neurology, 336,* 293–306.

32. McLaughlin, I. J., et al. (1990). Zinc in depressive disorder. *Acta Psychiatr. Scandinavia, 82,* 451–453.

33. Shaw, D. M., et al. (1988). Senile dementia and nutrition [letter]. *British Medical J., 288,* 792–793.

34. Gibson, Q. E., et al. (1988). Reduced activities of thiamine dependent enzymes in the brains and peripheral tissues of patients with Alzheimer's disease. *Archives of Neurology, 45,* 836–840.

35. Strachan, R. N., & Henderson, J. G. (1967). Dementia and folate deficiency. *Quarterly J. Medicine, 36,* 189–204; Perkins, A. J., et al.

(1999). Association of antioxidants and memory in multiethnic elderly sample using the Third National Health and Nutrition Examination Study. *Am. J. Epidemiol., 150,* 37–44.

36. Hoffman and Herbert (1990). Beware of cold remedies in the elderly. *Courtlandt Forum,* 28–41.

37. Yen, S. S. C. (1995). Replacement of DHEA in aging men and women: Potential remedial effects. *Ann. New York Acad. Sciences, 774,* 128–142; Mevril, C. R., et al. (1990). Reduced plasma DHEA concentrations in HIV infection and Alzheimer's disease. In M. Kalimi & W. Regleson (eds.), *The Biological Role of Dehydroepiandrosterone,* 101–105. New York: de Gruyter; Regleson, W., et al. (1994). Dehydroepiandrosterone (DHEA) – the 'mother steroid.' I. Immunologic action. *Ann. New York Acad. Sciences, 719,* 553–563.

38. Tabor, A. (2000). *Brain Health: Soy Benefits and Research,* 24. Winston-Salem, NC: Physician Laboratories.

39. Pan, Y., et al. (1999). Effect of estradiol and soy phytoestrogens on choline acetyltransferase and nerve growth factor mRNAs in the frontal cortex and hippocampus of female rats. *Proc. Soc. Exp. Biol. Med., 221* (2), 118–125.

40. Refat, S. L., et al. (1990). Effect of exposure of miners to aluminum powder. *Lancet, 336,* 1162–1165.

41. Council on Scientific Affairs (1985). Aspartame: Review on safety issues. *JAMA, 254* (3), 400–402; U. S. Department of Health and Human Services (1980). *Decision of the Public Board of Inquiry* (DHHS docket 75F–0335). Rockville, MD: Food & Drug Administration; Wurtman, R. J. (1983). Neurochemical changes following high-dose aspartame with dietary carbohydrates. *NEJM, 309,* 429–430; Yokogoshi, H., et al. (1984). Effects of aspartame and glucose administration on brain and plasma levels of large neutral amino acids and brain 5-hydroxyindoles. *Am. J. Clin. Nutr., 40* (1), 1–7; Aspartame Consumer Safety Network, P.O. Box 780634, Dallas, TX 75378. Tel: 214-352-4268.

42. McEwen, B. S., et al. (1999). Op. cit.

43. Connor, J. R., Melone, J. H., & Yuen, A. R. (1981). Dendritic length in aged rats' occipital cortex: An environmentally induced response. *Experimental Neurology, 73* (3), 827–830; Connor, J. R., Diamond, M. C., & Johnson, R. E. (1980). Aging and environmental influences on two types of dendritic spines in the rat occipital cortex. *Experimental Neurology, 70* (2), 371–379.

44. Eriksson, P., et al. (1998). Neurogenesis in the adult human hippocampus. *Nature Medicine, 4* (11), 1313–1317.

45. Diamond, M., et al. (1985). Plasticity in the 904-day male rat cerebral cortex. *Experimental Neurology, 87,* 309–317.

46. Hausdorff, J., et al. (1999). The power of ageism on physical function of older persons: Reversibility of age-related gait changes. *J. Am. Geriatric Soc., 47,* 1346–1349.

47. Langer, E. (1989). *Mindfulness,* 113. Reading, MA: Addison-Wesley.

Chapter 11: From Rosebud to Rose Hip: Cultivating Midlife Beauty

1. Fisher, G. J., et al. (1997). Pathophysiology of premature skin aging induced by ultraviolet light. *NEJM, 337* (20), 1419–1428.

2. Lopez-Torres, M., et al. (1998). Topical application of alpha-tocopherol modulates the antioxidant network and diminishes ultraviolet-induced oxidative damage in murine skin. *British J. Dermatology, 138,* 207–215; Biesalki, H. K., et al. (1996). Effects of controlled exposure of sunlight on plasma and skin levels of beta-carotene. *Free Radical Research, 24* (3), 215–224; Gollnick, H., et al. (1996). Systemic beta-carotene plus topical UV sunscreen are an optimal protection against harmful effects of natural UV sunlight. *European J. Dermatology, 6,* 200–205.

3. Perricone, N. V. (1997). Aging: Prevention and intervention. Part 1: Antioxidants. *J. Geriatric Dermatology, 5* (1), 1–2.

4. Perricone, N. V. (1993). The photoprotective and anti-inflammatory effects of topical ascorbyl palmitate. *J. Geriatric Dermatology, 1* (1), 5–10; Perricone, N. V., & DiNardo, J. (1996). Photoprotective and anti-inflammatory effects of topical glycolic acid. *Dermatologic Surgery, 22* (5), 435–437; Perricone, N. V. (1997). Topical vitamin C ester (ascorbyl palmitate). *J. Geriatric Dermatology, 5* (4), 162–170; Perricone, N. V. (2000). *The Wrinkle Cure.* Emmaus, PA: Rodale Press.

5. Serbinova, E., et al. (1991). Free radical recycling and intermembrane mobility in the antioxidant properties of alpha-tocopherol and alpha-tocotrienol. *Free Radical Biology & Medicine, 10,* 263–275.

6. Hargrove, J. T., et al. (1998). Absorption of estradiol and progesterone delivered via Jergens lotion used as hormone replacement therapy. Division of Reproductive Endocrinology, Dept. of Ob/Gyn, Vanderbilt Medical Center, Nashville, TN (Abstract no. 97.051).

7. Shaak, C. (in press). Restoration of early luteal phase hormone levels in menopausal women by transdermal application of progesterone, estradiol, and testosterone. Dr Shaak can be contacted about her ongoing research at WomanWell, 405 Great Plain Ave., Needham, MA 02492, US. Tel. 781-453-0321.

8. Schmidt, J., et al. (1998). Treatment of skin aging with topical estrogens. *International J. of Pharmaceutical Compounding, 2* (4), 270–274.

9. Saliou, C., et al. (1999). French *Pinus maritima* bark extract prevents ultraviolet-induced NF-KB-dependent gene expression in a human keratinocyte cell line. Abstract of a poster presentation at the Oxygen Club of California, 1999 World Congress.

10. Sinatra, S. (1998). *The Coenzyme Q_{10} Phenomenon.* Chicago: Keats Publishing.

11. Lopez-Torres, M., et al. (1998). Op. cit.; Eberlein-Konig, B., et al. (1998). Protective effect against sunburn of combined systemic ascorbic acid and vitamin E. *J. American Academy of Dermatology, 38,* 45–48.

12. Engels, W. D. (1982). Dermatological disorders: Psychosomatic illness review (No. 4 in the series). *Psychosomatics, 23* (12), 1209–1219; Bick, E.

(1968). Experience of the skin in early object relations. *International J. of Psychoanalysis, 49,* 484–486.

13. Strauss, J. S., & Pochi, P. E. (1963). The human sebaceous gland: Its regulation by steroidal hormones, and its use as an end organ for assaying androgenicity *in vivo. Recent Progress in Hormonal Research, 19,* 385–444.

14. Peck, G. L., et al. (1979). Prolonged remissions of cystic and conglobate acne with 13-retinoic acid. *NEJM, 300,* 329–333.

15. Engels, W. D. (1982). Op. cit.; Bick, E. (1968). Op. cit.; Kaplan, H. I., & Sadock, B. J. (eds.) (1989). *Comprehensive Textbook of Psychiatry* (5th ed., 1221). Philadelphia, PA: Lippincott, Williams & Wilkins.

16. DeVille, R. L., et al. (1994). Androgenic alopecia in women: Treatment with 2% topical minoxidil solution. *Arch. Dermatol., 130* (3), 303–307.

17. Lewenberg, A. (1996). Minoxidil-tretinoin combination for hair regrowth: Effects of frequency, dosage, and mode of application. *Advances in Therapy, 13* (5), 274–283.

18. Halsner, U. E., & Lucas, M. W. (1995). New aspects in hair transplantation for women. *Dermatol. Surg., 21* (7), 605–610.

19. Burkitt, D. P., et al. (1974). Dietary fiber and disease. *JAMA, 229* (8), 1068–1074; Braunwald, E. (ed.) (1987). *Harrison's Principles of Internal Medicine* (11th ed.). New York: McGraw-Hill.

20. Grismond, G. L. (1981). Treatment of pregnancy-induced phlebopathies. *Minerva Ginecol., 33,* 221–230.

21. Ries, W. (1976). Prevention of venous disease from nutritional-physiologic aspect. *ZFA, 31* (4), 383–388; Braunwald, E. (ed.) (1987). Op. cit.

22. Ako, H., et al. (1981). Isolation of fibrinolysis enzyme activator from commercial bromelain. *Arch. Int. Pharmacodyn., 254,* 157–167.

23. Stemmer, R. (1990). *Sclerotherapy of Varicose Veins.* Sigvaris Company (available from Ganzoni & Cie AG, St Gallen, Switzerland).

Chapter 12: Standing Tall for Life: Building Healthy Bones

1. Cummings, S., et al. (1985). Epidemiology of osteoporosis and osteoporotic fractures. *Epidemiology Review, 7,* 178–208.

2. Shipman, P., et al. (1985). *The Human Skeleton.* Cambridge, MA: Harvard University Press; Brown, J. (1990). *The Science of Human Nutrition.* New York: Harcourt Brace Jovanovich.

3. Lanyon, L. E. (1993). Skeletal responses to physical loading. In G. Mundy & J. T. Martin (eds.), *Physiology & Pharmacology of Bone, vol. 107,* 485–505. Berlin: Springer-Verlag.

4. Travis, J. (2000). Boning up: Turning on cells that build bone and turning off ones that destroy it. *Science News, 157,* 41–42.

5. Manolagas, S. C. (1995). Sex steroids, cytokines, and the bone marrow: New concepts on the pathogenesis of osteoporosis. *Ciba Foundation Symposium, 191,* 187–202.

6. Riggs, B., et al. (1986). In women dietary calcium intake and rates of bone loss from midradius and lumbar spine are not related. *J. Bone & Mineral Research, 1* (suppl.), 167; Genant, H. K., et al. (1985). Osteoporosis: Assessment by quantitative computed tomography. *Orthopedic Clinics of North America, 16* (3), 557–568.

7. Trotter, M., et al. (1974). Sequential changes in weight, density, and percentage weight of human skeletons from an early fetal period through old age. *Anatomical Record, 179,* 1–8.

8. Adams, P., et al. (1970). Osteoporosis and the effects of aging on bone mass in elderly men and women. *J. Medical News Series, 39,* 601–615.

9. Harris, S., et al. (1992). Rates of change in bone mineral density of the spine, heel, femoral neck and radius in healthy postmenopausal women. *Bone Mineralization, 17* (1), 87–95; Riggs, B., et al. (1985). Rates of bone loss in the appendicular and axial skeletons of women: Evidence of substantial vertebral bone loss before menopause. *J. Clinical Investigation, 77,* 1487–1491.

10. Fujita, T., et al. (1992). Comparison of osteoporosis and calcium intake between Japan and the United States. *Proc. Soc. Experimental Biology & Medicine, 200* (2), 149–152.

11. Frost, H. (1985). The pathomechanics of osteoporosis. *Clinical Orthopedics, 200,* 198–225.

12. Chappard, D., et al. (1988). Spatial distribution of trabeculae in iliac bones from 145 osteoporotic females. *Maturitas, 10,* 353–360; Biewener, A. A. (1993). Safety factors in bone strength. *Calcified Tissue International, 53* (suppl. 1), S68–S74.

13. Brown, S. (1996). *Better Bones, Better Body: Beyond Estrogen and Calcium.* Los Angeles: Keats Publishing.

14. Lees, B., et al. (1993). Differences in proximal femur bone density over two centuries. *Lancet, 341,* 673–675; Eaton, S., et al. (1991). Calcium in evolutionary perspective. *Am. J. Clinical Nutr., 54* (suppl.), 281S–287S.

15. Bauer, D. C., et al. (1993). Factors associated with appendicular bone mass in older women. *Ann. Internal Medicine, 118* (9), 647–665.

16. Rigotti, N. A., et al. (1984). Osteoporosis in women with anorexia nervosa. *NEJM, 311* (25), 1601–1605.

17. Prior, J., et al. (1990). Spinal bone loss and ovulatory disturbances. *NEJM, 323* (18), 1221–1227; Cann, C., et al. (1984). Decreased spinal mineral content in amenorrheic women. *JAMA, 251* (5), 626–629.

18. Schuckit, M. (1994). Section 5: Alcohol and alcoholism. In K. Isselbacher et al. (eds.), *Harrison's Principles of Internal Medicine, vol. 2* (13th edn, 2420). New York: McGraw-Hill.

19. Diamond, T., et al. (1989). Ethanol reduces bone formation and may cause osteoporosis. *Am. J. Medicine, 86,* 282–288; Bikler, D. D., et al. (1985). Bone disease in alcohol abuse. *Ann. Internal Medicine, 103,* 42–48.

20. Gold, P. W., et al. (1986). Responses to corticotropin-releasing hormone

in the hypercortisolism of depression and Cushing's disease: Pathophysiology and diagnostic implications. *NEJM, 314*, 1329–1335; Michelson, D., et al. (1996). Bone mineral density in women with depression. *NEJM, 335* (16), 1176–1181.

21. Tatemi, S., et al. (1991). Effect of experimental human magnesium depletion on parathyroid hormone secretion and 1,25-dihyroxyvitamin D metabolism. *J. Clin. Endocrinol. Metab., 73* (5), 1067–1072; Gaby, A., & Wright, J. (1988). *Nutrients and Bone Health.* Seattle, WA: Wright/Gaby Nutrition Institute.

22. Adinoff, A. D., & Hollister, J. R. (1983). Steroid-induced fracture and bone loss in patients with asthma. *NEJM, 309* (5), 265–268.

23. Hahn, T. J., et al. (1988). Altered mineral metabolism in glycocorticoid-induced osteopaenia: Effect of 25-hydroxyvitamin D administration. *J. Clinical Investigation, 64*, 655–665.

24. Crilly, R. G., et al. (1981). Steroid hormones, ageing and bone. *Clinical Endocrinology & Metabolism, 10* (1), 115–139.

25. Johnell, O., et al. (1979). Bone morphology in epileptics. *Calcified Tissue International, 28*(2), 93–97.

26. Franklin, J. A., et al. (1992). Long-term thyroxine treatment and bone mineral density. *Lancet, 340*, 9–13; Paul, T. L., et al. (1988). Long-term L-thyroxine therapy is associated with decreased hip bone density in pre-menopausal women. *JAMA, 259*, 3137–3141; Coindre, J. M., et al. (1986). Bone loss in hypothyroidism with hormone replacement: A histomorphometric study. *Arch. Intern. Med., 146*, 48–53.

27. Brincat, M. P., et al. (1996). A screening model for osteoporosis using dermal skin thickness and bone densitometry. In B. G. Wren (ed.), *Progress in the Management of the Menopause: The Proceedings of the 8th International Congress on the Menopause*, 175–178. Sydney: Parthenon Publishing Group.

28. Robins, S. P. (1995). Collagen crosslinks in metabolic bone disease. *Acta Orthopedica Scandinavia, 66* (266, suppl.), S171–S175; Garnero, P., et al. (1994). Comparison of new biochemical markers of bone turnover in late postmenopausal osteoporotic women in response to alendronate treatment. *J. Clin. Endocrinol. Metab., 79*, 1693–1700; Chesnut, C., et al. (1997). Hormone replacement therapy in postmenopausal women: Urinary N-telopeptide of type I collagen monitors therapeutic effect and predicts response of bone mineral density. *Am. J. Medicine, 102*, 29–37.

29. Cummings, S. R., et al. (in press). Regression to mean in clinical practice: Women who seem to lose bone density during treatment for osteoporosis usually gain if treatment is continued. *JAMA.* Cited in B. Ettinger (2000). Sequential osteoporosis treatment for women with postmenopausal osteoporosis. *Menopausal Medicine, Newsletter of the American Society for Reproductive Medicine, 8* (2), 3.

30. Munger, R. G. (1999). Prospective study of dietary protein intake and risk of hip fracture in postmenopausal women. *Am. J. Clin. Nutr., 69* (1), 147–152.

31. Potter, S. M., Baum, J. A., Teng, H., Stillman, R. J., Shay, N. F., & Erdman, J. W. (1998). Soy protein and isoflavones: Their effects on blood lipids and bone density in postmenopausal women. *Am. J. Clin. Nutr., 68* (6, suppl.), 1375S–1379S.

32. Bonfield, T. (1999, June 15). Research backs benefits of soy – postmenopausal women take note. *Cincinnati Enquirer.* This study, which was conducted by Dr Michael Scheiber, of the Obstetrics and Gynecology Department at the University of Cincinnati, and Dr Kenneth Setchell, director of mass spectrometry at Children's Hospital Medical Center, both in the US, demonstrated that eating three servings of soya foods per day containing a total of about 70mg of soya isoflavones had definite bone-building effects that may be as good as those of oestrogen.

33. Hegarty, V., et al. (2000). Tea drinking and bone mineral density in older women. *Am. J. Clin. Nutr., 71,* 1003–1007.

34. Watts, N. B., et al. (1995). Comparison of oral estrogens and estrogens plus androgen on bone mineral density, menopausal symptoms, and lipid-lipoprotein profiles in surgical menopause. *Obstetrics & Gynecology, 85,* 529–537.

35. Cummings, S., et al. (1998). Endogenous hormones and the risk of hip and vertebral fractures among older women. *NEJM, 339,* 733–738.

36. Riggs, B., & Melton, L. (1986). Involutional osteoporosis. *NEJM, 26,* 1676–1686.

37. Buchanan, J. R., et al. (1988). Early vertebral trabecular bone loss in normal premenopausal women. *J. Bone & Mineral Research, 3* (5), 583–587.

38. Carter, M. D., et al. (1991). Bone mineral content at three sites in normal perimenopausal women. *Clinical Orthopedics, 266,* 295–300; Harris, S., & Dawson-Hughes, B. (1992). Rates of change in bone mineral density of the spine, heel, femoral neck and radius in healthy postmenopausal women. *J. Bone & Mineral Research, 17* (1), 87–95.

39. Heaney, R. P. (1990). Estrogen-calcium interactions in the postmenopause: A quantitative description. *J. Bone & Mineral Research, 11* (1), 67–84.

40. Speroff, L. (1999, October 1). Treatment options for the prevention of osteoporosis. *Ob/Gyn Clinical Alert,* 46.

41. Lee, J. (1991). Is natural progesterone the missing link in osteoporosis prevention and treatment? *Medical Hypotheses, 35,* 316–318; Prior, J. (1991). Progesterone and the prevention of osteoporosis. *Can. J. Ob-Gyn & Women's Healthcare, 3* (4), 178–183; Lee, J. (1990). Osteoporosis reversal: The role of progesterone. *Clinical Nutritional Review, 10,* 884–889; Prior, M. C., et al. (1994). Cyclic medroxyprogesterone increases bone density: A controlled trial in active women with menstrual cycle disturbances. *Am. J. Medicine, 96,* 521–530; Adachi, J. D., et al. (1997). A double-blind randomized controlled trial of the effects of medroxyprogesterone acetate on bone density of women taking oestrogen replacement therapy. *British J. Obstet. Gynaecol., 104,* 64–70; Prior, J. C., et al. (1997).

Premenopausal ovariectomy-related bone loss: A randomized, double-blind, one-year trial of conjugated estrogen or medroxyprogesterone acetate. *J. Bone & Mineral Research, 12* (11), 1851–1863.

42. Leonetti, H., et al. (1999). Transdermal progesterone cream for vasomotor symptoms and postmenopausal bone loss. *Obstetrics & Gynecology, 94,* 225–228.

43. Abraham, G. (1991). The importance of magnesium in the management of primary postmenopausal osteoporosis: A review. *J. Nutritional Medicine, 2,* 165–178; Gaby, A., & Wright, J. (1990). Nutrients and osteoporosis: A review article. *J. Nutritional Medicine, 1,* 63–72.

44. Buckley, L. M., et al. (1996). Calcium and vitamin D3 supplementation prevents bone loss in the spine secondary to low-dose corticosteroids in patients with rheumatoid arthritis. A randomized, double-blind, placebo-controlled trial. *Ann. Internal Medicine, 125* (12), 961–968.

45. Nielson, B. E., et al. (1987). Effects of dietary boron on mineral, estrogen, and testosterone metabolism in postmenopausal women. *FASEB, 1,* 394–397.

46. Dawson-Hughes, G., et al. (1990). A controlled trial of the effects of calcium supplementation on bone density in postmenopausal women. *NEJM, 323,* 878–883.

47. McGuigan, J. (1994). Peptic ulcer and gastritis. In K. Isselbacher et al. (eds.), *Harrison's Principles of Internal Medicine, vol. 2* (13th edn, 1369). New York: McGraw-Hill.

48. Sources for this table are: US Department of Agriculture, *Composition of Foods,* handbooks no. 8 and 456 (Washington, DC: US Government Printing Office, 1963); J. A. Duke and A. A. Atchley, *Handbook of Proximate Analysis – Tables of Higher Plants* (Boca Raton: CRC Press, 1986); Leonard Jacobs, article in *East/West Journal,* May 1985; John Lee, 'Osteoporosis Reversal: The Role of Progesterone,' *International Clinical Nutrition Review,* vol. 10 (1990), 384–91; Judith Cooper Madlener, *The Sea Vegetable Book* (New York: Clarkson N. Potter, 1977); Nutrition Search, Inc., John Kirschmann, dir. comp., *Nutrition Almanac,* rev. ed. (New York: McGraw-Hill, 1979); US Department of Agriculture, *Nutritive Value of Foods,* handbook no. 72 (Washington, DC: US Government Printing Office, 1971); Mark Pedersen, *Nutritional Herbology* (Bountiful, UT: Pedersen, 1987); and Maine Coast Sea Vegetables Co., Shore Road, Franklin, ME 04634.

49. Chu, J. Y., et al. (1975). Studies in calcium metabolism, II. Effects of low calcium and variable protein intake on human calcium metabolism. *Am. J. Clin. Nutr., 28,* 1028–1035; Abelow, B., et al. (1992). Cross cultural association between dietary animal protein and hip fracture: A hypothesis. *Calcified Tissue International, 50,* 14–18.

50. Gillespie, L. (1999). *The Menopause Diet: Lose Weight and Boost Your Energy,* 36. Beverly Hills, CA: Healthy Life Publications.

51. Aiello, L., & Wheeler, P. (1995). The expensive tissue hypothesis: The brain and the digestive system in human and primate evolution. *Current*

Anthropology, 36 (2), 199–221; Lorenz, K., & Lee, V. A. (1997). The nutritional and physiological impact of cereal products in human nutrition. *Critical Reviews in Food Science & Nutrition, 8,* 383–456; Cassiday, C. M. (1980). Nutrition and health in agriculturalists and hunter-gatherers: A case study of two prehistoric populations. In R. F. Kandel, G. H. Pelto, & N. W. Jerome (eds.), *Nutritional Anthropology: Contemporary Approaches to Diet and Culture,* 117–145. Pleasantville, NY: Redgrave Publishing Company; Eaton, S. B., & Nelson, D. A. (1991). Calcium in evolutionary perspective. *Am. J. Clinical Nutrition, 54* (suppl.), 281S–287S; Goodman, A. H., Dufour, D., & Pelto, G. H. (2000). *Nutritional Anthropology: Biocultural Perspectives on Food and Nutrition.* Mountain View, CA: Mayfield Publishing. See also *The Paleopathology Newsletter,* published by the Paleopathology Association. Contact: Ms. Eve Cockburn, 18655 Parkside, Detroit, MI 48221–2208.

52. Caspit, A. (1994). Alendronate: An investigational agent for the prevention and treatment of osteoporosis. *Drug Therapy, 24,* 41.

53. Adami, S., et al. (1993). Treatment of postmenopausal osteoporosis with continuous daily oral alendronate in comparison with either placebo or intranasal salmon calcitonin. *Osteoporosis International, 3* (suppl. 3), S21–S27.

54. DeGroen, P. C. (1996). Esophagitis associated with the use of alendronate. *NEJM, 335,* 1016–1021.

55. Delmas, P., et al. (1997). Effects of raloxifene on bone mineral density, serum cholesterol concentrations, and uterine endometrium in postmenopausal women. *NEJM, 337,* 1641–1647.

56. Nelson, M., et al. (1994). Effects of high-intensity strength training on multiple risk factors for osteoporotic fractures: A randomized controlled trial. *JAMA, 272* (24), 1909–1914.

57. Nelson, M. (2000). *Strong Women Stay Young.* New York: Bantam.

58. Fiatarone, M., et al. (1994). Exercise training and nutritional supplementation for physical frailty in very elderly people. *NEJM, 330* (25), 1769–1775.

59. Rosen, C. et al. (1994). The effects of sunlight and diet on bone loss in elderly women from rural Maine. *Maine J. Health Issues, 1* (2), 35–48. (Study done by Michael Holick in Bangor, Maine.)

60. Vieth, R. (1999). Vitamin D supplementation, 25-hydroxyvitamin D concentrations, and safety. *Am. J. Clin. Nutr., 69,* 842–856. (Anyone who is serious about gathering more information on vitamin D and sunlight should read this impressive review article on the subject.)

61. Ibid.

62. Neer, R. M., et al. (1971). Stimulation by artificial lighting of calcium absorption in elderly human subjects. *Nature, 229,* 255.

63. Holick, M. F. (1995). Environmental factors that influence the cutaneous production of Vitamin D. *Am. J. Clin. Nutr., 61* (suppl. 3), 638S–645S.

64. Dawson-Hughes, B., et al. (1991). Effect of vitamin D supplementation

on wintertime and overall bone loss in healthy postmenopausal women. *Ann. Internal Medicine, 115* (7), 505–511.

65. McNeil, T. (1998, spring). The vitamin D guru: School of Medicine professor sees the light and spreads the news. *Bostonia,* 34–35.
66. Veith, R. (1999). Op. cit.
67. Berger, J. (1998). *Herbal Rituals,* 64–72. New York: St Martin's Press.
68. Weed, S. (1989). *Healing Wise: Wise Woman's Herbal,* 262. Woodstock, NY: Ashtree Publications.

Chapter 13: Creating Breast Health

1. Toikkanene, S., et al. (1991). Factors predicting late mortality from breast cancer. *European J. Cancer, 27* (5), 586–591.
2. Chen, C. C., et al. (1995). Adverse life events and breast cancer: Case-control study. *British Medical J., 311,* 1527–1530.
3. Levy, S., et al. (1987). Correlation of stress factors with sustained depression of natural killer cell activity and predicted prognosis in patients with breast cancer. *J. Clinical Oncology, 5,* 348–353.
4. Spiegel, D., et al. (1989). The effect of psychosocial treatment on survival of patients with metastatic breast cancer. *Lancet, 2* (8668), 888–891.
5. Prior, J. (1992). Critique of estrogen treatment for heart attack prevention: The Nurses' Health Study. *A Friend Indeed, 8* (8), 3–4; Schairer, C., et al. (2000). Menopausal estrogen and estrogen-progestin replacement therapy and breast cancer risk. *JAMA, 283* (4), 485–491.
6. Bulbrook, P. D., Swain, M. C., Wang, D. Y., et al. (1976). Breast cancer in Britain and Japan: Plasma oestradiol-17b, oestrone, and progesterone, and their urinary metabolites in normal British and Japanese women. *European J. Cancer, 12,* 725–735.
7. Seely, S., et al. (1983). Diet and breast cancer: The possible connection with sugar consumption. *Medical Hypotheses, 11,* 319–327; Kazer, R. (1995). Insulin resistance, insulin-like growth factor I and breast cancer: A hypothesis. *International J. Cancer, 62,* 403–406; Bruning, P., et al. (1992). Insulin resistance and breast-cancer risk. *International J. Cancer, 52,* 511–516.
8. Willett, W. C., et al. (1987). Moderate alcohol consumption and the risk of breast cancer. *NEJM, 316,* 1174–1180.
9. Ginsburg, E. (1996). Effects of alcohol ingestion on estrogens in post-menopausal women. *JAMA, 276* (21), 1747–1751.
10. Zhang, S., et al. (1989). A prospective study of folate intake and the risk of breast cancer. *JAMA, 281* (17), 1632–1637.
11. Ambrosone, C., et al. (1996). Cigarette smoking, N-acetyltransferase 2 genetic polymorphisms, and breast cancer risk. *JAMA, 276* (18), 1494–1501.
12. Martinsen, E. W. (1990). Benefits of exercise for the treatment of depression. *Sports Medicine, 9* (6), 380–389.

13. Coleman, B. C. (1999, March 10). Fatty diet and breast cancer: No link? *Portland Press Herald.*
14. Adlercreutz, H., et al. (1982). Excretion of the lignans enterolactone and enterodiol and of equol in omnivorous and vegetarian post-menopausal women and in women with breast cancer. *Lancet, 2* (8311), 1295–1299.
15. Goldin, B. R., Adlercreutz, H., et al. (1982). Estrogen excretion patterns and plasma levels in vegetarian and omnivorous women. *NEJM, 307,* 1542–1547.
16. Percival, M. (1997). Phytonutrients and detoxification. In *Clinical Nutrition Insights* (pp. 1–4). Published by the Foundation for the Advancement of Nutritional Education. Available from Metagenics North East, P.O. Box 848, Kingston, NH 03848.
17. Zava, D., & Duwe, G. (1997). Estrogenic and antiproliferative properties of genistein and other flavonoids in human breast cancer cells *in vitro. Nutrition & Cancer, 27* (1), 31–40.
18. Bagga, D., et al. (1997). Dietary modulation of omega-3/omega-6 polyunsaturated fatty acid ratios in patients with breast cancer. *J. Nat.Cancer Inst., 89* (15), 1123–1131.
19. Lockwood, K., et al. (1994). Partial and complete regression of breast cancer in patients in relation to dosage of coenzyme Q_{10}. *Biochemical & Biophysical Research Communications, 199* (3), 1504–1508.
20. Welch, H. G., & Black, W. C. (1997). Using autopsy series to estimate the disease 'reservoir' for ductal carcinoma in situ of the breast: How much more breast cancer can we find? *Ann. Internal Medicine, 127* (11), 1023–1028; Nielsen, M., et al. (1987). Breast cancer and atypia among young and middle-aged women: A study of 110 medicolegal autopsies. *British J. Cancer, 56* (6), 814–819.
21. Welch, H. G., & Black, W. C. (1997). Op. cit., 1023.
22. Moody-Ayers, S., et al. (2000). 'Benign' tumors and 'early detection' in mammography-screened patients of a natural cohort with breast cancer. *Arch. Intern. Med., 160* (8), 1109–1115.
23. Moore, F. (1978). Breast self-examination. *NEJM, 299* (6), 304–305.
24. Personal communication from Dana Wyrick. Dana Wyrick is a registered massage therapist who developed this self-massage routine for breast health after studying with lymphoedema therapy specialists in Europe and Australia, where the technique is far more common.
25. Kerlikowske, K., et al. (1993). Positive predictive value of screening mammography by age and family history of breast cancer. *JAMA, 270* (2), 444.
26. Veronesi, U., et al. (1997). Sentinel node biopsy to avoid axillary dissection in breast cancer with clinically negative lymph nodes. *Lancet, 349* (9069), 1864–1867.
27. National Council on Aging (1997). *Myths and Perceptions About Aging and Women's Health.* Washington, D.C.: Author; No author listed (1997). Assessing the odds. *Lancet, 350* (9091), 1563.

28. Ries, L. A. G., Eisner, M. P., Kosary, C. L., Hankey, B. F., Miller, B. A., Kleg, L., and Edwards, B. K. (eds.) (2000). *SEER Cancer Statistics Review, 1973–1993*. Bethesda, MD: National Cancer Institute; Black, W. C., et al. (1995). Perceptions of breast cancer risk and screening effectiveness in women younger than 50 years old. *J. Nat. Cancer Inst.*, *87*, 720–731.

29. Phillips, K. A. (1999). Putting the risk of breast cancer in perspective. *NEJM, 340* (2), 141–144.

30. Hirshaut, Y., & Pressman, P. (2000). *Breast Cancer: The Complete Guide* (p. 256). New York: Bantam.

31. American College of Obstetrics & Gynecology, Committee on Genetics (1996, October). *Breast–Ovarian Cancer Screening* (Committee Opinion no. 176). Washington, D.C.: Author.

32. Collins, F. S. (1986). BRCA1 – lots of mutations, lots of dilemmas. *NEJM, 334* (3), 186–188.

33. Weisberg, T. (1996, October). Genetic testing for breast cancer. *Maine Cancer Perspectives, 2* (4), 3.

34. Kesaniemi, Y. A. (unpublished data). Cited in A. Viitanen (1996), A new estrogen gel: Clinical benefits. In B. G. Wren (ed.), *Progress in the Management of the Menopause: The Proceedings of the 8th International Congress on the Menopause* (p. 168). Sydney, Australia: Parthenon.

35. LaVecchia, C., Negri, E., Franceschi, S., et al. (1995). Hormone replacement therapy and breast cancer risk: A cooperative Italian study. *British J. Cancer, 72*, 244–248.

36. Campagnoli, C., et al. (1999). HRT and breast cancer risk: A clue for interpreting the available data. *Maturitas, 33*, 185–190; Collaborative Group on Hormonal Factors in Breast Cancer (1997). Breast cancer and hormone replacement therapy: Collaborative reanalysis of data from 51 epidemiological studies of 52,705 women with breast cancer and 108,411 without breast cancer. *Lancet, 350*, 1047–1059.

37. Bhavani, B. R., et al. (1994). Pharmacokinetics of 17-ß-dihydroequilin sulfate and 17-ß-dihydroequilin in normal postmenopausal women. *J. Clin. Endocrinol. & Metab., 78*, 197–204.

38. Hargrove, J., & Eisenberg, E. (1995) Menopause. *Med. Clin. North Am., 79* (6), 1337–1363.

39. Campagnoli, C. (1999). Op. cit.; Collaborative Group on Hormonal Factors in Breast Cancer (1997). Op. cit.

40. Campagnoli, C. (1999). Op. cit.

41. Huang, Z., Willett, W. C., Colditz, G. A., Hunter, D. J., Manson, J. E., Rosner, B., Speizer, F. E., & Hankinson, S. E. (1999). Waist circumference, waist:hip ratio, and risk of breast cancer in the Nurses' Health Study. *Am. J. Epidemiol., 150* (12) 1316–1324. 'Furthermore,' they write, 'it has been proposed that abdominal adiposity is associated with an excess of androgen and increased conversion of androgen to estrogen in adipose tissue.' They also point out that hormone use by postmenopausal women probably raises hormone levels in all those women. '[A]s a

result, all postmenopausal hormone users were at increased risk of breast cancer regardless of central obesity,' they reason.

42. Schuurman, A. G., van den Brandt, P. A., & Goldbohm, R. A. (1995). Exogenous hormone use and the risk of postmenopausal breast cancer: Results from the Netherlands Cohort Study. *Cancer Causes Control, 6,* 416–424; Cobleigh, M., et al. (1994). Estrogen replacement therapy in breast cancer survivors: A time for change. *JAMA, 272* (7), 540–545.

43. Henrich, J. B. (1992). The postmenopausal estrogen/breast cancer controversy. *JAMA, 268,* 1900–1902; Wotiz, H. H., Beebe, D. R., & Muller, E. (1984). Effect of estrogen on DMBA-induced breast tumors. *J. Steroid Biochem., 20,* 1067–1075.

44. Drife, J. O. (1986). Breast development in puberty. *Ann. N.Y. Acad. Sci., 464,* 58–65; Dulbecco, R., et al. (1982). Cell types and morphogenesis in the mammary gland. *Proc. Natl. Acad. Sci. USA, 79,* 7346–7350; Long-acre, T., & Bartow, S. (1986). A correlative morphologic study of human breast and endometrium in the menstrual cycle. *Am. J. Surgical Path., 10* (6), 382–393; Weinberg, R. A. (1996, September). How cancer arises. *Scientific American,* 62–70.

45. Lemon, H. (1973). Oestriol and prevention of breast cancer. *Lancet, 1* (802), 546; Lemon, H. (1975). Estriol prevention of mammary carcinoma induced by 7,12-dimethyl-benzanthracene and procarbazine. *Cancer Res., 35,* 1341–1353; Lemon, H. (1980). Pathophysiologic considerations in the treatment of menopausal patients with oestrogens: The role of oestriol in the prevention of mammary cancer. *Acta Endocrinol., 1,* 17–27; Lemon, H., Wotiz, H., Parsons, L., et al. (1966). Reduced estriol excretion in patients with breast cancer prior to endocrine therapy. *JAMA, 196,* 1128–1136.

46. Bu, S. Z., et al. (1997). Progesterone induces apoptosis and upregulation of p53 expression in human ovarian carcinoma cell lines. *Cancer, J. American Cancer Society, 79* (10), 1944–1950.

47. Zava, D. T., & Duwe, G. (1997). Estrogen and antiproliferative properties of genistein and other flavonoids in human breast cancer cells *in vivo. Nutr. & Cancer, 27* (1), 31–40.

48. Cowan, A. D., et al. (1961). Breast cancer incidence in women with a history of progesterone deficiency. *Am. J. Epidemiol., 114* (2), 209.

49. Chang, K. J., et al. (1995). Influences of percutaneous administration of estradiol and progesterone on human breast epithelial cell cycle *in vivo. Fertil. & Steril., 63,* 785–791.

50. Badwe, R. A., et al. (1991). Timing of surgery during menstrual cycle and survival of premenopausal women with operable breast cancer. *Lancet, 337,* 1261–1264.

51. Hrushesky, W. (1996). Breast cancer, timing of surgery, and the menstrual cycle: Call for prospective trial. *J. Women's Health, 5* (6), 555–566.

52. Wren, B., & Eden, J. A. (1996). Do progestogens reduce the risk of breast cancer? A review of the evidence. *Menopause: The J. of the N. Am. Menopause Soc., 3* (1), 4–12.

53. McEwen, B. S., et al. (1999). Inhibition of dendritic spine induction on hippocampal ca-1 pyramidal neurons by nonsteroidal estrogen antagonist in female rats. *Endocrinology, 140,* 1044–1047; McEwen, B. S., & Wooley, C. S. (1994). Estradiol and progesterone regulate neuronal structure and synaptic connectivity in adult as well as developing brain. *Experimental Gerontology, 29,* 431–436; Wooley, C. S., & McEwen, B. S. (1993). Roles of estradiol and progesterone in regulation of hippocampal dendritic spine density during the estrous cycle in the rat. *J. Comparative Neurology, 336,* 293–306.

54. Timmerman, D., et al. (1998). A randomized trial on the use of ultrasonography or office hysteroscopy for endometrial assessment in postmenopausal patients with breast cancer who were treated with tamoxifen. *Am. J. Obstetrics & Gynecology, 179,* 62–70; Franchi, M., et al. (1999). Endometrial thickness in tamoxifen-treated patients: An independent predictor of endometrial disease. *Obstetrics & Gynecology, 93,* 1004–1008; Ramonetta, L. M., et al. (1999). Endometrial cancer in polyps associated with tamoxifen use. *Am. J. Obstetrics & Gynecology, 180,* 340–341.

55. Osborne, C. K. (1999). Questions and answers about tamoxifen. In *Tamoxifen for the Treatment and Prevention of Breast Cancer.* V. Craig, ed. Melville, NY: PRR; [no author] (1995). NSABP halts B-14 trial: No benefit seen beyond 5 years of tamoxifen use. *J. Nat. Cancer Inst., 87,* 1829.

56. Hemminki, K., et al. (1996). Tamoxifen-induced DNA adducts in endometrial samples from breast cancer patients. *Cancer Research, 56* (19), 4374–4377; Zimniski, S. J., et al. (1993). Induction of tamoxifen-dependent rat mammary tumors. *Cancer Research, 53,* 2937–2939.

57. Fisher, B. (1998). Tamoxifen for prevention of breast cancer: Report of the National Surgical Adjuvant Breast and Bowel Project P-1 Study. *J. Nat. Cancer Inst., 90* (18), 1371–1388.

58. Love, S. (1999, August 3). Wondering about a wonder drug. *New York Times.*

Chapter 14: Living with Heart, Passion, and Joy:
How to Listen to and Love Your Midlife Heart

1. Svendsen, Nanna Aida (1999, October). Personal letter, excerpted in *Health Wisdom for Women, 6* (10), 8. Used here with permission from the author.

2. Tremollieres, F. A., et al. (1999). Coronary heart disease risk factors and menopause: A study in 1,684 French women. *Atherosclerosis, 142* (2), 415–423.

3. National Center for Health Statistics (1996). *Vital Statistics of the United States. 1992. Vol. 11: Mortality, Part A* (DHHS Publication 96–1101). Hyattsville, MD: U.S. Dept. of Health and Human Services, Public Health Service.

4. American Heart Association (1997). *Heart and Stroke Statistical Update.* Dallas, TX: Author; Centers for Disease Control and Prevention, National Center for Health Statistics (1996). *Health, United States, 1995* (PHS Publication 96–1232). Hyattsville, MD: U.S. Dept. of Health and Human Services, Public Health Service; Leiman, J. M., Meyer, J. E., Rothschild, N., & Simon, L. J. (March 1997). *Selected Facts on U.S. Women's Health: A Chart Book.* New York: The Commonwealth Fund; Maynard, C., et al. (1992). Gender differences in the treatment and outcome of acute myocardial infarction. Results from the Myocardial Infarction Triage and Intervention Registry. *Arch. Intern. Med., 152* (5), 972–976.

5. *Selected Facts on U.S. Health,* Op. cit.

6. Clow, B. H. (1996). *Liquid Light of Sex: Kundalini Rising at Mid-life Crisis,* 103–104. Santa Fe, NM: Bear & Co.

7. Childre, D., & Martin, H. (1999). *The HeartMath Solution* (foreword). San Francisco: HarperSanFrancisco.

8. Skinner, J. (1993). Neurocardiology: Brain mechanisms underlying fatal cardiac arrhythmias. *Neurologic Clinics, 11* (2), 325–351.

9. Kudenchuk, P. J., et al. (1996). Comparison of presentation, treatment and outcome of acute myocardial infarction in men vs. women (The Myocardial Infarction Triage and Intervention Registry). *Am. J. Cardiology, 78* (1), 9–14.

10. Cooper, G. S. (1999). Menstrual and reproductive risk factors for ischemic heart disease. *Epidemiology, 10* (3), 255–259; Hazeltine, F. P., & Jacobson, B. (1997). *Women's Health Research: A Medical and Policy Primer,* 173. Washington, D.C.: APA Press.

11. Iribarren, C., et al. (2000). Association of hostility with coronary artery calcification in young adults: The CARDIA Study. *JAMA, 283* (19), 2546–2551.

12. Friedman, M., & Rosenman, R. (1974). *Type A Behavior and Your Heart.* New York: Alfred A. Knopf.

13. Webber, L. S., et al. (1979). Occurrence in children of multiple risk factors for coronary artery disease: The Bogalusa Heart Study. *Preventive Medicine, 8,* 407–418; Khoury, P., et al. (1980). Clustering and interrelationships of coronary heart disease risk factors in schoolchildren, ages 6–19. *Am. J. Epidemiol., 112,* 524–538.

14. Stampfer, M., et al. (2000). Primary prevention of coronary heart disease in women through diet and lifestyle. *NEJM, 343,* 16–22.

15. Mo-Suwan, L., & Lebel, L. (1996). Risk factors for cardiovascular disease in obese and normal school age children: Association of insulin with other cardiovascular risk factors. *Biomed. Environ. Sci., 9* (2–3), 269–275; Wing, R. R., & Jeffery, R. W. (1995). Effect of modest weight loss on changes in cardiovascular risk factors: Are there differences between men and women between weight loss and maintenance? *Int. J. Obes. Relat. Metab. Disord., 19* (1), 67–43.

16. Manson, J. E., et al. (1992). The primary prevention of myocardial infarction. *NEJM, 326* (21), 1406–1416; Mosca, L., et al. (1999). Guide to

preventive cardiology for women. AHA/ACC Scientific Statement Consensus panel statement. *Circulation, 99* (18), 2480–2484.

17. No authors listed (1998). Prevention of cardiovascular events and death with pravastatin in patients with coronary heart disease and a broad range of initial cholesterol levels. The Long-Term Intervention with Pravastatin in Ischaemic Disease (LIPID) Study Group. *NEJM, 339* (19), 1349–1357.

18. Manson, J. E., et al. (1990). A prospective study of obesity and risk of coronary heart disease in women. *NEJM, 332* (13), 882–889.

19. Wu, T., et al. (2000). Periodontal disease and risk of cerebrovascular disease: The first national health and nutrition examination survey and its follow-up study. *Arch. Intern. Med., 160* (18), 2749–2755; Hujoel, P. P., et al. (2000). Periodontal disease and coronary heart disease risk. *JAMA, 284* (11), 1406–1410.

20. American Cancer Society (1997). *Cancer Facts and Figures,* 5008. Atlanta: Author.

21. Hollenbach, K. A., et al. (1993). Cigarette smoking and bone mineral density in older men and women. *Am. J. Public Health, 83,* 1265–1270.

22. Berenson, G. S., et al. (1998). Association between multiple cardiovascular risk factors and atherosclerosis in children and young adults. *NEJM, 338,* 1650–1656.

23. Mann, D. (1996, May 2). Job stress can cause fatal MI. *Medical Tribune, Primary Care Edition,* 21; Suadicani, P., Hein, H. O., & Gyntelberg, F. (1993). Are social inequalities as associated with the risk of ischaemic heart disease a result of psychosocial working conditions? *Atherosclerosis, 101* (2), 165–175; Legault, S. E., et al. (1995). Pathophysiology and time course of silent myocardial ischemia during mental stress: Clinical, anatomical, and physiological correlates. *British Heart J., 73,* 242–249; Kaplan, G. A., & Keil, J. E. (1993). Socioeconomic factors and cardiovascular disease: A review of the literature. *Circulation, 88,* 1973–1998.

24. Castelli, W. P. (1988). Cardiovascular disease in women. *Am. J. Obstetrics & Gynecology, 158* (6), 1553–1560, 1566–1567; Lacroix, A. Z. (1994). Psychosocial factors in risk of coronary heart disease in women: An epidemiologic perspective. *Fertility-Sterility, 62* (suppl. 2), 133S–139S; Mahoney, L. T., et al. (1996). Coronary risk factors measured in childhood and young adult life are associated with coronary artery calcification in young adults: The Muscatine Study. *J. Am. Coll. Cardiol., 27* (2), 277–284; Schaefer, E. J., et al. (1994). Factors associated with low and elevated plasma HDL cholesterol and apolipoprotein A-I levels in the Framingham Offspring Study. *J. Lipid Research, 35* (5), 871–872; Garrison, R. J., et al. (1993). Educational attainment and coronary heart disease risk: The Framingham Offspring Study. *Prevention Medicine, 22* (1), 54–64.

25. Ferketich, A. K., et al. (2000). Depression as an antecedent to heart disease among women and men in the NHANES I Study. *Arch. Intern. Med., 160,* 1261–1268.

26. Jeppesen, J. (1997). Effects of low-fat high-carbohydrate diets on risk for ischemic heart disease in postmenopausal women. *Am. J. Clin. Nutr., 65* (4), 1027–1033.

27. Kearney, M. T., et al. (1997). William Heberden revisited: Postprandial angina – interval between food and exercise and meal composition are important determinants of time to onset of ischemia and maximal exercise tolerance. *J. Am. College of Cardiology, 29* (2), 302–307.

28. Crapo, P. A., et al. (1976). Plasma glucose and insulin responses to orally administered simple and complex carbohydrates. *Diabetes, 25* (9), 741–747; Crapo, P. A. (1977). Postprandial plasma-glucose and -insulin responses to different complex carbohydrates. *Diabetes, 26* (12), 1178–1183.

29. Modan, M., et al. (1985). Hyperinsulinemia: A link between hypertension, obesity and glucose intolerance. *J. Clin. Invest., 75,* 809–817.

30. Ridker, P. M., et al. (2000). C-reactive protein and other markers of inflammation in the prediction of cardiovascular disease in women. *NEJM, 342* (12), 836–843; Black, H. R. (1990). Coronary artery disease paradox: The role of hyperinsulinemia and insulin resistance and its implications for therapy. *J. Cardiovascular Pharmacology, 15* (suppl. 5), 26S–38S; Brindley, D. M., & Rolland, Y. (1989). Possible connections between stress, diabetes, obesity, hypertension, and altered lipoprotein metabolism that may result in arteriosclerosis. *Clinical Science, 77* (5), 453–461; DeFronzo, R., & Ferrannini, E. (1991). Insulin resistance: A multifaceted syndrome responsible for NIDDM, obesity, hypertension, dyslipidemia, and atherosclerotic cardiovascular disease. *Diabetes Care, 14* (3), 173–194; Eades, M., & Eades, M. D. (1996). *Protein Power.* New York: Bantam; Kazer, R. (1995). Insulin resistance, insulin-like growth factor I and breast cancer: A hypothesis. *International J. Cancer, 62,* 403–406; Lehninger, A. L. (1993). *Principles of Biochemistry.* New York: Worth; Jeppesen, J. (1997). Op. cit.

31. Tribble, D. L. (1999). AHA science advisory. Antioxidant consumption and risk of coronary heart disease: Emphasis on vitamin C, vitamin E, and beta-carotene: A statement for health care professionals from the American Heart Association. *Circulation, 99* (4), 591–595.

32. Anderson, J. W., et al. (1995). Meta-analysis of the effects of soy protein intake on serum lipids. *NEJM, 333* (5), 276–282.

33. Nelson, G. J., & Chamberlain, J. G. (1995). The effects of dietary alpha-linolenic acid on blood lipids and lipoproteins in humans. In Cunnane, S. C., & Thompson, L. U. (eds.). *Flaxseed in Human Nutrition.* Champaign, IL: AOCS Press; Nestel, P. J., Pomeroy, S. E., Sasahard, T., et al. (1997). Arterial compliance in obese subjects is improved with dietary plant n-3 fatty acid from flaxseed oil despite increased LDL oxidizability. *Arterioscler. Throm. Vasc. Biol., 17,* 1163–1170.

34. Witteman, J. C., et al. (1994). Reduction of blood pressure with oral magnesium supplementation in women with mild to moderate hypertension. *Am. J. Clin. Nutrition, 60* (1), 129–135.

35. Altura, B. M., et al. (1991). Cardiovascular risk factors and magnesium: Relationships to atherosclerosis, ischemic heart disease, and hypertension. *Magnes. Trace Elem., 10*, 182–192; Bostick, R. M. (1999). Relation of Ca+, vitamin D, and dairy food intake to ischemic heart disease mortality among postmenopausal women. *Am. J. Epidemiol., 149* (2), 151–161; Morrison, H., et al. (1996). Serum folate and risk of fatal coronary heart disease. *JAMA, 275* (24), 1893–1896; Stampfer, M. J., et al. (1993). Vitamin E consumption and the risk of coronary disease in women. *NEJM, 328*, 1444–1449; Yochum, L., et al. (1999). Dietary flavonoid intake and risk of cardiovascular disease in postmenopausal women. *Am. J. Epidemiol., 149* (10), 943–949; Kushi, L. H., et al. (1996). Dietary antioxidant vitamins and death from coronary heart disease in postmenopausal women. *NEJM, 334*, 1156–1162.
36. Digiesi, V., et al. (1990). Effect of coenzyme Q_{10} on essential hypertension. *Current Therapy Research, 47*, 841–845.
37. Ghirlanda, G., et al. (1993). Evidence of plasma CoQ_{10}-lowering effects by HMG-CoA reductase inhibitors: A double-blind, placebo-controlled study. *J. Clinical Pharmacology, 33*, 226–229.
38. Sinatra, S. (2000). *Heart Sense for Women*, 108. Washington, D.C.: Lifeline.
39. Singh, R. B., et al. (1999). Effect of hydrosoluble coenzyme Q_{10} on blood pressures and insulin resistance in hypertensive patients with coronary artery disease. *J. Human Hypertension, 13* (3), 203–208.
40. Yamagami, T., et al. (1977). Study of coenzyme Q_{10} in essential hypertension. In K. Folkers & Y. Yamamura (eds.), *Biochemical and Clinical Aspects of Coenzyme Q_{10}, vol. 1*, 231–242. Amsterdam: Elsevier.
41. Sinatra, S. (1998). *The Coenzyme Q_{10} Phenomenon*. Los Angeles: Keats Publishing.
42. Howard, A. N., et al. (1996). Do hydroxycarotenoids prevent coronary heart disease? A comparison between Belfast and Toulouse. *International J. Vitamin & Nutritional Research, 66*, 113–118.
43. Stephens, N. G., et al. (1996). Randomized controlled trial of vitamin E in patients with coronary disease. Cambridge Heart Antioxidant Study (CHAOS). *Lancet, 347*, 781–786.
44. Janson, M. (1997). Drug free management of hypertension. *Am. J. Natural Medicine, 4* (8), 14–17.
45. Fernandez, C., et al. (1992). L-carnitine in the treatment of chronic myocardial ischemia. An analysis of three multicenter studies and a bibliographic review. *Clinical Ter., 140* (4), 353–377; Kobyayashi, A., et al. (1992). L-carnitine treatment for congestive heart failure – experimental and clinical study. *Japan Circulation J., 56* (1), 86–94.
46. Gaziano, J. M. (1994). Antioxidant vitamins and coronary artery disease risk. *Am. J. Medicine., 97* (suppl.), 3S–18S, 3S–21S; Nenseter, M. S., Volden, V., Berg, T., et al. (1995). No effect of beta-carotene supplementation on the susceptibility of low-density lipoprotein to *in vitro* oxidation among hypercholesterolaemic postmenopausal women. *Scan. J.*

Clin. Lab. Invest., 55, 477–485; Riemersma, R. A., et al. (1991). Risk of angina pectoris and plasma concentrations of vitamin A, E, C, and carotene. *Lancet, 337* (8732), 1–5; Stampfer, M. J., Hennekens, C. H., Manson, J. E., et al. (1993). Vitamin E consumption and the risk of coronary disease in women. *NEJM, 328* (20), 1444–1449; Steinberg, E., et al. (1992). Antioxidants in the prevention of human atherosclerosis. *Circulation, 85* (6), 2238–2343; Street, D. A., Comstock, G. W., Salkeld, R. M., Schuep, W., & Klag, M. J. (1994). Serum antioxidants and myocardial infarction. Are low levels of carotenoids and alpha-tocopherol risk factors for myocardial infarction? *Circulation, 90* (3), 1154–1161.

47. Rimm, E. B. (1998). Folate and vitamin B_6 from diet and supplements in relation to risk of coronary heart disease among women. *JAMA, 279,* 359–364.

48. Leaf, A., et al. (1988). Cardiovascular effect of n-3 fatty acids. *NEJM, 318* (9), 549–557; von Schaky, C., et al. (1999). The effect of dietary omega-3 fatty acids in coronary atherosclerosis: A randomized, double-blind, placebo-controlled trial. *Ann. Internal Medicine, 130* (7), 554–562.

49. Hertog, M. G., et al. (1997). Antioxidant flavonols and coronary heart disease. *Lancet, 349* (9053), 699.

50. Jain, A. K., et al. (1993). Can garlic reduce levels of serum lipids? A controlled clinical study. *Am. J. Medicine., 94,* 632–635; Kleijnen, J., et al. (1989). Garlic, onions, and cardiovascular risk factors: A review of the evidence from human experiments with emphasis on commercially available preparations. *Br. J. Clin. Pharmacol., 28,* 535–544; Mader, F. H. (1990). Treatment of hyperlipidemia with garlic powder tablets. *Arzneim.-Forsch., 40,* 1111–1116; McMahon, F. G., & Vargas, R. (1993). Can garlic lower blood pressure? A pilot study. *Pharmacotherapy, 13* (4), 406–407.

51. Berger, J. (1998). *Herbal Rituals,* 132–138. New York: St Martin's Press.

52. Skrabal, F. (1981). Low sodium/high potassium diet for the prevention of hypertension: Probable mechanisms of action. *Lancet, 2* (8252), 895–900.

53. Alpers, G. W., et al. (1999). Antiplatelet therapy: New foundations for optimal treatment decisions. *Neurology, 53* (7, suppl. 4), 25S–31S; Antiplatelet Trialists' Collaboration (1994). Collaborative overview of randomised trials of antiplatelet therapy – 1: Prevention of death, myocardial infarction, and stroke by prolonged antiplatelet therapy in various categories of patients. *British Medicine J., 308,* 81–106; DeAbago, F. J., et al. (1999). Association between SSRIs and upper GI bleeding. *British Medicine J., 319,* 1106–1109; Easton, J. D., et al. (1999). Antiplatelet therapy: Views from the experts. *Neurology, 53* (7, suppl. 4), 32S–37S; Rong, Y., et al. (1994). Pycnogenol protects vascular endothelial cells from induced oxidant injury. *Biotechnol. Therapy, 5* (3–4), 117–126.

54. Hambrecht, R., et al. (2000). Effect of exercise on coronary endothelial function in patients with coronary artery disease. *NEJM, 342,* 454–460;

Goldman, E., (1999, November 1). Exercise equals estrogen for lowering heart risk. *Internal Medicine News, 16.*

55. Belardinelli, R., et al. (1998). Effects of moderate exercise training on thallium uptake and contractile response to low-dose dobutamine of dysfunctional myocardium in patients with ischemic cardiomyopathy. *Circulation, 97,* 553–561.

56. Lemole, J. (1999, February). Personal interview for *Health Wisdom for Women.*

57. Koh, K. K., Mincemoyer, R., Bui, M. N., et al. (1997). Effects of hormone replacement therapy on fibrinolysis in postmenopausal women. *NEJM, 336,* 683–690; Nasr, A., & Breckwoldt, M. (1998). Estrogen replacement therapy and cardiovascular protection: Lipid mechanisms are the tip of an iceberg. *Gynecol. Endocrinol., 12,* 43–59; Oparil, S. (1999). Arthur C. Corcoran Memorial Lecture: Hormones and vasoprotection. *Hypertension, 33,* 170–176; Pines, A., Mijatovic, V., van der Mooren, M. J., et al. (1997). Hormone replacement therapy and cardioprotection: Basic concepts and clinical considerations. *Eur. J. Gynecol. Reprod. Biol., 71,* 193–197; van der Mooren, M. J., Mijatovic, V., & van Baal, W. M. (1998). Hormone replacement therapy in postmenopausal women with specific risk factors for coronary artery disease. *Maturitas, 30,* 27–36; Rosano, G. (1996). 17-ß-estradiol therapy lessens angina in postmenopausal women with syndrome X. *J. Am. Coll. Cardiol., 28,* 1500–1505.

58. Clarkson, T. B., & Anthony, M. S. (1997). Effects on the cardiovascular system: Basic aspects. In R. Lindsay, D. W. Dempster, & V. C. Jordan (eds.), *Estrogens and Antiestrogens,* 89–118. Philadelphia: Lippincott-Raven; Gerhard, M., & Ganz, P. (1995). How do we explain the clinical benefits of estrogen? From bedside to bench. *Circulation, 92,* 5–8; Reis, S. E., Gloth, S. T., Blumenthal, R. S., et al. (1994). Ethinyl estradiol acutely attenuates abnormal coronary vasomotor responses to acetylcholine in postmenopausal women. *Circulation, 89* (1), 52–60; Sullivan, J. M. (1996). Hormone replacement therapy in cardiovascular disease: The human model. *British J. Obstet. Gynaecol., 103* (suppl. 13), 50S–67S.

59. Darling, G. M., Johns, J. A., McCloud, P. L., et al. (1997). Estrogen and progestin compared with simvastatin for hypercholesterolemia in post-menopausal women. *NEJM, 337,* 595–601; Davidson, M. H., Testolin, L. M., Maki, K. C., et al. (1997). A comparison of estrogen replacement, pravastatin, and combined treatment for the management of hyper-cholesterolemia in postmenopausal women. *Arch. Intern. Med., 157,* 1186–1192; Koh, K. K., Cardillo, C., Bui, M. N., et al. (1997). Vascular effects of estrogen and cholesterol-lowering therapies in hyperchole-sterolemic postmenopausal women. *Circulation, 99,* 354–360.

60. Barrett-Connor, E., Slone, S., Greendale, G., et al. (1997). The Post-menopausal Estrogen/Progestin Interventions Study: Primary outcomes in adherent women. *Maturitas, 30,* 27–36; Miyagawa, K., et al. (1997). Medroxyprogesterone interferes with ovarian steroid protection against

coronary vasospasm. *Nature Medicine, 3,* 324–327; The Writing Group for the PEPI Trial (1995). Effects of estrogen or estrogen/progestin regimens on heart disease risk factors in postmenopausal women. *JAMA, 273,* 199–208; Sarrel, P. M. (1995). How progestins compromise the cardioprotective effects of estrogen. *Menopause: The J. of the N. Am. Menopause Soc., 2* (4), 187–190.

61. Herrington, D., et al. (2000). Effects of estrogen replacement on the progression of coronary artery atherosclerosis. *NEJM, 343,* 522–529; Hulley, S., et al., for the Heart and Estrogen/Progestin Replacement Study (HERS) Research Group (1998). Randomized trial of estrogen plus progestin for secondary prevention of coronary heart disease in postmenopausal women. *JAMA, 280,* 605–613; No authors listed (2000, March 13). Estrogen replacement and atherosclerosis (ERA). Presented at the 49th annual meeting of the American College of Cardiology, Anaheim, CA.

62. This data is made available by the Data and Safety Monitoring Board (DSMB) (2000, May). The final data won't be made available until the end of the study. In: Postmenopausal hormone therapy and coronary heart disease: Abstract and commentary. *ObGyn Alert: A Monthly Update of Developments in Female Reproductive Medicine, 17* (1), 1–4.

63. Williams, J. K., & Adams, M. R. (1997). Estrogens, progestins, and coronary artery reactivity. *Nature Medicine, 3* (3), 273–274.

64. Grodstein, F., Stampfer, M. H., Manson, J. E., et al. (1996). Postmenopausal estrogen and progestin use and the risk of cardiovascular disease. *NEJM, 335,* 453–461.

65. Thorogood, M., Mann, J., Appleby, P., & McPherson, K. (1994). Risk of death from cancer and ischaemic heart disease in meat and non-meat eaters. *British Medicine J., 308* (6945), 1667–1670; Koh, K. (1999). Vascular effects of estrogen and cholesterol-lowering therapies in hypercholesterolemic postmenopausal women. *Circulation, 99,* 354–360; Sarrel, P. M. (1988). Effects of ovarian steroids on the cardiovascular system. In J. Ginsberg (ed.), *Circulation in the Female,* 117–141. Carnforth, Lancashire: Parthenon; Sarrel, P. M. (1995). How progestins compromise the cardioprotective effects of estrogen. *Menopause: The J. of the N. Am. Menopause Soc.,* 187–190.

66. Sarrel, P. M. (1994). Estrogen's actions in arteries, bone, and brain. *Sci. Med., 1,* 44–53; Sarrel, P. M. (1998). Cardiovascular aspects of androgens in women. *Seminars in Reprod. Endocrinol., 16* (2), 121–128.

67. Nabel, E. G. (2000). Coronary heart disease in women – an ounce of prevention. *NEJM, 343* (8), 572–574.

68. Fitzgerald, F. T. (1986). The therapeutic value of pets. *Western J. Medicine, 144,* 103–105.

69. Ibid.

70. Friedmann, E., Katcher, A., Lunch, J. J., & Thomas, S. A. (1980). Animal companions and the one-year survival of patients after discharge from a coronary care unit. *Public Health Reports, 95,* 307–312.

71. Beck, A., & Katcher, A. (1983). *Between Pets and People: The Importance of Animal Companionship.* New York: Putnam; Katcher, A., & Beck, A. (1983). *New Perspectives on Our Lives with Companion Animals.* Philadelphia: University of Pennsylvania Press.

Resources

NOTE: The phone numbers and addresses listed in this section were current as of the publication date of the book.

General Resources

Women's Health Resources from Christiane Northrup, MD

Christiane Northrup, MD, FACOG, PO Box 199, Yarmouth, ME 04096, website: www.drnorthrup.com.

Dr Northrup's interactive website (www.drnorthrup.com) is the best place to find regularly updated information on her lectures and other resources. Dr Northrup also welcomes your letters. Many of her readers' questions are answered in her monthly newsletter, *Health Wisdom for Women* (see below).

MEDICAL AND EDUCATIONAL LITERATURE FOR WOMEN

Women's Bodies, Women's Wisdom: Creating Physical and Emotional Health and Healing (Piatkus, 1998). Available through www.drnorthrup.com or www.piatkus.co.uk

This ground-breaking book is now completely revised, offering up-to-date information on the entire range of women's health problems. With over 1.2 million copies now in print, and translated into eight languages, Dr Northrup's first book has been described as contemporary medicine at its best, combining new technologies with natural remedies and the miraculous healing powers within the body itself.

Health Wisdom for Women. Information about ordering Dr Northrup's monthly newsletter can be obtained by calling 207-846-3626 or by visiting www.drnorthrup.com. Or write to Dr Northrup at the above address for an order form.

Every month, Dr Northrup provides a forum for discussing safe, effective, and natural solutions to women's health problems. With her characteristic compassion, she presents the most up-to-date information on topics from help for hot flushes to choosing the best foods for your body. She also answers readers' health questions, shares personal success stories from readers, and recommends further reading. Newsletter subscribers also have access to Dr Northrup's monthly Wisdom Wire telephone message, a health care provider referral service, and a wide range of products and services designed to help women live their lives more fully and healthily.

AUDIOTAPES

Igniting Intuition: Unearthing Body Genius – Six Ways to Create Health, Happiness, and Almost Everything Else in Your Life. By Christiane Northrup, MD, and Mona Lisa Schulz, MD, PhD. Six-tape audio programme available through www.drnorthrup. com or Hay House, Inc., PO Box 5100, Carlsbad, CA 92018-5100, tel. 800-654-5126, fax 800-650-5115, website: www.hayhouse.com.

Dr Christiane Northrup and Dr Mona Lisa Schulz teach you powerful, energising, and life-changing tools for personal growth – how to use your body's own unique intuitive language to help you heal body, mind, and soul. With over thirty years of combined medical practice between them, Drs Northrup and Schulz describe the seven emotional centres that are associated with the major organ systems in the body, and show how both good health and illness communicate information you can use to change your life. With wit and wisdom, they teach you how to recognise the patterns associated with disease so that you can change the conditions of the cells themselves by changing your thoughts, your relationships, and your activities.

Body Talk: No-Nonsense, Common-Sense Solutions to Create Health and Healing. By Christiane Northrup, MD, and Mona Lisa Schulz, MD, PhD. Six-tape audio programme available through www.drnorthrup. com or Hay House, Inc. (address above).

In *Igniting Intuition*, Drs Schulz and Northrup explored the basics of how intuition is wired in the body and brain. The *Body Talk* tape series decodes the language of intuition further, with particular focus on practical and effective solutions to health concerns.

Empowering Women: Six Empowered Women Bring You Positive Words of Wisdom and Inspiration! Six-tape audio programme available through www.drnorthrup.com or Hay House, Inc. (address above).

Filled with inspiration, knowledge, and heart, this audio programme – compiled from the 'Empowering Women' lectures – includes six powerful speakers: Louise L. Hay; Caroline Myss, PhD; Christiane Northrup, MD; Susan Jeffers, PhD; Doreen Virtue, PhD; and Mona Lisa Schulz, MD, PhD. Learn how to empower your life and turn your dreams into reality.

Women's Bodies, Women's Wisdom: Creating Physical and Emotional Health and Healing. Live lecture by Dr Christiane Northrup. Two-tape set available through www.drnorthrup.com or Hay House, Inc. (address above). Inspired by her best-selling book of the same name, these audiocassettes explore the unity of mind and body and the powerful role of the human spirit in creating health.

Creating Health – Two-Cassette Tape Set. By Dr Christiane Northrup. Available through www.drnorthrup.com or Sounds True at 800-333-9185.
By learning to trust in your body's intuitive wisdom, you can control most of the factors that go into creating your health. What you learn may surprise you (for example, that the heart and uterus produce the same chemicals as the brain does; they are in effect 'thinking organs'). Contains a wealth of subtle, simple techniques for engaging with your body, drawing from your inner wisdom, and taking the action necessary to create the health you want.

Creating Health Series – Six-Cassette Tape Set. By Dr Christiane Northrup. Includes: *Creating Health* (described above), plus *Premenstrual Syndrome, Menopause, Whole Nutrition,* and *Creating Breast Health* (described below). Now available in two formats: archive edition in durable polyvinyl case (ISBN 1-56455-244-6) or new, compact bookshelf edition (ISBN 1-56455-698-0). Available through www.drnorthrup. com or Sounds True at 800-333-9185.

Premenstrual Syndrome. Cassette tape. Available through www. drnorthrup.com or Sounds True at 800-333-9185.
Straightforward answers to a wide range of questions about premenstrual syndrome. Dr Northrup discusses the connections between the oestrous cycle and sex drive, how diet and exercise can help control PMS symptoms, the links between alcoholic families and PMS, and much more. A way to view your menstrual cycle as part of the life-giving power that is a woman's special gift.

Creating Breast Health. Cassette tape. Available through www.drnorthrup. com or Sounds True at 800-333-9185.
The medical profession stresses the importance of breast examinations, yet so often these 'early detection' programmes create nothing but fear in women. Here Dr Northrup discusses how to stop fearing your breasts, optimise your breast health through diet and nutrition, cope with a family history of breast disease, and transform the routine breast self-examination into a positive experience.

Women's Health Resources in the UK

Woman to Woman, Dr Sara Miller, 12 Chapel Hill, Backwell Farleigh, North Somerset BS48 3PP, tel. 01275 464149.
Holistic health care for women offering face-to-face or telephone consultations, and weekend or shorter workshops on women's health and spirituality.

Educational Organisations

Women's Resource Centre, London Women's Centre, Unit 100, 134–146 Curtain Road, London EC2A 3AR, tel. 020 7729 4011.
A central point of contact, a directory and information exchange for London women and women's groups, giving support and referral on a range of issues and information on current events and activities.

The Amarant Centre, 80 Lambeth Road, London SE1 7PW, tel. 020 7401 3855.
The Amarant Trust is a registered charity set up to help women with menopause problems. (Based only in London.)

CHAPTER 2:
The Brain Catches Fire at Menopause

Toxic Emotions/Forgiveness

SUGGESTED READING
Casarjian, R. (1992). *Forgiveness: A Bold Choice for a Peaceful Heart.* New York: Bantam Books.
Hay, L. L. (1998). *Heal Your Body: The Mental Causes for Physical Illness and the Metaphysical Way to Overcome Them.* Carlsbad, CA: Hay House, Inc.
Levine, S. (1989). *Healing into Life and Death.* New York: Doubleday and Co., Inc.
Northrup, C. (1998). *Women's Bodies, Women's Wisdom.* London: Piatkus Books.
Schulz, M. L. (1998). *Awakening Intuition.* New York: Harmony Books.
Smedes, L. B. (1996). *Forgive and Forget: Healing the Hurts We Don't Deserve.* New York: HarperCollins Publishers, Inc.

CHAPTER 3:
Coming Home to Yourself

Career Counselling

SUGGESTED READING
Wright, B. (1999). *Careershift: How to Plan and Develop a Successful Career.* London: Piatkus Books.

Deliberate Creating

Jerry and Esther Hicks, PO Box 690070, San Antonio, TX 78269, tel. 210-755-2229.
Jerry and Esther Hicks publish books and tapes containing spiritual messages on everything from how to create deliberate intent and how to discover your life purpose to the value of your relationships with others. I have enjoyed their material for many years. Write or ring for a catalogue, or visit their website at www.abraham-hicks.com.

Feng Shui

SUGGESTED READING
Collins, T. K. (1996). *The Western Guide to Feng Shui: Creating Balance, Harmony, and Prosperity in Your Environment.* Carlsbad, CA: Hay House.
Collins, T. K. (1999). *The Western Guide to Feng Shui – Room by Room.* Carlsbad, CA: Hay House.

Financial Independence

SUGGESTED READING
Dominguez, J., and Robin, V. (2000). *Your Money or Your Life: Transforming Your Relationship with Money and Achieving Financial Independence.* New York: Viking Penguin.
Orman, S. (1999). *The Courage to Be Rich: Creating a Life of Material and Spiritual Abundance.* New York: Penguin/Putnam.

Proprioceptive Writing

Metcalf/Simon Proprioceptive Writing Workshop. Drs Metcalf and Simon can be contacted at the Proprioceptive Writing Centers, 88 Lexington Ave., Mezz. D, New York, NY 10016, tel. 212-213-5402.
Proprioceptive writing is a therapy that uses writing to explore the psyche. A meditational writing practice that has the power to open the heart and clear the mind, it was developed twenty years ago by Linda Trichter Metcalf and Tobin Simon after a decade of teaching writing to college students. I personally worked with them privately and in group settings for seven years.

CHAPTER 4:
This Can't Be Menopause, Can It?

Salivary and Adrenal Hormone Testing for Adrenal and Ovarian Function

Wisdom Hormone Program. For more information or to order a salivary hormone test kit, call 800-705-5559.
The Wisdom Hormone Program is an alliance between the *Health Wisdom for Women* newsletter and Aeron Labs to bring individualised hormone replacement solutions to newsletter subscribers and other interested women.

Aeron LifeCycles Laboratory, 1933 Davis Street, Suite 310, San Leandro, CA 94577, tel. 800-631-7900, website: www.hrtdoctor.com.
Tests for a panel of hormones, including oestrogen, progesterone, testosterone, DHEA, and cortisol, via saliva sampling, are available to health care providers. Aeron Labs conducts regular CME-approved courses for physicians on individualised hormone replacement.

Higher Nature Ltd, Burwash Common, East Sussex TN19 7LX, tel. 01435 882880.
Arrange salivary testing in UK, with Aeron LifeCycles laboratory. It may be cheaper if you go via a holistic doctor, who can also help you interpret your results.

The Doctor's Laboratory, 55 Wimpole Street, London W1G 7DF, tel. 020 7460 4800, fax 020 7460 4848, e-mail: tdl@tdlplc.co.uk, website: www.tdlplc.co.uk
Test for free (unbound) testosterone levels. You have to be referred by a medical practitioner.

Relaxation Techniques

SUGGESTED READING
Domar, A. D., and H. Dreher (1997). *Healing Mind, Healthy Woman: Using the Mind-Body Connection to Manage Stress and Take Control of Your Life.* New York: Delta.
Dr Domar offers a wide range of stress reduction approaches that help women manage the biochemical effects of stress. Audiotape programmes of her techniques are also available.
Domar, A. D., and H. Dreher (1997). *Self-Nurture: Learning to Care for Yourself as Effectively as You Care for Everyone Else.* New York: Viking.

CHAPTER 5: *Hormone Replacement Therapy*

See Chapter 4 Resources for information on salivary and adrenal hormone testing.

Progesterone Cream

Progesterone cream (1.5–3 per cent strength) is currently available in the UK under the trade names ProGest and ProJuven. If your doctor does not want to prescribe it for you, contact the Natural Progesterone Information Service.

Higher Nature Ltd, Burwash Common, East Sussex TN19 7LX, tel. 01435 882880.
UK distributors – will provide information to medical practitioners only.

Natural Progesterone Information Service, PO Box 24, Buxton, Derbyshire, SK17 9FB. Send a large SAE with a first-class stamp for a list of prescribing private doctors and a patient information pack.

Progesterone cream (2 per cent strength) is available from a number of different sources in the US. I have personally used the following preparations and find them all comparable in quality and effectiveness.

ProGest Cream, by Women's Group Formulas. This is the first brand I ever used or recommended. Available from Emerson Ecologics, 7 Commerce Drive, Bedford, NH 03110, tel. 800-654-4432, fax 800-718-7238. Outside the United States, tel. 01-603-656-9778, fax 01-603-656-9797, website: www.emersonecologics.com.

FemGest, by Bio-Nutritional Formulas. This is a brand I also recommend to my patients and newsletter subscribers. Available from Emerson Ecologics (see address above).

DHEA (dehydroepiandrosterone)

Pharmaceutical-grade DHEA is available from Emerson Ecologics (see address above). I recommend sublingual 5-mg DHEA capsules manufactured by Douglas Laboratories. Suggested dose: one to four capsules daily.

The Nutri Centre, The Hale Clinic, 7 Park Crescent, London W1B 1PF, tel. 020 7436 5122, fax 020 7436 5171, e-mail: enq@nutricentre.com, website: www.nutricentre.com.
Offer professional advice and carefully prepared and researched supplements including DHEA (which is only available on prescription in UK).

CHAPTER 6:
Foods and Supplements to Support the Change

Nutrition

Institute for Optimum Nutrition, Blades Court, Deodar Road, London SW15 2NU, tel. 020 8877 9993.
Provides information on health through food and nutrition, helping 'people reach their maximum potential for health and well-being by balancing body chemistry and cooperating with nature'.

Soil Association, Bristol House, 40–56 Victoria Street, Bristol BS1 6BY, tel. 0117 929 0661, www.soilassociation.org.
Provides information on sources of organic fruit and vegetables.

Women's Nutritional Advisory Service, PO Box 268, Lewes, East Sussex BN7 2QN, tel. 01273 487366.

Herbs
Many quality herbal supplements are available. Some of my favourite suppliers are listed here.

SUPPLIERS

Revival Herbs, available from Physicians Laboratories, PO Box 242368, Charlotte, NC 28224. For more information, including references and research documentation, call 800-500-8053. Outside the United States, call 01-336-722-2337. Their website (you can place orders online or send e-mail) is www.revivalfarm.com.
Revival herbs are organically grown, harvested by hand, and immediately processed with a proprietary liquid-extraction process. The liquid extract is then concentrated, standardised, and encapsulated into a vegetable capsule. This delivery system combines the quality, absorption, and bioavailability of a liquid extract with the convenience and purity of a capsule. It has been documented that liquid extracts are very well absorbed and more bioavailable than powdered herb capsules or tablets. The encapsulated herbal liquid extract is an easy way to take herbs.
    The following Revival herbs are available: kava kava for relaxation; St John's wort for improved mental outlook; ginkgo and gotu kola for improved memory and concentration; echinacea and goldenseal for healthy immune function; milk thistle seed for healthy liver function; nettle leaf for relief of allergy symptoms; valerian root for restful sleeping; Siberian ginseng for stress, low energy levels, and fatigue.

Hambledon Herbs, Court Farm, Milverton, Somerset TA4 1NS, tel. 01823 401205.
Supplier of loose, dried, mostly organic herbs.

Argyll Herbs Direct, 9 Chancellors Pound, Redhill, Bristol BS40 5TZ, tel. 01934 863353, e-mail: enquiries@argyllherbsdirect.com, website: www. argyllherbsdirect.com.
Herbal tablets and capsules, fluid extracts, teas, individual advice and consultations. Will dispense a menopausal mixture for your own needs.

Emerson Ecologics, 7 Commerce Drive, Bedford, NH 03110, tel. 800-654-4432, fax 800-718-7238. Outside the United States, tel. 01-603-656-9778, fax 01-603-656-9797, website: www.emersonecologics.com.
Emerson Ecologics provides highest-quality nutritional supplements, antioxidants, vitamins, minerals, herbs, standardised herbal extracts, green foods, and essential fatty acids from the world's leading manufacturers of professional supplements. They currently offer over three thousand quality natural products.

SPECIFIC HERBAL PRODUCTS

Black cohosh. The rhizome of *Cimicifuga racemosa* has been used by Native Americans for centuries in much the same way as the Chinese have used dong quai. It is used for the treatment of menopausal ailments due to increasing ovarian insufficiency, mild postoperative functional deficits after ovariectomy or hysterectomy, PMS, and juvenile menstrual disorders. Many different preparations are available. I recommend Black Cohosh Pro, 40mg twice a day, from Emerson Ecologics (see address above). Remifemin is another widely used brand available in many natural food stores. Take as directed.

Women's Phase II. Women's Phase II is a combination of dong quai, licorice root, burdock, wild yam, and motherwort. This formula was developed by Dr Tori Hudson, a naturopathic physician and professor at the Bastyr University of Natural Health Sciences. It has been tested clinically and found to help relieve many common menopausal symptoms. Available from Transitions for Health, 621 S.W. Alder Street, Suite 900, Portland, OR 97205-3627, tel. 800-888-6814 or 503-226-1010, fax 503-226-6455, website: www.transitionsforhealth.com.

Women's Menocaps (also known as Women's Hormone Balance/ Menopause Formula). These capsules contain the highest-quality wild-crafted dong quai, burdock, *Vitex agnus-castus,* black cohosh, motherwort, and licorice. Wise Woman Herbals was founded by Dr Sharol Tilgner, a naturopathic physician who formulates all of the company's products and was the former head of the pharmacy at the National College of Naturopathic Medicine. Available from Emerson Ecologics (see address above).

Soya

Information regarding soya can be obtained at the website www. soyfoods. com. The intent of this site is to promote the consumption of soya foods throughout the world by providing reliable, scientifically based information about health benefits, taste-tested recipes that include nutritional information, and other resources for consumers, dietitians, journalists, scientists, and soya foods companies.

Revival Soy Products. Available from Physicians Laboratories, PO Box 242368, Charlotte, NC 28224. For a free sample, call 888-983-6286. For more information, including references and research documentation, call 800-500-8053. Outside the United States, call 01-336-722-2337, website (you can place orders online or send e-mail): www.revivalsoy.com. The following soya products are available:

Revival Soy. Of all the numerous soya products on the market, my favourite is Revival, a meal replacement drink that contains 20g of protein and >160mg of soya isoflavones per serving, the equivalent of six servings of soya. Gram for gram, Revival soya contains more isoflavones than, say, soya milk simply because it is made from whole, genetically pure soya beans and is six times more concentrated than most other soya products. This healthy, protein-based meal replacement won't cause weight gain and has many benefits for both men and women.

Digestive Aid Enzyme. If you experience any flatulence (wind), constipation, or bloating with soya, this supplement has fifteen times the strength of the leading retail digestive enzyme.

Revival Soy Coffee. Caffeine-free and organically grown, one cup delivers about 10–15mg of isoflavones to supplement your diet. Flavours available include French vanilla, hazelnut, mocha, almond amaretto, original roast, and dark roast. A breakfast blend of half soy coffee and half Colombian coffee is also available.

Natural Soy, by Natural Prevention. Certified organic, certified GMO-free fermented soya powder. Three tablespoons contain 40mg soya isoflavones. Can be mixed in milk or juice or sprinkled over cereal. Available from Emerson Ecologics (see address p. 546).

Flax (Linseed)

The Flax Council of Canada endeavours to provide general flax facts of interest to consumers, as well as more specialised information for nutritionists, dietitians, food producers, manufacturers, and flax growers. Contact them at 465-167 Lombard Avenue, Winnipeg, Manitoba R3B 0T6, Canada, tel. 204-982-2115, fax 204-942-1841, website www.flaxcouncil.ca, e-mail flax@flaxcouncil.ca.

FiProFlax (ground flax), cold-milled by Oakmont Labs from premium-quality flax with a high oil content, is available through Emerson Ecologics, (see address p. 546).

Pizzey's Whole Flaxseed is specially selected for its superior flavour and quality. The seed is cleaned and sized, with only the plumpest seeds being selected. Pizzey's Whole Flaxseed can be ordered through Emerson Ecologics (see address p. 546).

Dakota Flax Gold. This is an organic flaxseed grown at Heintzman Farms in South Dakota. Contact Heintzman Farms, R.R. 2, Box 265, Onaka, SD 57466. Question and information line: 605-447-5813. Credit card orders only: 1-888-333-5813. Fax orders: 605-447-5855. Website: www. heintzman-farms.com or www.flaxgold.com. A 'jet kit' is available that consists of three bags of flaxseed, an electric grinder, and a bottle of flaxseed oil capsules to use when travelling.

ChanoVita UK Ltd, Everitt Close, Wellingborough NN8 2QE. Organically grown golden linseed (flaxseed) specially cracked to aid absorption of the polyunsaturated fatty acids.

SUGGESTED READING
Bennett, M. (1998). *The Flaxseed Revolution: Nature's Source of Omega-E's, Lignans, and Fiber.* Optimal Healthspan Publications.

Traditional Chinese Medicine (TCM)

Acupuncture, used alone or in conjunction with herbs, is very effective for relieving hot flushes, insomnia, night sweats, anxiety, restlessness, emotional instability, moodiness, menstrual cramps, and excessive bleeding. It's ideal to get a referral to an acupuncturist from your doctor, but if you can't find one this way, contact:

British Acupuncture Council, 63 Jeddo Road, London W12 9HQ, tel. 020 8735 0400.
They have a directory and register of qualified practitioners.

British Medical Acupuncture Society, 12 Marbury House, Higher Whitley, Warrington, Cheshire WA4 4QW, tel. 01925 730492.

CHINESE HERBS

Your best option for obtaining Chinese herbs is to see a good practitioner of Chinese medicine, but if that's not an option where you live, you can purchase them from:

Quality Life Herbs, PO Box 565, Yarmouth, ME 04096, tel. 207-842-4929, fax 207-846-3168. Quality Life Herbs is run by my personal acupuncturist, Fern Tsao, and her daughter Maureen, both experts in the use of Chinese herbs. All the Chinese herbs mentioned in this book, as well as numerous others, are available through mail order from Quality Life Herbs. Their products meet the highest standards possible for effectiveness and quality. I have been referring patients with a wide variety of conditions to Fern for many years, with excellent results.

Dong quai (also known as dang gui, tang kuei, or angelica). Dong quai is the foundation of almost all menopausal formulations and can be taken indefinitely. Sometimes called angelica root, it can be found in many herb shops and health food stores. It is also processed into capsules, tablets, and tinctures, although I would avoid alcohol-based tinctures. The recommended dosages for most over-the-counter dong quai preparations are probably too low to be helpful. Increasing the dosage to four or five of the tiny pills twice per day is unlikely to cause any problems, but it's always best to be under the supervision of a certified herbalist or Chinese medicine practitioner if you're going to do this. Available from:

Enzymatic Therapy, 825 Challenger Drive, Green Bay, WI 54311, tel. 800-783-2286, website www.enzy.com, or Quality Life Herbs (address above).

Joyful Change. I highly recommend this formula because it addresses menopausal symptoms at their root and helps rebalance the body. Dosage is three tablets two times per day before meals. Available from Quality Life Herbs (address above).

Yunnan bai yao (also known as yunna pai yao). This formula stops or slows excessive bleeding but should not be used long term. It also doesn't address the root cause of the problem. Still, it is very helpful for temporarily controlling the flooding, or heavy bleeding, so common in perimenopausal women. Recommended dosage: one or two capsules four times daily. Available from Quality Life Herbs (address above).

Xiao Yao Wan Plus. This is a Chinese nutritional supplement that helps women with PMS, menstrual cramps, and perimenopausal symptoms. This supplement contains paeonia, a well-known female tonic. Recommended dosage: four or five tablets four times per day, beginning two weeks before period is due and continuing to the first day of bleeding. It may take up to three months to experience optimal results. Available from Quality Life Herbs (address above).

Acuherb, Chinese Medicine Centre, 30 Carlyon Avenue, Harrow, HA2 8SX, tel. 020-8423-4554, fax 020-8357-1811.
Doctors trained in Western medicine and TCM; some herbal preparations can be bought directly.

CHAPTER 7: The Menopause Food Plan

Dietary Supplements

COENZYME Q_{10}

C_0Q_{10} **Q-Gel Forte,** manufactured by Designs for Health. Recommended dose: 10–100mg/day. Available from Emerson Ecologics (see address p. 546).

PharmaNord make a good brand of Q_{10} – 30mg and 100mg strengths – available at Boots the Chemist, Holland & Barrett, and health food shops.

DOCOSAHEXAENOIC ACID (DHA)

Recommended dose: 100–400mg per day. Made from algae, Neuromins is my first choice for taking this oil in supplement form. Consumers who would like more information on DHA can write to the DHA Information Center, attention Dean Skandalis, 6840 Dobbin Road, Columbia, MD 21045; or call their consumer line on 888-652-7246.

Neuromins Pro, manufactured by Murdock Madaus Schwabe, is available through Emerson Ecologics (see address p. 546).

Martek Biosciences Neuromins Products. To order Martek Neuromins Products, write to 6840 Dobbin Road, Columbia, MD 21045, call 800-662-6339, or visit their website at www.martekbio.com.

METABOLIC BOOSTERS

L-carnitine or **acetyl-L-carnitine.** Usual dose: 500–4,000mg/day. Available from Emerson Ecologics (see address p. 546).

Chromium picolinate. Usual recommended dose is 200–700mcg/day. I recommend the chromium picolinate manufactured by Douglas Labs, available in a dose of 250mcg. I also recommend the chromium picolinate manufactured by Progressive Labs, which is available in a dose of 200mcg. Both are available from Emerson Ecologics (see address p. 546). This supplement is also widely available in drugstores and natural food stores.

Keto Burner Shake. Kick-start metabolic fat burning with this high-protein nutrient complex. Containing only 2g of carbohydrates and 24g of protein per serving, this shake is designed to maximise energy, extend appetite satisfaction, and support protein synthesis to help preserve and build lean muscle tone. Available from Life Services Supplements, tel. 800-542-3230. Outside the United States and Canada, tel. 01-732-922-0099. Or log on to their website at www.lifeservices.com.

Keto Bar. Available from Life Services Supplements (address above), this low-carbohydrate, high-protein snack is perfect for anyone decreasing carbohydrate intake and switching from fat storage to fat burning. Keto Bars have just 4g of carbohydrates and 19g of energising protein – great any time you experience sugar cravings, lethargy, or between-meal hunger. I keep these in the freezer and cut off a bite now and again.

MULTIVITAMINS/MINERALS

Ultra-Preventive III. Available from Emerson Ecologics (see address p. 546).

Biocare Ltd, Lakeside, 180 Lifford Lane, Kings Norton, Birmingham B30 3NU, tel. 0121 433 3727, fax 0121 433 3879. A good range of excellent vitamins and minerals.

Higher Nature Ltd, Burwash Common, East Sussex TN19 7LX, tel. 01435 882880. Contact for a comprehensive product list.

PROANTHOCYANIDINS
These powerful antioxidants are found in grape pips and pine bark. Recommendations: start with 1mg per pound of body weight per day, divided into three doses. After two weeks, cut back to 40–80mg per day.

Pycnogenol, manufactured by Advanced Medical Nutrition, and **OPC Grape Gold,** manufactured by ORT, are available from Emerson Ecologics (see address p. 546). Many excellent brands of OPCs are also available at natural food stores.

Proflavenol is available from USANA, tel. 888-953-9595. For more information, log on to their website at www.usana.com.

PROBIOTICS
Probiotic supplements provide gastrointestinal (GI) nutritional support by augmenting naturally occurring intestinal bacteria. The intestinal micro-ecosystem typically carries up to four hundred strains of bacteria. From the point of view of intestinal health, a product that provides bacteria for multiple probiotic 'niches' makes sense. These flora may become depleted in a number of ways, including antibiotic therapy, poor diet, and disease. Probiotics are useful for individuals bothered by flatulence and bloating, and may also be used when taking an antibiotic to prevent yeast infection. Be sure to take a probiotic whenever you're on antibiotics, but take them at different times of the day, so the antibiotic won't kill off the new friendly bacteria. Continue to take the probiotic for a week or so after you've finished your course of antibiotics. That way you'll be much less likely to get a yeast infection or GI upset from the antibiotic.

I recommend **PB 8 Probiotic** or **Spectra Probiotic,** manufactured by NF Formulas, Inc. These products do not require refrigeration to maintain their potency, as most others do. Take as directed on the bottle. PB 8 is available at health food shops. Spectra Probiotic is available through Emerson Ecologics (see address p. 546).

Biocare Ltd, Lakeside, 180 Lifford Lane, Kings Norton, Birmingham B30 3NU, tel. 0121 433 3727, fax 0121 433 3879. Do a range of probiotic formulations, which are dairy free.

Digestive Aids

ENTERIC-COATED PEPPERMINT OIL
Most of the studies performed have utilised enteric-coated peppermint oil at a dosage of 0.2ml twice daily between meals.

Pepogest, manufactured by Nature's Way, is available through Emerson Ecologics (see address p. 546).

DEGLYCYRRHIZINATED LICORICE (DGL)
Recommended dose for the solid extract is 1/4–1/2 teaspoon two to three times a day. Please note that the cortisol-like activity of this herb may cause a problem in people prone to hypertension. If you are taking licorice root, your blood pressure should be monitored to ensure that it stays stable.

Gaia Herbs Licorice Root Solid Extract is available at health food stores. **Wise Woman Herbals Licorice Root Solid Extract** and **Douglas Labs Licorice Root Max-V** (deglycyrrhizinated dried root, capsule form) are available from Emerson Ecologics (see address p. 546).

SeaCure. Manufactured by Proper Nutrition, Inc., SeaCure is a concentrated fish protein that is gaining increasing recognition for its nutritional benefits in a wide range of disease conditions. Recommended for all digestive dysfunctions, eg Crohn's disease, irritable bowel syndrome, and ulcerative colitis. Also helpful after chemotherapy for nutritional support and immune system support. It is certified to be free of mercury and other heavy metals. Recommended dose is three capsules in the morning and three capsules in the afternoon. Available from Emerson Ecologics (see address p. 546).

Sea Plasma. Manufactured by BioCare Ltd (see address page 551), Sea Plasma is a phyto-plankton which provides a highly nutritious food, without contaminants, which is 85–90 per cent digestible and includes a concentrated source of natural beta-carotene.

Audiotape Programmes

Weight Loss. Guided-imagery audiotape by Belleruth Naperstak. Available from Health Journeys, 891 Moe Drive, Suite C, Akron, OH 44310, tel. 800-800-8661, website: www.healthjourneys.com.
Designed to reduce the craving for food, increase confidence, safely speed up the body's metabolism, help the body convert fat into energy, reinforce positive behaviour change, and teach relaxation skills. Side B has affirmations.

CHAPTER 8:
Creating Pelvic Health and Power

See Chapter 5 Resources for information on progesterone.

Menstrual Pain

Bupleurum (Xiao Yao Wan, also known as Hsiao Yao Wan). Xiao Yao Wan Plus is a Chinese nutritional supplement that helps women with PMS, menstrual cramps, and perimenopausal symptoms. This supplement contains paeonia, a well-known female tonic. Available from Quality Life Herbs, PO Box 565, Yarmouth, ME 04096, tel. 207-842-4929, fax 207-846-3168.

Menastil, for menstrual pain. Made of pure essential oils, Menastil's active ingredient is calendula oil. The United States Food and Drug Administration and the Homeopathic Pharmacopoeia US recognise this pure grade of calendula oil for the temporary relief of menstrual pain, as a non-prescription, over-the-counter, topically applied homeopathic product. Available from Menastil Products, Dept 711, PO Box 901, Westborough, MA 01581, tel. 508-366-6311, fax 508-366-1121.

Castor oil packs. Saturate a piece of flannel with castor oil and apply directly to the area to be treated. On the side opposite the skin, lay a sheet of plastic, then apply a hot-water bottle. Use for 30–60 minutes five times weekly, or as directed by a practitioner.

Cold-pressed castor oil and **wool flannel** are available through Emerson Ecologics (see address p. 546).

Fomentek hot-water bag, available from Women to Women, 3 Marina Road, Yarmouth, ME 04062, tel. 207-846-6163.

Heavy Bleeding/Iron Deficiency

Iron EAP2. Iron EAP2 is an organic compound which is highly absorbable and hypoallergenic. It is therefore well suited to those who are sensitive to iron supplements. It does not have gastrointestinal side effects. Available from Biocare, see page 551.

Iron Drops. Manufactured by Levine Health, Iron Drops is a nonconstipating, impressively bioavailable form of iron. Recommended dose: 1.5ml (cc) twice per day. Available from Emerson Ecologics (see address p. 546).

Yunnan bai yao. This herbal combination is superb for helping flooding problems. Available from Quality Life Herbs, P.O. Box 565, Yarmouth, ME 04096, tel. 207-842-4929, fax 207-846-3168.

Prepare for Surgery

Note: Avoid taking vitamin E for two weeks preoperatively and one week postoperatively. It may enhance bleeding.

Health Journeys for People Undergoing Surgery. Guided-imagery audiotape by Belleruth Naperstak. Available from Health Journeys, 891 Moe Drive, Suite C, Akron, OH 44310, tel. 800-800-8661, website: www. healthjourneys.com.
A two-tape set designed to help the listener imagine a successful surgery experience, surrounded by protection and support, with the body cooperating fully by slowing down blood flow and speeding up its mending capacity. Side B has affirmations. Tape 2 has continuous music to be taken into the operating room (the same music that underscores the imagery on Tape 1). This was the title that was studied so successfully at the Cleveland Clinic, Kaiser Permanente, and University of California at Davis Medical Center in the US.

Prepare for Surgery, Heal Faster. Book and relaxation/healing audiotape by Peggy Huddleston. Available through Dr Huddleston's website, www.healfaster.com.
I found Peggy Huddleston's book very beneficial in my own recovery from surgery. Her work has helped thousands of others, as well.

Urological Problems

Probiotics. To treat recurrent vaginal yeast infections, I recommend **PB 8 Probiotic** or **Spectra Probiotic,** manufactured by NF Formulas, Inc. (See Chapter 7 Resources for more information.)

Vaginal Weights

Ask at your local chemist who may stock or be able to obtain weights.

FemTone Weights. Available from As We Change catalogue, 6255 Ferris Square, Suite F, San Diego, CA 92121-3232, tel. 858-456-8333. Ask for offer AX004. Or access their website at www.aswechange.com.

Kegel Weights. Available from the Self-Care catalogue, 104 Challenger Drive, Portland, TN 37148, tel. 800-345-7889 or 800-422-8811. Ask for product A5770.

Kegel (Exercise) Kones and Perineal Exerciser. Manufactured by Milex Products, 5915 Northwest Highway, Chicago, IL 60631, tel. 800-621-1278. Available from doctors by prescription in the US.

Contiform. Available from chemists or suppliers Bard Ltd, Forest House, Tilgate Forest Business Park, Brighton Road, Crawley, West Sussex RH11 9BP, tel. 01293 527888. Confidential Women's Health Adviser, tel. 01293 606741.

Educational Resources
National Institute on Aging, Building 31, Room 5C27, 31 Center Drive, MSC 2292, Bethesda, MD 20892, tel. 301-496-1752, website: www.nih.gov/nia/, e-mail niainfor@access.digex.net.
National Kidney and Urologic Diseases Information Clearinghouse, 3 Information Way, Bethesda, MD 20892-3580, website: www.niddk. nih.gov/health/kidney/nkudic.htm, e-mail nkudic@info.niddk.nih.

CHAPTER 9: Sex and Menopause

Suggested Reading
Barbach, Lonnie G. (2000). *For Yourself: The Fulfillment of Female Sexuality.* New York: Signet Books.
Covington, S. (1992). *Awakening Your Sexuality: A Guide for Recovering Women and Their Partners.* HarperSanFrancisco.
Love, P., and J. Robinson (1994). *Hot Monogamy: Essential Steps to More Passionate, Intimate Lovemaking.* New York: Dutton, 1994. The *Hot Monogamy* tape series is available from Sounds True, 735 Walnut Street, Boulder, CO 80302, tel. 800-333-9185.
Masters, M., and V. Johnson (1966). *Human Sexual Response.* New York: Little, Brown and Co.
Ogden, G. (1999). *Women Who Love Sex: An Inquiry into the Expanding Spirit of Women's Erotic Experience.* Cambridge, MA: Womanspirit Press. Gina Ogden is a sexuality researcher and therapist who is a pioneer in

exploring the fullness of women's sexuality. Her delightful and insightful work reenvisage the entire field.

Vaginal Lubricants

Women's Group Formulas Vaginal Lubricant. This is a personal lubricant with moisturising properties. It may also be used as a lubricant for tampons, rectal thermometers, and douches. It is clear, water-based, unscented, flavourless, and non-staining. The following ingredients have been added to create a superior lubricant that helps promote tissue health and comfort: marigold, chamomile, ginseng, aloe vera gel, black walnut leaf, vitamin E, and black cohosh. Available from Emerson Ecologics (see address p. 546).

Sylk is available in many health food shops. For further information, call Geneva Marketing at 203-853-4773.

CHAPTER 10: Nurturing Your Brain

Refer to Chapter 3 Resources for information on feng shui, and Chapter 6 Resources for information on herbs.

Insomnia

Cuddle Ewe Underquilt. The Cuddle Ewe is a wool underquilt that goes on top of your mattress, between it and your sheets. This natural product supports the body and may substitute for a new mattress. Even though the Cuddle Ewe is made of wool, it's cool in the summer and warm in the winter. Available by calling 1-800-705-5559. Ask for offer 61FF520.

Melatonin. Melatonin helps the body adjust to different time zones. Recommended dosage: 1–3mg. I recommend **Melatonin Source Naturals,** available by calling 800-816-2333, as well as **Douglas Laboratories'** and **Advanced Medical Nutrition's** sublingual melatonin, both of which are available through Emerson Ecologics (see address p. 546).

Seasonal Affective Disorder/Light Therapy
Women with SAD are often helped by light therapy. Full-spectrum lighting can also help PMS, perimenopausal symptoms, and ovulatory and other menstrual cycle disturbances. It can also increase serotonin levels.

Light for Health, 942 Twisted Oak Lane, Buffalo Grove, IL 60089, tel. 800-468-1104, fax 847-459-4492, website: www. lightforhealth.com.
Light for Health manufactures high-quality full-spectrum lighting in the form of UL-approved light boxes, fluorescent tubes, and compact fluorescents.

Verilux Company, 9 Viaduct Road, Stamford, CT 06907, tel. 800-786-6850, website: www.verilux.net.
Verilux supplies lighting for the horticulture, exotic animal, and museum markets. They carry a full line of full-spectrum lights, both bulbs and fluorescent tubes. I have personally used their Happylite light box for several years and highly recommend it.

The SAD Box Company, Unit 48, Marlow Road, Stokenchurch, High Wycombe, Bucks. HP14 3QJ, tel. 01494 484852.

Suggested Reading
Goodrich, J. (1995). *Natural Vision Improvement.* Berkeley, CA: Celestial Arts.
Liberman, J. (1993). *Light: Medicine of the Future.* Santa Fe, NM: Bear and Co.

Supplements for Brain Support

5-HTP. 5-HTP is a precursor to serotonin, a neurohormone needed for melatonin production, appetite regulation, and mood regulation. 5-HTP is a natural product extracted from the seeds of *Griffonia simplicifolia,* unlike tryptophan, which is produced synthetically or through bacterial fermentation. Recommended dose is 100–200mg three times per day. Advanced Medical Nutrition's 5-HTP in 50-mg capsules is available through Emerson Ecologics (see address p. 546). Also available from Enzymatic Therapy, tel. 800-783-2286; Web Vitamins, tel. 800-919-9122; or Solgar Vitamins, tel. 800-945-2246. In the UK, contact: The Nutri Centre (see address p. 544) or any supplier of Solgar products.

Chai hu long gu muli wang. According to traditional Chinese medicine, most menopausal problems are due to liver and kidney *yin* deficiency, so strengthening energy in these organs will eliminate imbalances. This combination moves the liver *chi* and sedates the spirit. It is helpful for moodiness, emotional instability, outbursts of anger, and feelings of frustration. It is also beneficial for insomnia. It can be taken indefinitely and is commonly used by the general population in China, not just menopausal women. Available from Quality Life Herbs, PO Box 565, Yarmouth, ME 04096, tel. 207-842-4929, fax 207-846-3168.

DHA (docosahexaenoic acid). Refer to Chapter 7 Resources for more information.

Ginkgo biloba. Refer to Chapter 6 Resources for more information. Recommended dosage is 40mg three times per day.

St John's wort (0.3% hypericin). More than twenty double-blind clinical studies have shown that St John's wort is as effective as standard antidepressants at relieving symptoms of depression, but is much better tolerated and has fewer side effects. The herb's active ingredient is hypericin, which increases levels of brain neurotransmitters that maintain normal mood and emotional stability. Available from the Revival Herb Farm (tel. 800-500-2055, website: www.revivalfarm.com) and in health food shops. For the Revival brand, take one capsule per day. For other brands, take 300mg three times per day, or as directed on the bottle. (The Revival brand is so absorbable and bioavailable that you may need far less to notice results.)

Effervescent Inositol. Effervescent Inositol is well tolerated in doses as large as 18–20g per day, without side effects. In addition to inositol, Effervescent Inositol contains vitamins B_3 and B_6, as well as magnesium. It's best to take it with food. Available from Advanced Nutritional Research, tel. 888-436-7200. In the UK, contact Higher Nature Ltd, Burwash Common, East Sussex TN19 7BR, tel. 01435 882880.

Pregnenolone. Pregnenolone is a precursor to DHEA. Recommended starting dose is 10–50mg per day, but it has been safely used in doses as high as 100–200mg per day; start low and gradually increase if needed. Douglas Laboratories' PREG5 (sublingual 5-mg tablets) is available through Emerson Ecologics (see address p. 546).

Proanthocyanidins. Refer to Chapter 7 Resources for more information.

CHAPTER 11: From Rosebud to Rose Hip

Skin Care
The following are balanced, non-drying cleansers:
    Dove Beauty Bar
    Oil of Olay Beauty Bar
    Neutrogena Non-Drying Cleansing Lotion
    Nutritive Cleanser with Alpha-Lipoic Acid (N. V. Perricone, MD,
        Cosmeceuticals)
    Sensé Gentle Daily Cleanser (USANA)

N. V. Perricone, MD, Cosmeceuticals. Available by calling Clinical Creations at 888-823-7837; outside the United States, call 01-203-379-0726. Or log on to their website at www.clinicalcreations.com.
Cosmeceuticals is the only line of skin care products that is researched, created, patented, and marketed by a board-certified dermatologist research scientist.

The line is based on the use of antioxidant regimens, including vitamin C ester (ascorbyl palmitate), alpha-lipoic acid (ALA), and DMAE (dimethylaminoethanol), which reduce the threat of free radicals. Though Dr Perricone makes a wide range of products, which he continually updates as more research becomes available, I'd recommend that you start with the following:

Vitamin C Ester Cream. Use every night. It thickens collagen and also helps heal skin inflammation.

Face Firming Activator. This contains ALA and DMAE, and it works rapidly. Results may be visible in as little as twenty minutes. The DMAE helps firm sagging skin, while the ALA increases circulation, tightens pores, and evens out skin tone. ALA also helps alleviate puffiness around the eyes and smooths skin on the neck.

Sensé. USANA Health Sciences, Inc. To order, call 888-953-9595. For more information, log on to their website at www.usana.com.
This full skin-care line contains a wide range of highly effective antioxidants. The products have also been formulated so they don't cause irritation, even in those with sensitive skin. The Sensé line contains plant oils (calendula, orange peel, and ginseng), vitamin A, and fat-soluble forms of oligomeric proanthocyanidins (OPCs) and proline, both of which have been shown to help thicken collagen. In addition, the Sensé products contain boron nitrate, which gives skin a healthy glow. Malic, lactic, and glycolic acids give the beauty serum exfoliating properties as well. Clinical trials with the new USANA products have shown a substantial increase in skin moisture and a decrease in wrinkles and fine lines.

If you want to begin a trial of the Sensé line with just two products, I'd recommend the day cream, **Daytime Protective Emulsion,** and the beauty serum, **Night Renewal**, at night.

Internal Hair and Skin Care

Bilberry *(Vaccinium myrtillus).* Dose is 160mg per day for general prevention of varicose veins, and up to 480mg per day to treat varicose veins that already exist. Bilberry is widely available in health food shops and through Emerson Ecologics (see address p. 546).

Shou wu pian, a Chinese herbal supplement for hair growth, is available from Quality Life Herbs, P.O. Box 565, Yarmouth, ME 04096, tel. 207-842-4929, fax 207-846-3168.

Rosacea

Betaine Hydrochloride (betaine HC1). Advanced Medical Nutrition's capsules contain 648mg pure betaine HC1. NF Formulas capsules contain 628mg betaine HC1 plus the digestive enzyme pepsin. Both are available through Emerson Ecologics (see address p. 546), or contact Biocare Ltd, Lakeside, 180 Lifford Lane, Kings Norton, Birmingham B30 3NU, tel. 0121 433 3727, fax 0121 433 3879 for vegetable capsules of HC1 200mg with pepsin 100mg, the 2:1 ratio being the ideal balance. The low potency allows for individual adjustment as required.

Surgery

See Chapter 8 Resources for information on preparing for surgery.

CHAPTER 12: Standing Tall for Life

Bone Density Testing

The Osteoporosis Screening Service, 169 The Broadway, Thorpe Bay, Essex SS1 3EX, tel. 0800-371989. Runs clinics countrywide, providing ultrasound bone density screening at a reasonable price. You can self-refer.

TDL, The Doctors Laboratory, 58 Wimpole Street, London W1M 8LQ, tel. 020 7460 4800, fax 020 7460 4848, e-mail: tdlplc@tdlplc.co.uk, website: www.tdlplc.co.uk. Dpd (Dexoxypyridinoline) assay. Needs a doctor's referral.

National Osteoporosis Society, Camerton, Bath BA2 0PJ, tel. 01761 471771, Helpline: 01761 472721. A registered charity which provides help and information for both non-sufferers and sufferers of osteoporosis.

Supplements for Bone Health

CALCIUM SUPPLEMENTS

Microcrystalline hydroxyapatite is a good source of bone-building calcium that is made from whole bone matrix. Osteoguard 1:1 offers calcium and magnesium in a 1:1 ratio, which is the most effective form, and also contains boron and vitamin K. Recommended dose of Osteoguard 1:1 is three tablets per day. Available through Emerson Ecologics (see address p. 546).

USANA Calcium/Magnesium Plus. Calcium/Magnesium Plus contains calcium citrate, chelated magnesium, boron, and vitamin D_3. I take three in the morning and three at night. Combined with the USANA vitamins and minerals (see page 552), it gives me 1,000mg of calcium per day from supplements. Available by calling 888-953-9595. For more information, visit their website at www.usana.com.

Biocare Ltd, Lakeside, 180 Lifford Lane, Kings Norton, Birmingham B30 3NU, tel. 0121 433 3727, fax 0121 433 3879. Do several products in the ratio magnesium 1:2 calcium, in easily absorbable and utilisable forms, eg Osteoplex, mag 1:2 cal.

HERBAL INFUSIONS

Hambledon Herbs, Court Farm, Milverton, Somerset TA4 1NF, tel. 01823 401205.

Argyll Herbs Direct, 9 Chancellors Pound, Redhill, Bristol BS40 5TZ, tel. 01934 863353, e-mail: enquiries@argyllherbsdirect.com, Website: www. argyllherbsdirect.com.

Strength Training

SUGGESTED READING
Nelson, M., and S. Wernick (2000). *Strong Women Stay Young.* New York: Bantam.
Nelson, M., and S. Wernick (2000). *Strong Women, Strong Bones: Everything You Need to Know to Prevent, Treat and Beat Osteoporosis.* London: Piatkus.

Pilates. For more information on finding a certified instructor or a training programme in your area, or on obtaining Pilates method materials, visit the Pilates website at www.pilates-studio.com.

SUGGESTED READING
Siler, B. (2000). *The Pilates Body: The Ultimate At-Home Guide to Strengthening, Lengthening, and Toning Your Body – Without Machines.* New York: Broadway Books.
Winsor, M. (1999). *The Pilates Powerhouse.* Cambridge, MA: Perseus Books.

CHAPTER 13: Creating Breast Health

See Chapter 8 Resources for more information on where to obtain supplies for castor oil packs.

Breast Cancer Organisations

BACUP, 3 Bath Place, Rivington Street, London EC2A 3JR, tel. 020 7696 9003. Offers a cancer information and counselling service.

Breast Cancer Care, Kiln House, 210 New King's Road, London SW6 4NZ, tel. 020 7384 2984.
Glasgow branch, 46 Gordon Street, Glasgow G1 3PU, tel. 0141 221 2244.

A free service of practical advice, information and support to women concerned about breast cancer. Volunteers who have had breast cancer themselves assist the staff in providing emotional support nationwide.

Breast Cancer Care, Kiln House, 210 New King's Road, London SW6 4NZ, tel. 020 7384 2984.
Offers free help, information and support to women with breast cancer and other breast related problems. Has a national network of volunteers.

Bristol Cancer Help Centre, Grove House, Cornwallis Grove, Clifton, Bristol BS8 4PG, tel. 0117 980 9500, Helpline: 0117 980 9505, fax 0117 923 9184, e-mail: info@bristolcancerhelp.org, website: www.bristolcancerhelp.org. The centre aims to meet the needs of cancer patients and their families by offering help with the physical, emotional, psychological and spiritual problems experienced by people diagnosed as having cancer. Telephone counselling, day and residential courses, bookshop and register of support groups countrywide.

Cancer Relief Macmillan Fund, 89 Albert Embankment, London SE1 7UQ, tel. 020 7840 7840.
The Macmillan service provides home-care nurses and financial grants for people with cancer and their families.

Lymphoedema Support Network, tel. 020 7351 0990.
Information and telephone support.

Rage, tel. 020 8460 7476.
Breast support and guidance for women who have sustained radiotherapy damage after treatment for breast cancer.

The Woman's National Cancer Control Campaign, Suna House, 128–130 Curtain Road, London EC2A 3AR, tel. 020 7729 2229.
Information and advice on early detection of breast and cervical cancer. Help and advice for those being treated for or who may have cancer.

Supplements for Breast Health

Coenzyme Q_{10}. See Chapter 7 Resources for more information.

Flaxseed. See Chapter 6 Resources for more information.

CHAPTER 14:
Living with Heart, Passion, and Joy

Depression
See Chapter 10 Resources for more information.

Forgiveness
See Chapter 2 Resources for more information.

Supplements for Heart Health
Many of the sources for dietary supplements recommended for heart health
are detailed in Chapter 7 Resources.

Hawthorn (*Crataegus* spp.). Widely available in health food shops as berries
for tea infusions. Also available in pill form. If you prefer to take this in pill
form, look for a standardised extract, a product that contains 10 per cent
procyanidins or 1.8 per cent vitexin-4''-rhamnoside. Take 100–250mg three
times per day. Nature's Way and Enzymatic Therapy are reliable brands.
Nature's Way products are available through Emerson Ecologics (see address
p. 546). To order from Enzymatic Therapy, contact Enzymatic Therapy, 825
Challenger Drive, Green Bay, WI 54311, tel. 800-783-2286, website:
www.enzy.com.

L-carnitine. See Chapter 7 Resources for more information.

Proanthocyanidins. See Chapter 7 Resources for more information.

Tocotrienols. Tocotrienols are a vitamin E fraction. Vitamin E consists of
alpha, beta, delta, and gamma tocopherols plus alpha, delta, and gamma
tocotrienols. Allergy Research Group tocotrienols (mixed tocotrienols) are
available through Emerson Ecologics (see address p. 546).

Vitamin E. Recommended dose: 200–800IU per day. Douglas Laboratories'
Natural Vitamin E Complex (mixed tocopherols) is available through
Emerson Ecologics (see address p. 546).

Biocare Ltd, Lakeside, 180 Lifford Lane, Kings Norton, Birmingham B30
3NU, tel. 0121 433 3727, fax 0121 433 3879, do a range of vitamin E capsules,
including some as vegicaps, suitable for vegetarians.

Homocysteine-plasma total testing. TDL, The Doctors Laboratory, 58
Wimpole Street, London W1M 8LQ, tel. 020 7460 4800. Requires a doctor's
referral.

About the Author

Christiane Northrup, MD, trained at Dartmouth Medical School and Tufts New England Medical Center. She is a board-certified obstetrician/gynaecologist with over twenty years of clinical and medical teaching experience. As past president of the American Holistic Medical Association, and current Clinical Assistant Professor of Obstetrics and Gynecology through the University of Vermont College of Medicine's programme at Maine Medical Center, she appreciates the need for a partnership between the best of conventional and complementary medicine. Dr Northrup is the author of the *New York Times* best-selling book *Women's Bodies, Women's Wisdom,* editor of the monthly newsletter *Health Wisdom for Women,* and host of four successful public television specials. Her work has been featured on *The Oprah Winfrey Show, The Today Show, The View,* and *Good Morning America.* She and her family live in Maine.

Visit Dr Northrup's website at www.drnorthrup.com.

About the UK Editor

Sara Miller, MRCS, LRCP, MBBS, DCH, MCOH, MNFSH is a holistic physician, healer, psychosynthesis counsellor and workshop facilitator. Always passionate about woman's health issues she has, over the years, incorporated an interest in complementary medicines and the psychological and spiritual aspects of health into her work with women.

Sara runs Woman to Woman, a holistic health care clinic for women in Bristol. She is also on the staff of the Bristol Cancer Help Centre and is tutor for the College of Healing, West Malvern. Sara is a member of the British Holistic Medical Association and the Medical and Scientific Network.

Index

Note: Page numbers in *italics* refer to illustrations, page numbers in **bold** refer to tables.